TRENDS IN KIDNEY CANCER RESEARCH

HORIZONS IN CANCER RESEARCH
VOLUME 18

HORIZONS IN CANCER RESEARCH

Volume 1: Prostate Cancer
John N. Lucas (Editor)
ISBN 1-59454-100-0
Volume 2: Trends in Ovarian Cancer Research
A. P. Bardos (Editor)
ISBN 1-59454-023-3
Volume 3: Percutaneous Cryotherapy of Renal Cell Carcinoma under an Open MRI System
Junta Harada, Kazuo Miyasaka and Sajio Sumida (Editors)
ISBN 1-59454-169-8
Volume 4: Focus on Colorectal Cancer Research
Julia D. Martinez (Editor)
ISBN 1-59454-101-9
Volume 5: Focus on Leukemia Research
Rafael M. Romero (Editor)
ISBN 1-59454-093-4
Volume 6: Progress in Bladder Cancer Research
A. M. Mallory (Editor)
ISBN 1-59454-129-9
Volume 7: Trends in Prostate Cancer Research
John N. Lucas (Editor)
ISBN 1-59454-265-1
Volume 8: Tumor Budding in Colorectal Cancer Recent Progress in Colorectal Cancer Research
Tadahiko Masaki (Editor)
ISBN 1-59454-189-2
Volume 9: Trends in Breast Cancer Research
Andrew P. Yao (Editor)
ISBN 1-59454-134-5
Volume 10: Trends in Leukemia Research
Rafael M. Romero (Editor)
ISBN 1-59454-311-9
Volume 11: Liver Cancer: New Research
Felix Lee (Editor)
ISBN 1-59454-182-5
Volume 12: Focus on Lung Cancer
Robert L. Carafaro (Editor)
ISBN 1-59454-082-9
Volume 13: Treatment of Ovarian Cancer
A. P. Bardos (Editor)
ISBN 1-59454-022-5
Volume 14: Focus on Kidney Cancer Research
Kelvin R. Nunez (Editor)
ISBN 1-59454-110-8
Volume 15: Focus on Pacreatic Cancer Research
Maxwell A. Loft (Editor)
ISBN 1-59454-270-8
Volume 16: Peritoneal Carinomatosis from Ovarian Cancer
Kostantinos N. Chatzigeorgiou and John N. Bontis (Editors)
ISBN 1-59454-398-4
Volume 17: Trends in Pacreatic Cancer Research
Maxwell A. Loft (Editor)
ISBN 1-59454-524-3
Volume 18: Trends in Kidney Cancer Research
Kelvin R. Nunez (Editor)
ISBN 1-59454-141-8

TRENDS IN KIDNEY CANCER RESEARCH

HORIZONS IN CANCER RESEARCH
VOLUME 18

KELVIN R. NUNEZ
EDITOR

Nova Biomedical Books
New York

For permission to use material from this book please contact us:
Telephone 631-231-7269; Fax 631-231-8175
Web Site: http://www.novapublishers.com

Library of Congress Cataloging-in-Publication Data
Available upon request.

ISBN 1-59454-141-8

Published by Nova Science Publishers, Inc. ✢New York

CONTENTS

PREFACE

Kidney cancer usually occurs in older adults and constitutes about 2% of all adult cancers (more frequent in men than women). It is also known as nephrocarcinoma, renal cell carcinoma, hypernephroma, and Grawitz's tumor. This book includes within its scope the prevention, risk factors, symptoms, diagnosis, treatment, and rehabilitation of kidney cancer. Leading-edge scientific research from throughout the world is presented.

Angiogenesis describes the development of new blood vessels and is a prerequisite for the progressive growth of solid tumors and their metastases. New vessels are necessary for the supply of the tumor over a size of a few mm^3 with oxygen and nutrition. If a tumor becomes hypoxic, whereupon the tumor cells begin to secrete pro-angiogenic factors that bind to specific receptors on the surface of surrounding endothelial cells. Subsequent the endothelial cells proliferate and create a new tumor blood vessel. These new vessels are growing into the tumor tissue and produce optimal conditions for tumor growth and metastasis. The inhibition of tumorangiogenesis is currently an auspicious approach in cancer research as discussed in chapter one.

PTK787/ZK222 584 (PTK/ZK) has been developed as a potent inhibitor of all three VEGF-receptor tyrosine kinases. PTK/ZK is based on a phthalazine scaffold and is active against VEGF receptor tyrosine kinases (IC_{50} = 37 nM for VEGFR-2 and 77 nM for VEGFR-1). PTK/ZK has antiproliferative effects on cells that express VEGF receptors. In pre-clinical studies, PTK/ZK was tested in a variety of rodent models, using either human tumors in immune-deficient mice, or rodent syngenic tumors. Results showed that PTK/ZK inhibited the growth of the subcutaneous xenografts and reduced the number of microvessels in the interior of the tumors. In two syngenic models, B16 F10 melanoma and M5076 reticulosarcoma, significant inhibition of the primary tumor was seen.

Objectives in chapter two are as follows: No reliable tumor-markers for renal cell carcinoma (RCC) for use in clinical routine are present. Increased plasma levels of Transforming Growth Factor-ß1 (TGF-ß1) were described as tumor-marker and prognostic factor in RCC. The aim of the study was to test the clinical utility of TGF-ß1 as a tumor-marker for localized and metastatic RCC.

The material and methods used are as follos: Active and latent TGF-ß1 levels were determined in plasma of patients with localized (n=39) and metastatic (n=17) RCC. A new developed, highly sensitive ELISA, specific for the isoform ß1, was used. Active TGF was directly measured in the EDTA plasma. To determine the amount of latent TGF-ß1, which is bound predominantly at α2-Macroglobulin, an optimized activation procedure came to application.

The results are: 100 patients with various nonmalignant urological diseases were recruited as control group and showed median concentrations of 20106 ng/L (2631-52285 ng/L) for active TGF-ß1. Patients with localized RCC showed median concentrations of 16790 ng/L (6204-54834 ng/L) for active TGF-ß1. A significant difference between these groups was not detectable. Patients with metastatic disease showed median concentrations of 34421 ng/L (6800-48960 ng/L) for active TGF-ß1. In comparison to the localized RCC group a statistically significant difference was found ($p<0.01$). Control of TGF-ß1 levels after operative therapy on day 1, 5, 10 and during follow-up without evidence of disease showed no significant differences.

The conclusion for chapter two indicates: In contrast to other studies our results show that TGF-ß1 is not a useful tool for the diagnosis of localized RCC. In the face of higher TGF-ß1 plasma levels in metastatic disease TGF-ß1 may be useful in early detection of RCC recurrence or to control success of therapy in case of metastases (i.e. immunochemotherapy).

Before new agents for treatment of metastatic renal cell carcinoma (RCC) are developed, immunotherapy with cytokines (interferon-α or interleukin-2) remains a standard treatment option. The overall impact of immunotherapy on survival of metastatic RCC patients is small. However, long lasting remissions are achieved in some patients. Given the great variability in natural course of metastatic RCC, it is important to define patients with good or bad prognosis and those likely to benefit from immunotherapy with cytokines. Traditional clinical and laboratory prognostic factors (performance status, time from initial diagnosis, lactate dehydrogenase, hemoglobin level, etc.) are not sufficient for this purpose. Therefore, identification of new prognostic and predictive factors in advanced RCC is necessary. In the retrospective study in chapter three, the authors analyzed the impact of pre-treatment levels of peripheral blood lymphocyte subsets (CD3+, CD19+, CD16&56+, CD4+, CD8+, CD4+CD45ROhigh and CD8highCD57+) on survival of advanced RCC patients treated and non-treated with interferon-α2b (IFN). Percentages and absolute levels of lymphocyte subsets in peripheral blood were determined in 85 consecutive advanced RCC patients using flow cytometry. Sixty patients with known IFN treatment status were selected for survival analysis. Thirty-two of these 60 patients were treated with IFN and 28 patients were non-treated. Survival of IFN-treated and non-treated patients was analyzed by testing gradually different cut-of levels of each lymphocyte subset. Of all lymphocyte subsets analyzed, only the CD8highCD57+ lymphocytes ('cytotoxic/ regulatory' CD8+ lymphocytes) were found to be significant in determining survival of IFN-treated and non-treated RCC patients. Non-treated patients with < 30% CD8highCD57+ lymphocytes in CD8+ subset survived significantly longer compared to patients with ≥ 30% CD8highCD57+ lymphocytes in CD8+ subset (median survival 23.5 months and 6 months, respectively; $p = 0.01$). Treatment with IFN increased overall survival only in the latter subgroup of advanced RCC patients (median survival increased from 6 to 18.5 months; $p = 0.02$), whereas in the former group, a trend towards decreased survival after treatment with IFN was observed (median survival 23.5 months and 13.6 months for non-treated and treated patients, respectively; $p = 0.11$). Thus, theirr results suggest that percentage of CD8highCD57+ lymphocytes in the

CD8+ subset may have a prognostic significance for advanced RCC patients and may have a predictive value in patient selection for survival benefit due to treatment with IFN.

PAR(proteinase-activated receptor)-type thrombin receptors are members of a novel family of seven-transmembrane G-protein coupled receptors. The discovery of this receptor subclass has provided a framework for understanding how the coagulation proteinase thrombin communicates with cells. Recent studies provided evidence for the crucial role of PARs in tumor development and progression. Renal carcinomas belong to a coagulation type tumors where the tumor cells are associated with intact coagulation pathway that leads to thrombin formation. Therefore, investigation of PARs in this tumor entity is highly important on the definition of their significance in malignancy. In chapter four, the present knowledge of PAR-type thrombin receptors in renal carcinoma cells is summarized. After an overview including PAR structure and their effects in different tumor cell types; PAR characterization on RNA, protein, signaling and cellular level in renal carcinoma cells (permanent human renal carcinoma cell line A-498 and primary cultures obtained from surgically resected renal cell carcinomas) is described. A potential role of PAR-type thrombin receptors in renal cell carcinoma prognosis and therapy is discussed.

N-nitroso compounds act as alkylating agents, and several such compounds are present in tobacco smoke and are detectable in patients treated with diuretics for hypertension and after long-term dialysis treatment for end-stage kidney disease. Rat kidney tumors of various histological types, morphologically resembling their human counterparts, are inducible by *N*-nitroso compounds, thus providing direct evidence to link tobacco smoking and renal dialysis to kidney tumors in humans. These carcinogen-induced rat kidney tumors are also useful for identification of molecular mechanisms of renal tumorigenesis. As seen in humans, alterations in the *von Hippel-Lindau* (*VHL*) gene have been frequently detected in rat kidney tumors of the clear cell phenotype and are rare in eosinophilic renal epithelial tumors, mesenchymal tumors, and nephroblastomas in rats. When rat non-clear cell kidney tumors are examined for VHL protein, almost all tumors show down-regulation of the protein in comparison with adjacent non-neoplastic tissues. This finding suggests that reduction of wild-type VHL protein can also contribute to kidney tumor development regardless of histology as discussed in chapter five. Further analysis of human renal cell carcinomas confirms that down-regulation of VHL protein occurs more frequently than *VHL* gene mutations. Differential localization of VHL protein has been also observed using various antibodies against different VHL epitopes and has been associated with tumor characteristics and patients' survival. In contrast to the significance of protein alteration, clinical utility of *VHL* gene mutational status has not been consistently demonstrated, even though many tumorigenic and angiogenic factors are up-regulated in kidney tumors or cancer cells carrying *VHL* gene alterations. The broad implications of VHL protein for renal tumorigenesis are further highlighted by the discovery of differential expression of VHL protein variants in different organs in rats.

Chinese-herb nephropathy (CHN) is a progressive interstitial fibrosis associated with the use of *Aristolochia* species, a Chinese herb regularly replacing *Stephania tetrandra*, *Akebia*, *Asarum*, *Clematis* and *Cocculus* species in herbal remedies and containing nephrotoxic and carcinogenic aristolochic acids (AA). Moderate to end-stage renal disease (ESRD) may develop, requiring renal replacement therapy by dialysis or transplantation. Experimental models reproducing the clinical entity are available in rabbits and rats.

Aristolochic acids are powerful carcinogens in animal experiments. Removal of the native kidneys and ureters in CHN patients with ESRD has confirmed a high prevalence of upper urinary tract carcinoma (46 %). Tissue samples contained AA-related DNA adducts, which are not only specific markers of prior exposure to AA but are also involved in the tumorigenesis.

In chapter six, the authors took the opportunity of planned nephroureterectomies in our 41 end-stage CHN patients treated by dialysis (N=10) or renal transplantation (N=31) to assess the diagnostic value of urinary cytologic tests prior to surgery. Fresh voided urine samples were available in 37 cases (4 hemodialysed patients were anuric). Cystoscopy with bilateral ureteral brushings and random bladder biopsies (if no bladder lesions were visible) were performed. Cytologic data were compared to histologic findings in the surgical specimens. All preoperative bladder biopsies were normal, except in 5 patients with mild-to-moderate dysplasia and one with superficial pTa bladder cancer. Neoplastic lesions were almost equally distributed between the renal pelvis and ureters. Of the 37 voided urine samples, 3 only showed atypia in relation with upper urinary tract carcinoma, whereas 18 patients had cancer diagnosed histologically. By contrast, bilateral ureteral brushings enabled to detect 14 out of 26 malignant lesions (in those 18 patients) by cytologic examinations. According to these results, specificity of cytologic analyses on voided urine and brushing samples were 100% and 96%, respectively and sensitivity 17% and 54%, respectively. In this specific population where the urinary output from native kidneys was impaired by terminal renal failure, the sensitivity of cytologic analysis of voided urine was much less helpful as compared to what could be expected in the general population.

In summary, exposure to *Aristolochia* species is associated with the development of renal interstitial fibrosis (CHN) and urothelial cancer in humans. Cystoscopy with ureteral brushings should be considered as a first-line screening procedure in patients with renal failure at risk of developing upper urinary tract carcinoma.

In chapter 7, it is discussed how aggressive resection of the vena cava infiltrated by malignancy may yield good results.

The case presented is of a 61-year-old Japanese man who underwent right adrenalectomy for non-hormonal cortical adenoma with indeterminate malignant potential at the age of 51, then right nephrectomy for recurrent and invasive growth of the initial tumor diagnosed as adrenal cortical carcinoma at the age of 56, was admitted to our hospital for another recurrence in August, 1998. He tolerated resections of the liver and inferior vena cava for the invasiveness. He had been alive and well for 4 years since the last surgery, but eventually died of metastases to the spine, hepatic hilum and lung in August 2003. Besides the surgeries, no any other chemotherapy or radiation therapy as an adjuvant or main strategy was given throughout the entire disease course.

The conclusion indicates since this patient with adrenal cortical carcinoma survived the curative resections for 14 years, aggressive surgery can yield a good quality of life and long survival for a patient who had resections of slow-growing malignancy and subsequent recurrences.

The purpose of chapter eight is as follows: Despite interleukin-2 and interferon treatments, the survival of metastatic renal carcinoma patients remains poor. Unlike treatment toxicity, the quality of life of these patients has seldom been investigated.

The materials and methods used in this chapter are as follows: Quality of life was evaluated on patients of the CRECY trial randomized to intravenous interleukin 2 or subcutaneous interferon, or a combination of both drugs. Investigators had initially hypothesized that quality of life was better in patients receiving interferon alone. Quality of life was assessed using a 17-item questionnaire investigating 4 domains of everyday life: health, relationships, inner life, material conditions. The degree of importance or satisfaction attributed by patients to each parameter, and the degree of change experienced were measured. Questionnaires were given 12 weeks after treatment start; 182 patients returned the questionnaire. Results were submitted to different correlation tests, principal component analyses, and survival analyses.

The results of chapter eight indicate the following: Contrary to expected findings, no difference was revealed between interferon or interleukin-2 patients. Overall, quality of life seems relatively poor. The profiles of satisfaction and change are close: relationships were judged positive and improved, whereas physical activities were labeled negative and worse. No significant correlation was found with patients' features, except age.

In conclusion of chapter eight, the authors demonstrate that patients with metastatic renal carcinoma receiving cytokines, either subcutaneous interferon at home or intravenous interleukin-2 in the hospital, have equally impaired quality of life.

Radical nephrectomy is a conventional method of treating patients with renal cell carcinoma. The implementation of clinical pathways has been used to monitor health outcomes. Recently, many advantages of web-based technologies have been reported. Therefore, this study in chapter nine develops a web-based clinical pathway for radical nephrectomy and applies it to improve patient care quality.

The web-based clinical pathway for radical nephrectomy was a daily special form that scheduled consultation, discharge plan, elimination, medication, nutrition, psychosocial support, teaching, laboratory test, treatment, and variance times. Daily patient activities were tracked via the web-based clinical pathway. The clinical pathway variations were identified and recorded using the Internet. Following patient discharge, the web-based clinical pathway was completed and the results were stored on the web server. The analyzed data, including variations, then were e-mailed to the clinical physicians and nurses for reference.

From July 2000 to August 2001, 63 consecutive patients with renal cell carcinoma were treated using the web-based clinical pathway for radical nephrectomy. After implementing the web-based clinical pathway, the mean hospital stay reduced significantly from 11.4 to 9.9 ($p = 0.0063$) days compared to before clinical pathway implementation. Average admission charges also reduced significantly ($p = 0.0075$). The percentage of patients with variances reduced from 38.3% to 23.8% ($p = 0.232$) compared to the first-year paper-based pathway. Notably, no significant differences were noted in variances between the web-based and paper-based pathways. However, the variance detection time in the web-based implementation was significantly ($p = 0.0162$) less than that in the paper-based pathway.

A previous report confirmed the improvement in care quality when using a paper-based clinical pathway. The web-based clinical pathway improved care quality by a quantity equal to that reported for the paper-based pathway in 2002. In this study, one of the four quality indicators was continuously improved ($p = 0.0006$) in the implementing web-based pathway. Additionally, the web-based clinical pathway captured the data directly in an electronic format, facilitating and accelerating analysis.

Implementation of a web-based clinical pathway for radical nephrectomy can improve health outcomes by reducing mean hospital stay and average admission charges, and by improving care quality. Such a web-based pathway is as efficient as the paper-based pathway. However, the web-based clinical pathway is superior to the paper-based pathway in variance detection.

The successful excision of a renal cell carcinoma (RCC) invading the inferior vena cava (IVC) remains a technical intraoperative challenge and requires careful preoperative surgical management planning. Although a radical operation remains the mainstay of the therapy for RCC, optimal management of patients with RCC causing IVC tumor thrombus remains unresolved. In chapter ten, the authors review their experience over the past 12 years with 18 patients who had RCC causing IVC tumor thrombus.

Between July 1990 and October 2001, 18 patients with RCC with IVC tumor thrombus underwent surgical treatment. The mean patient age was 54.2 years and the male to female ratio was 1. The cephalad extension of the tumor was infrahepatic in 9 patients, intrahepatic in 6, and suprahepatic with right atrial extension in 3 patients. All tumors were resected via the inferior vena cava isolation and, when necessary, extended hepatic mobilization and Pringle maneuver, with primary or patch closure of the vena cavotomy. Cardiopulmonary bypass (CPB) and deep hypothermic circulatory arrest (DHCA) were used in 3 patients.

Results: The mortality rate was 5.5 % (1 patient was lost on the 11th postoperative day). Complications occurred in 5 patients. The remaining 17 patients (94.4 %) were successfully discharged from the hospital. Two of them died of tumor progression at the 43rd and 54th postoperative months. The 10-year Kaplan-Meier survival estimate was 75.6, with a mean follow-up of 64.1 months. The presence of lymph node metastases and perinephric spread seemed to possess an adverse effect on the survival in our patients. Although the groups in this series included small numbers of patients, there was no significant difference in survival with regard to the different levels of tumor thrombus extension into the vena cava.

Surgical treatment is the preferred approach to patients with RCC and IVC tumor thrombi as it provides markedly better results when compared with the other therapeutical modalities. The authors' experience confirms that RCC with extension into the IVC is a potentially curable condition provided complete removal is achieved. The level of extension of the tumor thrombus dictates the surgical techniques used for successful removal of the tumor thrombus. The treatment of patients with caval involvement and metastatic disease at presentation needs to be carefully individualized. We believe that complete surgical excision of the tumor and the resulting thrombus and metastases, if present, with appropriate preoperative staging and a well-planned surgical approach, using CPB and DHCA when necessary, provide an acceptable long-term survival with a good quality of life expectation.

Renal cell carcinoma (RCC) is known to be resistant against a couple of cytostatics. This phenomenon, called multidrug resistance (MDR), is explained in chapter eleven first of all by an increase in transport of cytostatics out of RCC or by an enhanced cleavage of these substances in the tumour cells. In the past, attention was focussed on both mechanisms to overcome MDR. Unfortunately, the therapeutic benefit was low in most cases. Therefore, a new trial was tested: the possibility to stimulate the uptake of cytostatic drugs into RCC.

The experiments were started on the basis of the following findings: Organic anions like p-aminohippurate (PAH) are transported across the basolateral membrane of the renal proximal tubule, a mechanism indirectly coupled to sodium via Na^+/α-ketoglutarate co-transport. For about two decades it has been known that the renal excretion capacity of PAH can be stimulated by a suitable treatment schedule *in vivo*. The PAH excretion into urine increases, e.g. after T_3 treatment, by about 60%. In further *in vitro* investigations on renal cortical slices it could be demonstrated that PAH accumulation capacity was significantly increased after *in vivo* stimulation with T_3. Both renal transport capacity and the effect of stimulatory pre-treatment on renal function are age dependent: renal excretion capacity of 10-day-old rats is immature, however, in young rats the extent of stimulation of renal transport processes is often larger than in adult animals.

The next step was the creation of an *in vitro* model suitable to stimulate the accumulation of PAH in renal cortical slices of immature and adult rats. For this goal, tissue slices were incubated for 24 hours in Williams medium E containing different concentrations of hormones. After this incubation period, slices were placed in PAH containing Cross-Taggart medium and PAH uptake into kidney tissue was measured for two hours. In both age groups, the accumulation capacity after 24 hours incubation reaches about 40 - 60 % of that of acute two hours incubation experiments (slice to medium ratios [$Q_{S/M}$] after two hours of incubation: immature rats: 9.5 ± 0.4; adults: 11.4 ± 0.3). After 24 hours incubation with dexamethasone the PAH uptake capacity significantly increases concentration dependently: 10- and 55-day-old rats: 26 and 36 % increase, respectively. It was concluded that 1.) a stimulation of tubular transport capacity can be performed *in vitro*, and 2.) discrepancies between *in vitro* and *in vivo* stimulation exist concerning PAH accumulation in rat renal cortical slices.

Then the *in vitro* accumulation of PAH was investigated in "intact" human renal cortical slices of normal kidney tissue and in tissue slices of human renal cell carcinoma (RCC). In principle, the accumulation capacity is comparable in renal tissue slices of man and rat ($Q_{S/M}$ between 4 and 8). In man, sex differences in accumulation capacity do not exist. But accumulation capacity drops with age. Tissue slices of RCC are unable to accumulate PAH. Surprisingly, in tumours of stage pT1, PAH uptake is lowest, perhaps as a sign of PAH transport out of the cells. There is no difference between peripheral and central parts of RCC. Age and sex are without influence on PAH uptake in RCC tissue slices. Interestingly, the accumulation capacity of "intact" tissue of kidneys infested with RCC also depends on the severity of the tumour (stage, diameter), but not on the formation of metastases.

The aim of the next experimental approach was to test whether or not the accumulation of PAH can be increased in intact human renal cortical slices obtained from tumour-bearing kidneys of patients suffering from RCC. As in rat's renal tissue slices, in intact human kidney tissue PAH uptake capacity increased significantly after 24 hours incubation in dexamethasone-containing medium (56%). The stimulatory effect became significant already after 12 hours incubation. In additionally performed experiments, it was shown that incubation in T_3-containing medium has different effects: In man, T_3 does not influence PAH accumulation capacity of renal cortical slices whereas in rats the PAH accumulation is significantly lower after 24 hours incubation with T_3.

Thereafter, the response of RCC on dexamethasone or T_3 was investigated using tissue slices *ex vivo*. By this approach the PAH accumulation capacity of RCC should be stimulated as a prerequisite for testing the uptake of anti-tumour drugs. RCC samples were incubated for 24 hours in Williams medium E containing dexamethasone or T_3. Thereafter, the slices were placed in PAH containing a Cross-Taggart medium and $Q_{S/M}$ for PAH uptake was measured. As expected, in intact human renal cortical slices, $Q_{S/M}$ was about 3 and increased in dexamethasone-containing medium up to 150%, whereas T_3 did not influence the PAH accumulation. Despite the fact that in RCC the PAH accumulation was completely abolished ($Q_{S/M} \sim 1$), after administration of dexamethasone the accumulated amount of PAH increased significantly also in RCC tissue up to 190%. T_3 was without effect in RCC, too. The dexamethasone-mediated stimulation could be differentiated into responder and non-responder. Altogether, moderate stimulation of tubular transport capacity can be shown *ex vivo* in human RCC, too. The response of RCC on dexamethasone was considered as a basis for new therapeutic strategies to overcome MDR in RCC.

The final aim of the study was to test the accumulation of anticancer drugs (methotrexate = MTX, cisplatin = CP, Tomudex®, topotecan) in intact kidney and in RCC. Kidney tissue slices were incubated in Williams medium E containing dexamethasone, T_3, or EGF. Thereafter slices were placed in anticancer drug containing Cross-Taggart medium and the drug uptake into kidney tissue was measured. As described above, in intact kidney the uptake of PAH (= reference substance) increased significantly only after incubation in dexamethasone, but not in T_3 or EGF. On the other hand, only the accumulation of MTX, but not of CP, Tomudex®, and topotecan, was significantly enhanced after pre-treatment both in intact tissue and in RCC. Discrepancies between the effects of dexamethasone and T_3 and/or EGF indicate different modes of action of these substances at the cellular level.

Unfortunately, the uptake of a variety of anticancer drugs cannot be stimulated effectively in RCC. Evidently the transport of these drugs out of the tumour cells or their metabolism within the tumour is more effective than their uptake. Furthermore, the doses necessary to stimulate the uptake of cytostatics is too high and, therefore, side effects on intact cells must be considered. Thus the therapeutic approach of hormonal stimulation of the uptake of cytostatics cannot be recommended as yet.

The members of the IAP family, including survivin, have recently emerged as modulators of an evolutionarily conserved step in apoptosis. Survivin is present during embryonic and fetal development, but is generally down-regulated in normal adult tissues. However, it becomes reexpressed in a variety of cancers. During tumorigenesis, survivin expression is inversely correlated with apoptosis inhibition and positively correlated with proliferation and angiogenesis. Chapter twelve reviews the relationships between survivin expression and diagnosis, progression, or prognosis in transitional cell carcinoma (TCC). A regards survivin expression in normal samples, no survivin is detected in urine or in transitional cells in the urinary bladder and upper urinary tract. As regards diagnosis, survivin expression has been detected with high sensitivity in urine samples, using ELISA; therefore, this noninvasive test is well suited to bladder cancer, and a disease with high rates of recurrence. However, the relevance of survivin expression to the progression or prognosis of TCC remains controversial.

In: Trends in Kidney Cancer Research
Editor: Kelvin R. Nunez, pp. 1-14

ISBN 1-59454-141-8

Chapter I

PTK787/ZK222584, A SPECIFIC VEGF-RECEPTOR TYROSINE KINASE INHIBITOR, IN THE TREATMENT OF RENAL CELL CARCINOMA

Joachim Drevs
Tumor Biology Center at the Albert Ludwigs University, Freiburg, Germany

ABSTRACT

Angiogenesis describes the development of new blood vessels and is a prerequisite for the progressive growth of solid tumors and their metastases. New vessels are necessary for the supply of the tumor over a size of a few mm^3 with oxygen and nutrition.

Because of the dependence on a functional blood vessel system for tumor survival and growth, tumor vessels developed to interesting key targets in oncology. One approach is the inhibition of tumor vessel formation by antiangiogenic agents, e.g. inhibitors of vascular endothelial growth factor (VEGF) and its receptors, MMP-inhibitors or endothelial cell adhesion inhibitors. Unlike, the aim of vascular targeting agents is to influence the function of the already existing tumor vasculature system. The pivotal point for this therapeutic approach is the difference in the physiology of immature tumor vessels and mature normal vessels.

There has been both hope and disappointment in the clinical efficacy of antiangiogenic therapy during the past decade. Despite evidence in preclinical models that antiangiogenic therapy could completely inhibit tumor growth, no convincing clinical trial evidence to support this principle was reported until recently, when Hurwitz et al. demonstrated that the addition of bevacizumab, a monoclonal antibody against VEGF, to standard chemotherapy with FOLFIRI could improve response rates and survival in patients with metastatic colorectal cancer. This trial was the first to convincingly demonstrate that antiangiogenic therapy added to standard chemotherapy was of clinical benefit for patients. This trial has renewed enthusiasm in the field of antiangiogenic therapy, and the findings on PTK/ZK and its surrogates are thus particularly important.

INTRODUCTION

Angiogenesis describes the development of new blood vessels and is a prerequisite for the progressive growth of solid tumors and their metastases. New vessels are necessary for the supply of the tumor over a size of a few mm^3 with oxygen and nutrition. If a tumor becomes hypoxic, whereupon the tumor cells begin to secrete pro-angiogenic factors that bind to specific receptors on the surface of surrounding endothelial cells. Subsequent the endothelial cells proliferate and create a new tumor blood vessel. These new vessels are growing into the tumor tissue and produce optimal conditions for tumor growth and metastasis. The inhibition of tumorangiogenesis is currently an auspicious approach in cancer research.

Because of the dependence on a functional blood vessel system for tumor survival and growth, tumor vessels developed to interesting key targets in oncology. One approach is the inhibition of tumor vessel formation by antiangiogenic agents, e.g. inhibitors of vascular endothelial growth factor (VEGF) and its receptors, MMP-inhibitors or endothelial cell adhesion inhibitors. Unlike, the aim of vascular targeting agents is to influence the function of the already existing tumor vasculature system. The pivotal point for this therapeutic approach is the difference in the physiology of immature tumor vessels and mature normal vessels. Tumor neovasculature can be selectively targeted by vascular targeting agents due to altered adhesion molecule expression, altered coagulation control, increased permeability, immature endothelial and consequential poorly formed vessels.

Various angiogenic factors produced by solid tumors have been identified and their roles in the formation of new blood vessels have been elucidated. Vascular endothelial growth factor (VEGF) is one of the most potent endothelial cell-specific angiogenic factors with a key role in tumor angiogenesis. VEGF is also known to increase vascular permeability. Its specificity for endothelial cells is explained by the enhanced expression of its two tyrosine kinase receptors, VEGF-R1 (FLT-1) and VEGF-R2 (KDR), on endothelial cells of tumor vessels and VEGF-R3 on lymphatic vessels. These receptors are mainly expressed on proliferating cells. Neovascularization is directly stimulated by an increase in proliferation and migration of the endothelial cells, and indirectly due to an increase in permeability of the vessels. The latter leads to a release of plasma proteins, which in turn generates an adequate environment for the new vessel growth. VEGF is produced by tumor cells; the expression in tumors is up-regulated in comparison to that of normal tissue. Several VEGF antagonists have been developed which have lead to very promising results in vitro and in vivo in animal models.

PTK787/ZK222584 (PTK/ZK) has been developed as a potent inhibitor of all three VEGF-receptor tyrosine kinases (Table 1). PTK/ZK is based on a phthalazine scaffold and is active against VEGF receptor tyrosine kinases (IC_{50} = 37 nM for VEGFR-2 and 77 nM for VEGFR-1). PTK/ZK has antiproliferative effects on cells that express VEGF receptors. In pre-clinical studies, PTK/ZK was tested in a variety of rodent models, using either human tumors in immune-deficient mice, or rodent syngenic tumors. Results showed that PTK/ZK inhibited the growth of the subcutaneous xenografts and reduced the number of microvessels in the interior of the tumors. In two syngenic models, B16 F10 melanoma and M5076 reticulosarcoma, significant inhibition of the primary tumor was seen.

PRECLINICAL DATA

There are numerous animal models of renal cell carcinoma described in the literature. Nevertheless, many of them are not useful for translational research.

Drug-induced tumors are mainly used to investigate tumor pathogenesis and biochemical and molecular mechanisms. Hormone-induced tumors have the disadvantage of a hormone dependence that is not analogous to that found in human renal cell carcinoma.

Nevertheless, two rat models have been established. The Eker model is characterized by unpredictable changes in the immune system whereas the White model has an uptake rate of 30% only and an unpredictable time to develop metastases (Rangel and Pontes 237-46;White, Previte, and Olsson 629-31;Hillman, Droz, and Haas 77-80).

Furthermore, two mouse models have been developed for renal cell carcinoma, the MKT-CDI and the RAG tumor. Both models are characterized by uptake rates <100% and are therefore rarely been used or described in the literature.

In order to investigate novel therapeutic strategies, such as anti-angiogenic therapy, as well as evaluation of novel diagnostic strategies, the murine renal cell carcinoma (RENCA) is a particularly suitable animal model. In this model, primary kidney tumors are induced by subcapsular renal injection of RENCA cells into syngenic Balb/c mice. Subsequently metastases in the lung, lymph nodes and peritoneum develop. The RENCA model has been used extensively for investigating the potential efficacy of treatments for renal tumors (Sufrin and Murphy 9-14)(Sayers et al. 5414-20) (Wiltrout et al. 9-16) (Nishisaka et al. 308-14). RENCA cells were originally obtained from a tumor that arose spontaneously in the kidney of BALB/c mice. Female BALB/c mice are usually used at 6-8 weeks of age (approximate weight 20 g). The injection of 10^6 RENCA cells in 0.2 ml aliquots into the subcapsular space of the left kidney has to be performed through a flank incision after the animals are anaesthetized. The injection of 10^6 RENCA cells in syngenic BALB/c mice induce progressive development of a primary tumor mass in the left kidney. One week after application, the primary tumor is macroscopically visible. At 10 days spontaneous metastases develop in the regional lymph nodes, in the lung and the peritoneum. The mean survival time of RENCA-bearing mice is approximately 32 days when 10^6 RENCA cells were injected.

The RENCA model was used to assess antitumor and antimetastatic efficacy of PTK/ZK. The optimal daily oral dose of PTK/ZK in animals is known to be 50mg/kg. The use of this dose in the RENCA model significantly decreased primary tumors by 61 and 67% after 14 and 21 days, respectively. Reductions of 98 and 78% in lung metastases were also observed after 14 and 21 days, respectively. The drug decreased vessel density, detected by immunohistochemical staining using an anti-CD31 antibody, in primary tumor as well as metastatic tumor tissues by approximately 60%.

In addition, the DNA-binding fluorescent dye Hoechst 33342 (H33342) was used to observe changes of PTK/ZK on VEGF-induced vascular permeability and to investigate its mode of action. H33342 was injected via one of the lateral tail veins at a dose of 20 mg/kg. This dose was chosen because it was well below the toxic limit for this compound and allowed easy identification of labeled cells in histological sections. Mice were killed one minute after injection. Significant reduction of vessel density in PTK/ZK-treated animals by 58% as shown by immunohistochemical technique could be confirmed. Sections of primary tumors from treated animals exhibited a shift of vessel diameters towards larger lumen as compared to control animals. Vascular lumen enclosed by the halos was quantified using a square scoring system. A significant decrease of the number of small vessels (diameter <62.5 μm) by 76% could be observed under therapy, whereas a significant increases of the number of large vessels (diameter >62.5 μm) by 582% occurred. In summary, a decreased abundance of microvessels accompanied by a shift to larger vessels could be detected by fluorescent dye technique.

Kinase	Specification	IC 50 [nM]
KDR (VEGF-R2)	VEGF-R2	37 ± 2
FLT-1 (VEGF-R1)	VEGF-R1	77 ± 12
Flk (mouse VEGF-R2)	Mouse VEGF-R2	270 ± 40
FLT-4 (VEGF-R3)	VEGF-R3	664
c-Kit		730 ± 50
PDGF-R		580 ± 80
c-Met		> 8.000
FGF-R1		> 10.000
EGF-R		> 10.000
v-Abl		> 10.000
c-Crc		> 10.000
PKC-α		> 10.000
TEK		14.000

Figure 1.

Further investigations on the targeted structure included vascular corrosion casting. Here, the RENCA mice were thoracotomized in deep anesthesia, an olive tipped cannula was inserted into the ascending aorta and 30 ml of body warm saline was perfused in order to rinse the vascular system. Vessels were fixed by an infusion of 25 ml bodywarm glutaraldehyde. The final casting was performed by the application of 5-15 ml of Mercox diluted with methylmetacrylate. After having sacrified the animal, polymerization of casting medium took place. Primary tumors were taken and tissue was dissolved. Casts of the primary tumors were coated with gold for electron microscopy. Microvascular corrosion casting is an established method to investigate vascular patterns of almost all organs. In the past evaluation of these specimens using scanning electron microscope (SEM) pictures had not allowed for quantitation, because depth could not be taken into account. However, SEM stereo images pairs allowed for quantitative 3 dimensional measurements. Therefore, three-dimensionally reconstructed scanning electron microscope images (Stereoscan 180, Cambridge instruments) were used for quantitative assessment of vessel diameters, inter-vessel distances and inter-branch distances.

(a). 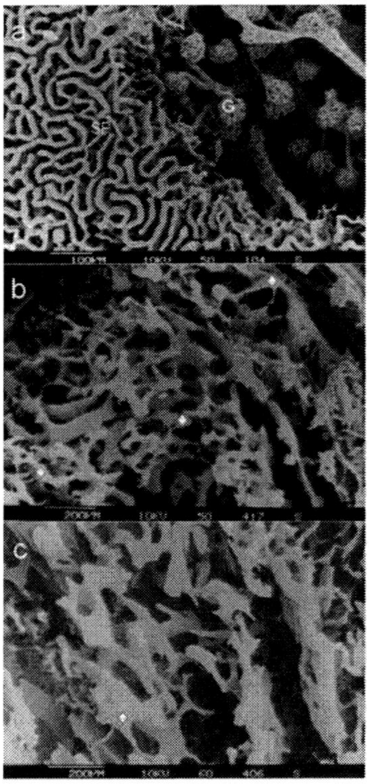

(b). 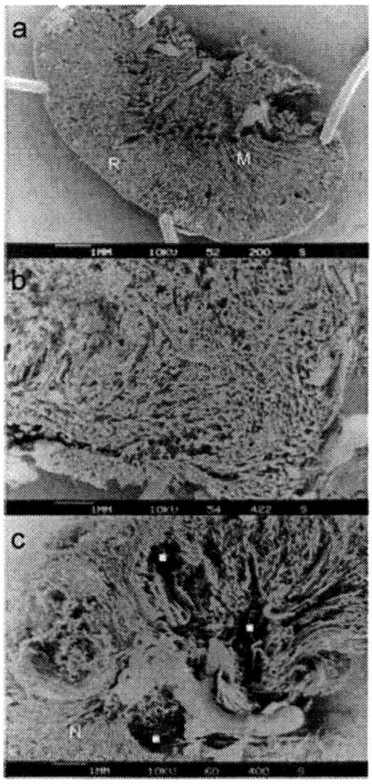

Figure 2.

Low power magnifications revealed the characteristic features of tumor vascularity in all primary RENCA tumors which was in striking contrast to the well organized vascularity in kidneys of healthy mice (Figure 2). Primary tumors showed a low or missing vessel hierarchy, heterogeneous vascular density and the presence of evasates and of blind ending vessels. The vessels in the PTK/ZK-treated group were found to have 26% larger diameter than the vessels of the controls confirming the observations made with the fluorescent dye technique. Mean inter-vessel distance was increased by 20 % in the PTK/ZK-treated animals. The reduction of mean inter-branch distance in treated animals was not significant. In summary, the vessels in primary tumors of the PTK/ZK-treated group were smaller in number but larger in diameter as compared to the control group.

Taken together, these results are interpreted as a PTK/ZK-induced decrease in tumor microvessels followed by reactive dilation of the remaining vessels indicating a feed back system by the hypoxic primary tumor.

Clinical Data

PTK/ZK has already entered phase III trials for the treatment of metastatic colon cancer (CONFIRM-1 and CONFIRM-2).

Two phase I studies have been conducted administering PTK/ZK on a continuous basis to patients with advanced cancer. In the first, PTK/ZK was administered on a once daily schedule and in the second, on a twice daily schedule. The latter was done to try and exploit the theoretical advantage of maintaining drug levels above a threshold known to interfere with VEGF receptor signaling. The majority of patients in these studies have had advanced colorectal cancer. The primary objectives of the studies were to determine the optimum dose and schedule of PTK/ZK administration, to characterize the pharmacokinetic profile of the drug, to assess the safety and tolerability of the drug and where possible efficacy. A modified Fibonacci trial design was used whereby cohorts of three patients were enrolled at escalating dose levels. All patients had to have metastatic and measurable disease, good performance status and adequate hematological, renal and hepatic function. PTK/ZK was administered continuously as capsules on a 28 day cycle. The starting dose was chosen based on 1/10 the LD_{10} in rats. Expansion of the cohort occurred if at least one dose limiting toxicity was encountered during the first 28 day cycle. If 2 DLTs were seen then no further dose escalation was permitted. The maximum tolerated dose (MTD) was defined as one dose level below that where at least 2 or more patients experienced dose limiting toxicity. Full pharmacokinetic sampling was performed on days 1, 15 and 28. Patients were encouraged to take their capsules at the same time each day followed by a 2 hour fast. DCE-MRI was performed at baseline, day 2 and at the end of cycle 1, 2 3, 4 and thereafter every second cycle. Patients were evaluable for the MTD determining aspect of the study if they completed the first 28 days administration of PTK/ZK. For a patient to have a minor response or stable disease demonstrated on MRI, this had to be confirmed 4 weeks later by the subsequent MRI.

PTK/ZK was orally administered as monotherapy in single doses of 50, 150, 300, 500, 750, 1.000, 1.500 and 2.000 mg/day or twice daily doses of 300, 500, 750, 1.000, 1.200 and 1.500 mg/day (n = 3/cohort). The average T_{max} was 1.6 h and average terminal half-life was 5.9 h. Stable disease was observed in approximately 50% of the evaluable patients with a median duration of 4.3 months (range, 3 to 12 months). Median overall survival by Kaplan-Meier analysis was 11.6 months. No hematological toxicity has been demonstrated in the twice daily PTK/ZK phase I study, non-hematological adverse events have been seen. The dose limiting toxicity is light-headedness and nausea and vomiting. The light-headedness comes on very quickly after administration of the capsules and is transient or reversible with a dose reduction of PTK/ZK. The spectrum of light-headedness varies from some mild 'dizziness' to patients being bed-bound with nausea, ataxia and dysarthria. In two patients with pre-existing hypertension, grade 3 hypertension which responded to anti-hypertensive medication, was demonstrated. Transient elevation in liver transaminases has been seen in 4 patients. In the single dose studies, side effects of lethargy, light-headedness and liver transaminase increase occurred. No dose limiting toxicity could be assessed. At doses of >1000 mg, tumor hypoxia was observed and the optimal dose was defined by surrogates to be 1250mg.

In an additional trial, designed for the assessment of changes on blood flow velocity as detected by color Doppler imaging, PTK/ZK was orally administered as monotherapy in single doses of 300, 500, 750, 1.000 and 1.200 mg/day (n = 3/cohort). Efficacy data as well as toxicity data could be confirmed.

One study detailed a phase I trial in patients (n = 20) with recurrent glioblastoma, a poor-prognosis population associated with overexpression of VEGF, where the primary endpoint was to determine the safety and tolerability of PTK/ZK. Patients were treated with single doses of 150, 500, 1000, 1500 and 2000 mg PTK/ZK per day. Dose expansion was performed at 1200 mg/day and 1500 mg/day. Dose-limiting toxicity was found to be confusion, speech impairment secondary to cerebral edema, fatigue, nausea and vomiting at 2.000 mg/day. Of 31 patients evaluable for response, 3% experienced a partial response and 65% had stable disease.

PTK/ZK has also been evaluated in combination with chemotherapy in patients with recurrent glioblastoma. Here, dose-limiting toxicity for PTK/ZK in combination with temozolomide (TMZ) was dizziness at 1.500 mg/day PTK/ZK. Two of 21 evaluable patients had a partial response and 9 patients had stable disease with a median time to progression of 15.0 weeks.

In view of encouraging phase I results in a subgroup analysis of patients with colorectal cancer, PTK/ZK was investigated in combination with chemotherapy for advanced colorectal cancer. Pre-clinical xenograft rodent models confirmed that PTK/ZK in combination with 5-FU had an additive effect on tumor growth inhibition. No excess toxicity was seen in the animal models although PTK/ZK is a substrate and inhibitor of several cytochrome P_{450} isoenzymes. In particular it is metabolized predominantly by CYP3A4. In view of this observation it was postulated that PTK/ZK could interfere with the clearance of a co-administered drug; either by decreasing the clearance of the drug or even auto-inducing metabolism of the drug. Since Oxaliplatin undergoes spontaneous non-enzymatic conversion and is not a substrate of cytochrome P_{450} isoenzymes a two-arm phase I study was designed using PTK/ZK in combination with FOLFOX (5-Fluorouracil, Leucovorin Oxaliplatin) or FOLFIRI (5-FU, Leucovorin, Irinotecan). The objectives of this phase I study were to characterize the safety, tolerability and pharmacokinetic profile of oral PTK/ZK when administered on a once daily dosing schedule in combination with standard dose chemotherapy to patients at first presentation of advanced colorectal cancer.

First data from these phase I/II trials were presented in May 2003. Oral PTK/ZK was administered once-daily in escalating doses, first-line therapy in combination with FOLFOX4 (oxaliplatin [85 mg/m^2 q 2 weeks] plus leucovorin [200 mg/m^2 via 2-hour infusion] and 5-fluorouracil [400 mg/m^2 bolus folowed by 600 mg/m^2 over 22 hours] on days 1 and 2 q 2 weeks) or FOLFIRI (irinotecan [180 mg/m^2 q 2 weeks] plus leucovorin [200 mg/m^2 via 2-hour infusion] and 5-fluorouracil [400 mg/m^2 bolus folowed by 600 mg/m^2 over 22 hours] on days 1 and 2 q 2 weeks).

A total of 35 patients were treated with escalating doses of PTK/ZK plus FOLFOX4 and 23 patients were treated at the expansion dose of 1.250 mg/day. The majority of adverse events were mild-to-moderate; dose-limiting toxicities were grade 3 fatigue and ataxia, as well as syncope at 1.500 mg/day and neurotoxicity (dizziness and light-headedness) at 2.000 mg/day. Of 21 evaluable patients, 9 (43%) patients had a partial response and 8 (38%) had stable disease. Median time to progression was 11 months (95% confidence intervals = 8.7, 12.0 months). Overall survival at one year was 79% with a median survival of 14 months (95% confidence intervals = 12.7, 21.0 months).

In combination with FOLFIRI, 16 patients have been enrolled and treated at doses of 500, 1.000, and 1.250 mg/day PTK/ZK. Median time on study was more than 6 months. PTK/ZK in combination with FOLFIRI was generally well-tolerated and the incidence and severity of adverse events were consistent with the previously-reported safety profile of irinotecan. Two dose-limiting toxicities were observed: grade 3 fatigue at 500 mg/day and grade 3 hypertension at 1.000 mg/day. Of 11 evaluable patients, 4 (36%) had a partial response and 4 (36%) had stable disease. Enrollment onto the trial had been ongoing for 14 months at the time of the report and all enrolled patients were still alive.

First data from a phase I/II trial of PTK/ZK monotherapy for the treatment of metastatic renal cell carcinomas were presented in May 2003. Here, PTK/ZK was administered orally, once-daily at 300, 750, 1.000, 1.200, and 1.500 mg/day to a total of 19 patients in the escalation phase. 30 patients were enrolled at the dose-expansion phase of 1.200 mg/day to evaluate the biologic activity and additional safety. More than 50% of patients had received prior systemic therapy. No dose-limiting toxicity was reached up to 1.500 mg/day PTK/ZK. Toxicities observed were grade 3 headache at 1,000 mg/day and grade 3 hypertension at 1.500 mg/day. Among 49 evaluable patients, 8 (19%) had measurable tumor regression and 25 (60%) had stable disease with a median time to progression of 5.3 months (95% confidence intervals = 3.7, 7.4 months). Overall survival at 1 year was 66.7%.

IMAGING DATA

When measuring response to chemotherapy and radiotherapy, conventional MRI and computerized tomography (CT) are excellent tools to demonstrate reduction in cross sectional tumor size. Intuitively, rapid involution of tumors was not envisaged with angiogenesis inhibitors and so surrogate marker of efficacy was sought. DCE-MRI with gadolinium chelate is a useful technique to study the pathophysiology of tumors particularly with respect to vascular perfusion and permeability. Since successful VEGF inhibition with PTK/ZK can reduce both tumor vascular perfusion and permeability, it was postulated that dynamic contrast-enhanced magnet resonance imaging (dceMRI) would be a valuable surrogate assessment of efficacy.

The MRI enhancement is due to increasing gadolinium concentration, largely in the extravascular and extracellular space and depends on tumor perfusion, tumor vascularity and tumor vascular permeability. Gadolinium diffuses passively from the blood vessel into the extracellular space at a rate proportional to the concentration difference. Once in the extracellular space it disperses freely without binding and will efflux back into the vascular space in a similar manner with a similar rate constant. Ki or Ktrans is an objective measurement quantifying the rate constant for this process.

Initially, animal studies using the RENCA model were conducted to evaluate the dceMRI technique under treatment with PTK/ZK. Contrast agents bolus application prior to placing the animals in the magnet was performed via tail vein. MRI experiments were carried out on a Bruker DBX 47/30 spectrometer at 4.7 T equipped with self-shielded 20 cm bore gradient system 21 days after RENCA tumor cell application into the left kidney of Balb/c mice. During the MRI experiments the animals had to be anesthesized to avoid movement artifacts. They were positioned on a cradle in supine position inside of a 40mm resonator. The exact position of the animal was assessed by a scout imaging sequence (Figure 3).

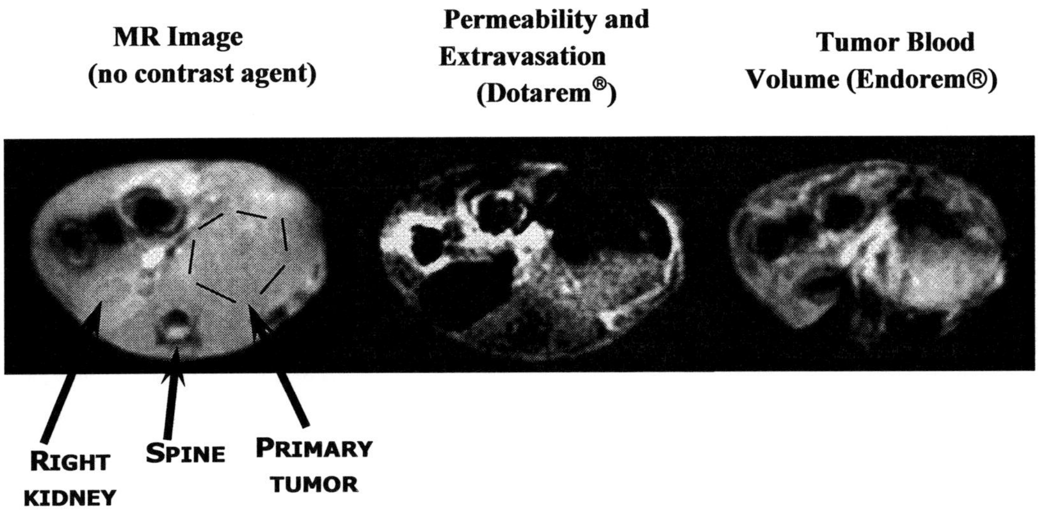

Figure 3.

Gradient recalled echo imaging sequences had been used for determination of blood vessel permeability. Acquisition parameters were: Repetition delay TR = 20 ms, echo delay TE = 3.1 ms, number of averages NA = 8, image matrix = 128^2, field-of-view FOV = 3.5x3.5 cm, slice thickness = 1.5 mm. 64 sequential images with a time resolution of 20 s had been recorded. After the 10th repetitive image a bolus application of 30 µl Dotarem® was given manually by the tail vein during approximately 20 s. Relative GdDOTA concentration in tumor tissue was calculated from the MR images as [GdDOTA] = $(S/S_0\text{-}1)$ (cf methods).

Vessel permeability, detected by which is known to correlate with the maximal slope, was significantly decreased by 52% in PTK/ZK-treated animals. Astonishingly, no significant difference between treated and untreated animals could be detected with regard to extravasation, represented by the maximal uptake of the contrast agent.

Partial tumor blood volume was assessed by gradient recalled echo imaging sequence with the following measuring parameters: Repetition delay TR = 10.7 ms, echo delay TE = 3.1 ms, number of averages NA = 2, image matrix = 128x64, field-of-view FOV = 3.5x3.5 cm, slice thickness = 2 mm. 40 sequential images with a time resolution of 1 s have been recorded. 60 µl Endorem® were injected into the tail vein during acquisition of image 11 using a spectrometer-controlled infusion pump. Relative tumor blood volume was estimated by: TBV = $-\ln(S/S_0)$ (cf methods). Comparing maximal Endorem® uptake in primary tumors of untreated animals with PTK/ZK-treated animals, a significant increase in treated animals by 44% became apparent reflecting an increased partial blood volume under therapy.

In addition, color Doppler imaging studies were performed. Animals, still anesthesized for dceMRI examination, underwent color Doppler imaging ultrasound. Primary tumors were located in all animals using a high end sonograph having a direct-contact high-frequency ultrasound transducer. The left renal artery was detected by color Doppler imaging and measurements of systolic and diastolic blood flow velocity and resistance index were performed. To rule out a systemic effect of PTK/ZK, blood flow velocity was additionally determined in the abdominal aorta. Heart rates were also assessed.

Direct comparison of systolic blood flow velocity in the left renal artery of PTK/ZK-treated with vehicle-treated animals revealed no difference. However, taking the values from a control vessel (abdominal aorta) into account, reduction of systolic blood flow velocity in the PTK/ZK-treated animals by 44% could be observed.

In summary, a significant decrease in tumor vascular permeability occurred in primary RENCA tumors in response to daily oral 50 mg/kg doses of PTK/ZK as measured by dceMRI. In addition, an increased blood volume was detected by dceMRI as well as a decreased blood flow velocity in the tumor-feeding renal artery was measured by Doppler sonography that could be explained by the corrosion cast findings on increased diameter in the remaining blood vessels.

The dceMRI technique as well as the color Doppler ultrasound were therefore translated into the initial clinical trials with PTK/ZK to assess optimal biological doses. Analyses published were mainly performed in a subgroup of 24 patients with liver metastases from colorectal cancer. The median age of the group was 60 ranging from 41-74 years. All patients had performance status of 0 or 1 despite being heavily pre-treated; the median number of previous courses of chemotherapy for advanced disease was three, with one patient having had five regimens. PTK/ZK was rapidly absorbed following oral administration with a peak plasma concentration achieved in 1 to 2.5 hours. The terminal half-life was 4-6 hours and steady state appeared to be reached at day 15. Figure 4 demonstrates the reduction of enhancement of a liver metastasis, 30 hours after administration of PTK.

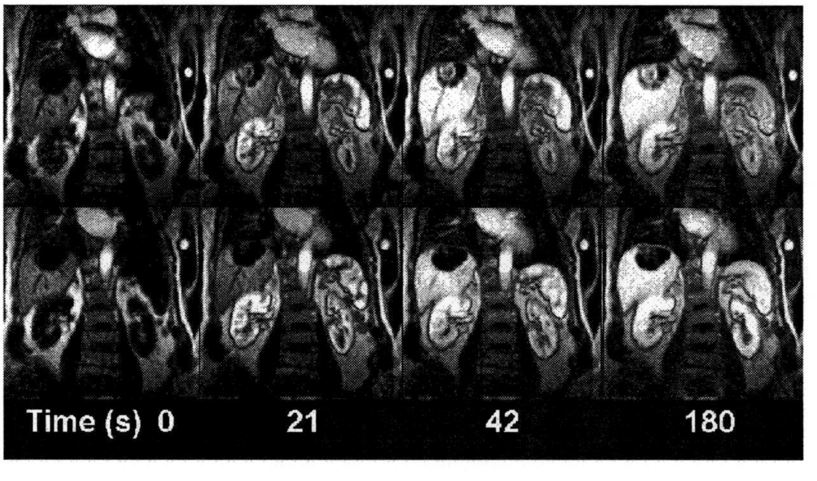

Figure 4.

The enhancement parameter Ki was measured as a percentage of baseline. At the lowest doses of PTK/ZK there was little change in Ki at day 2. A dose-dependent reduction in tumor vascular surface area and vessel wall permeability was observed. Twenty-four patients with liver metastases had a mean surface area reduction of 58% on day 2 on doses of > 750 mg. Furthermore, PTK/ZK monotherapy reduced tumor perfusion and vascular permeability, as determined by dynamic contrast-enhanced magnetic resonance imaging, and slowed tumor growth. There was a correlation with the pharmacokinetic parameters AUC and C_{min} and reduction in Ki at days 2 and 28. Of the 16 patients evaluable for response, 8 had progressive disease, and 8 had either stabilization or minor responses. Importantly, a 60% reduction from baseline in tumor perfusion and vascular permeability was significantly correlated with positive clinical outcome ($P = .004$).

In patients with liver metastases treated with PTK/ZK and analyzed by color Doppler imaging technique, a decrease of blood flow velocity in liver metastases by 60% could be observed on day 28.

Soluble Marker

Actually, VEGF and bFGF (basic fibroblast growth factor) can be detected as tumor surrogates, whereas sFLT-1 (soluble variant of VEGF-receptor 1), sKDR (soluble variant of VEGF-receptor 2), sTIE-2 (soluble variant of angiopoetin-receptor 2) and sE-Selectin (soluble E-Selectin) can be detected as endothelial cell surrogates. All markers can be assessed easily by ELISA technique. Soluble markers of tumor angiogenesis were already shown to be useful in prognosis of different malignancies like colon cancer or multiple myeloma. In patients with multiple myeloma, measurements of sFLT-1 and sTie2 under treatment with thalidomide revealed a correlation with adverse prognostic tumor markers (LDH), changes in dceMRI and survival.

Therefore, dceMRI was not only studied as a surrogate marker but also soluble biomarkers in the early phase I trials with PTK/ZK. These included markers of angiogenesis (plasma levels of VEGF and bFGF) and markers of activated endothelial cells (serum levels of sFLT-1, sTIE-2 and sE-Selectin). Here, plasma VEGF as well as bFGF increased up to 5-fold at doses of 1000 mg or higher in responders (partial response or stable disease). This increase of VEGF could reflect increasing tumor hypoxia under treatment with PTK/ZK. The occurrence of these findings in responders supports the hypothesis of an angiogenic phenotype.

Anti-angiogenesis is a new biological treatment technique, which is assessable for biological activity by dceMRI and soluble marker. Nevertheless, all used imaging techniques as well as all used soluble markers are experimental surrogates used in clinical trials with experimental compounds. To increase knowledge and validity of the methods used for the assessment of antiangiogenic treatment, preclinical and clinical studies designed for their evaluation must be performed.

Summary

There has been both hope and disappointment in the clinical efficacy of antiangiogenic therapy during the past decade. Despite evidence in preclinical models that antiangiogenic therapy could completely inhibit tumor growth, no convincing clinical trial evidence to support this principle was reported until recently, when Hurwitz et al. demonstrated that the addition of bevacizumab, a monoclonal antibody against VEGF, to standard chemotherapy with FOLFIRI could improve response rates and survival in patients with metastatic colorectal cancer. This trial was the first to convincingly demonstrate that antiangiogenic therapy added to standard chemotherapy was of clinical benefit for patients. This trial has renewed enthusiasm in the field of antiangiogenic therapy, and the findings on PTK/ZK and its surrogates are thus particularly important.

Although PTK/ZK inhibits primary tumor growth and metastasis and vessel density in tumor tissue in different animal models, tumor reduction was not generally observed, which is not the case for competitors like ZD6474 (AstraZeneca plc) which has additional activity against the EGF receptor tyrosine kinase. However, the preclinical work up of the compound compared to the competitors was more complete, and included anatomical and mechanistic analysis. This complete preclinical work up was transferred to phase I trials with innovative diagnostics allowing a better interpretation of the optimal biological dosing of PTK/ZK. Soluble marker analyses as well as dynamic contrast-enhanced MRI allowed the identification of 1.000 to 1.250 mg as the optimal biologically active dose. A toxicity profile could be described and clinical efficacy was demonstrated by long-term disease stabilization. In summary, the phase I trials demonstrate a promising therapeutic index for the drug. The questions left unanswered from the phase I/II studies are the interpretation of the diagnostics, which are still experimental. Why the VEGF serum levels increase under a VEGF-receptor inhibiting therapy and why dramatic changes in extravasation can be observed already after 30 h of treatment with PTK/ZK remain unclear.

The differing response rates among the patients to antiangiogenic drugs at all might be explained by their different angiogenic phenotypes. The regulation of angiogenesis in humans is obviously much more complex than previously thought. It must be presumed that neovascularization is controlled by the combined effects of several factors with different mechanisms. New receptor/ligand systems are increasingly being described and could be further important regulators of angiogenesis. Tumor entities being more sensitive to an antiangiogenic therapy then others turned out to be colon cancer, renal cell carcinoma, glioblastoma and hematological malignancies.

Proper end points of antiangiogenic compounds may have to differ from those of standard chemotherapy agents. The success of conventional chemotherapy is measured by objective response rates. Improved survival or duration of stable disease may be more appropriate end points for antiangiogenic substances. From actual trials, surrogate markers like dceMRI and soluble angiogenesis markers turn out to be predictive for biological activity, defining optimal biological doses far below below the MTD.

The ability to avoid acquired drug resistance is regarded to be one of the advantages of antiangiogenic drugs over other forms of anticancer therapy because of the nature of their cellular target: the genetically stable endothelial cells rather than rapidly mutating, genetically unstable cancer cells. Recently there is accumulating preclinical and clinical evidence that a number of antiangiogenic drugs or strategies can lose there activity over time. This can be caused by several possible mechanisms, e.g. an overexpression of other pro-angiogenic factors that may antagonize the function of the antiangiogenic agents if only one such factor is the target of an antiangiogenic therapy. For this reason the combined application of angiogenesis inhibitors might be a promising future strategy. An inhibition of various receptor/ligand systems could be effective due to different mechanisms of action within the angiogenesis process. In addition application of antiangiogenic drugs in an adjuvant setting might be the most promising option especially in kidney cancer or colorectal cancer.

REFERENCES

[1] Drevs J, Mross K, Reusch P, Peng B, Ball H, Henry A, Laurent D, Dugan M, Marmé D, Unger C (1999): Phase I dose escalation, pharmacokinetic (pk) study of a novel vascular endothelial growth factor (VEGF) receptor inhibitor, PTK787/ZK 222584 (PTK/ZK). *Eur J Canc* 35, p283

[2] Morgan B, Drevs J, Steward W, Lee L, Dilea C, Pfister C, Mietlowski W, Zirrgiebel U, Marmé D, Mross K, Unger C, Thomas A, Laurent D, Henry A, Dugan M (2002): Defining the biological active dose for PTK787/ZK222 584, a vascular endothelial growth factor (VEGF) receptor inhibitor, based on the assessment of two biomarkers [dynamic contrast enhanced MRI (DCEMRI) and plasma VEGF levels] in two phase I studies. *EJC* 38(7), a237, p75

[3] Wood JM, Bold G, Stover D, Hofmann F, Buchdunger E, Mestan J, Towbin H, Schnell C, Mett H, O'Reilly T, Cozens R, Rösel J, Siemeister G, Menrad A, Schirner M, Thierauch KH, Schneider MR, Drevs J, Martiny-Baron G, Marmé D (2000): Pharmacological profile of a novel, potent and orally active inhibitor of VEGF receptor tyrosine kinases. *Cancer Res* 60(8), p2178-2189

[4] Drevs J, Hofmann I, Hugenschmidt H, Madjar H, Müller M, Wood J, Martiny-Baron G, Unger C and Marmé D (2000): Effects of PTK787/ZK 222584, a specific inhibitor of VEGF-receptor tyrosine kinases, on primary tumor, metastasis, vessel density and blood flow in a murine renal cell carcinoma model. *Cancer Res* 60(17), p4819-4824

[5] Drevs J, Müller-Driver R, Wittig C, Fuxius S, Esser N, Hugenschmidt H, Konerding MA, Allegrini PR, Wood J, Hennig J, Unger C and Marmé D (2002): PTK787/ZK 222584, a specific VEGF-receptor tyrosine kinase inhibitor, effects the anatomy of the tumor vascular bed and the functional vascular properties as detected by dyMRI. *Cancer Res* 62(14), p4015-22

[6] Morgan B, Thomas AL, Drevs J, Hennig J, Buechert M, Jivan A, Horsfield M, Mross K, Henry A, Pfister C, Fuxius S, Unger C, O'Byrne K, Cherryman G, Laurent D, Lee L, Dugan M, Marmé D and Steward WP (2003): Dynamic contrast enhanced magnetic resonance imaging as a surrogate marker for efficacy of the VEGF inhibitor PTK787/ZK 222584 (PTK/ZK) in patients with liver metastases from colorectal cancer: Phase 1 trial. *JCO* 21(21):3955-3964

[7] Drevs J, Zirrgiebel U, Schmidt-Gersbach CIM, Mross K, Medinger M, Lee L, Pinheiro J, Wood J, Thomas AL, Unger C, Henry A, Steward WP, Laurent D, Lebwohl D, Dugan M, Marmé D (2005): Soluble Markers for the Assessment of Biologic Activity With PTK787/ZK222 584 (PTK/ZK), a Vascular Endothelial Growth Factor Receptor (VEGFR) Tyrosine Kinase Inhibitor in Patients With Advanced Colorectal Cancer From Two Phase I. *Annals Oncol*, 16(4):558-65

[8] Mross K, Drevs J, Laurent D, Dugan M, Henry A, Medinger M, Steward WP and Unger C (2005): Phase I study of PTK787/ZK 222584, a specific VEGF receptor tyrosine kinase inhibitor, in patients with advanced colorectal cancer. *Eur J Cancer*, 41(9):1291-9

[9] Lee L, Sharma S, Morgan B, Allegrini P, Schnell C, Brueggen J, Cozens R, Horsfield M, Guenther C, Steward WP, Drevs J, Lebwohl D, Wood J, McSheehy PM (2005): Biomarkers for assessment of pharmacologic activity for a vascular endothelial growth factor (VEGF) receptor inhibitor, PTK787/ZK 222584 (PTK/ZK): translation of biological activity in a mouse melanoma metastasis model to phase I studies in patients with advanced colorectal cancer with liver metastases. *Cancer Chemother Pharmacol* 20:1-11

In: Trends in Kidney Cancer Research
Editor: Kelvin R. Nunez, pp. 15-22

ISBN 1-59454-141-8

Chapter II

Tumor Growth Factor-ß1 (TGF-ß1) Plasma Levels in Patients with Localized and Metastatic Renal Cell Carcinoma

A. Hegele*, Z. Varga, R. von Knobloch, A. Heidenreich, R. Hofmann
Department of Urology and Pediatric Urology, Medical School,
Philipps University, Marburg,Germany
J. Kropf and B. Kosche
Department of Clinical Chemistry, Medical School,
Philipps University, Marburg,Germany

Abstract

Objectives: No reliable tumor-markers for renal cell carcinoma (RCC) for use in clinical routine are present. Increased plasma levels of Transforming Growth Factor-ß1 (TGF-ß1) were described as tumor-marker and prognostic factor in RCC. The aim of the study was to test the clinical utility of TGF-ß1 as a tumor-marker for localized and metastatic RCC.
Material & Methods: Active and latent TGF-ß1 levels were determined in plasma of patients with localized (n=39) and metastatic (n=17) RCC. A new developed, highly sensitive ELISA, specific for the isoform ß1, was used. Active TGF was directly measured in the EDTA plasma. To determine the amount of latent TGF-ß1, which is bound predominantly at α2-Macroglobulin, an optimized activation procedure came to application.
Results: 100 patients with various nonmalignant urological diseases were recruited as control group and showed median concentrations of 20106 ng/L (2631-52285 ng/L) for active TGF-ß1. Patients with localized RCC showed median concentrations of 16790 ng/L (6204-54834 ng/L) for active TGF-ß1. A significant difference between these

* Corresponding author: Dr. Med. Axel Hegele, Department of Urology, Philipps-University, Baldingerstraße, 35043 Marburg–Germany. Tel: +49-6421-2862513; Fax: +49-6421-2865590; E-Mail: lexaelegeh@aol.com

groups was not detectable. Patients with metastatic disease showed median concentrations of 34421 ng/L (6800-48960 ng/L) for active TGF-ß1. In comparison to the localized RCC group a statistically significant difference was found ($p<0.01$). Control of TGF-ß1 levels after operative therapy on day 1, 5, 10 and during follow-up without evidence of disease showed no significant differences.

Conclusions: In contrast to other studies our results show that TGF-ß1 is not a useful tool for the diagnosis of localized RCC. In the face of higher TGF-ß1 plasma levels in metastatic disease TGF-ß1 may be useful in early detection of RCC recurrence or to control success of therapy in case of metastases (i.e. immunochemotherapy).

INTRODUCTION

Renal cell carcinoma (RCC) represents the third most common urological tumor after prostate and bladder cancer. It is diagnosed between the ages of 50 and 70 years often found during abdominal sonography as incidental cancer (1). A lot of different factors (i.e. cigarette smoking, asbestos exposure, obesity) seem to influence development of RCC maybe as a cofactor (2,3). 30% of the patients are initially presented with metastatic disease and poor prognosis. Despite of radical surgery 40% will metastasize during future clinical course (4). To date only few tumor markers for RCC have been evaluated (5,6,7,8). Because of low sensitivity and specificity levels none of these markers were used in clinical routine. In the face of these data it seems to be necessary to identify reliable serological markers for early detection and monitoring after radical surgery during follow-up.

Various different immunomodulators are produced by tubular and renal cancer cells (9). Transforming growth factor-ß1 (TGF-ß1), one of these immunomodulators, represents a cytokine with multiple functions as for example the regulation of cell proliferation and differentiation, promotion of wound healing and suppression of the immune system by interacting with a number of different binding proteins and receptors (10). TGF-ß1 is an isoform of the 25-kDa polypeptide TGF-ß and has been suggested a tumor-specific marker for RCC (11). TGF-ß1 is mainly synthesized in bone matrix and the α-granules of platelets and can modulate lymphocyte activation and may therefore locally influence an immune response in RCC by suppressing immunological effects against tumor and promotion of metastases (12,13). So determination of TGF-ß1 in different stages of RCC may prove to be of clinical benefit. Various different immunoassays for detection have been described, but reference values as well as sample handling procedures differ greatly (14,15). For measuring TGF-ß1 levels we have developed a new, sensitive enzyme linked-immunosorbent assay (ELISA), which is specific for TGF-ß1. This assay which applies optimized activation procedure for TGF-ß1 has been described in connection with other commercially available assays (16). The aim of the present study was to introduce the new detection assay and to evaluate the clinical suitability of TGF-ß1 in plasma as a tumor marker for different stages of RCC and postoperative follow-up.

Material and Methods

To evaluate the value of TGF-ß1 in the diagnosis of localized and metastatic RCC blood samples were collected from 39 patients (19 women, 20 men, mean age 61.5 years) with localized RCC prior to surgical therapy (radical nephrectomy, tumor enucleation). Peripheral blood samples were collected in EDTA-supplemented tubes and processed for plasma within 3 hours. After centrifugation (2000rpm, 10 min) and removal of supernatant plasma the samples were stored at -70 °C. Physical examination, chest X-ray, intravenous urography, abdominal sonography, CT/MRI were used for clinical staging. In metastatic disease, additional examinations were performed. TGF-ß1 was also measured on days 1 (n=31), 5 (n=31), 10 (n=21) and 3-6 months (n=18) after surgical treatment. During surgery (n=10) blood was obtained from the renal vein and a distant peripheral vein in order to proof any tumor specific secretion of TGF-ß1. We also measured the TGF-ß1 plasma levels of 17 patients with metastatic disease (2 women, 15 men, mean age 63 years). Out of this group 11 patients presented with multiple pulmonary metastases, 4 patients with pulmonary and bone metastases, 1 patient with bone and cerebral metastases, 1 patient with pulmonary and thyroid gland metastases. 100 patients (27 women, 73 men, mean age 57.2 years) with various benign urological diseases (i.e. urinary incontinence, benign prostatic hyperplasia, hypospadia) and without malignancies in medical history were recruited as a control group. For measuring TGF-ß1 levels we have developed a new, sensitive enzyme linked-immunosorbent assay (ELISA), which is specific for TGF-ß1. The applied assay was thoroughly tested and the advantages of the new test in comparison with other assays has recently been published (16).

Statistical analysis was performed using nonparametric Kruskal-Wallis ANOVA test (SPSS® Software). A p-value <0.05 was accepted as statistically significance.

Results

The intra-assay variance was evaluated by 20-fold determination of on sample. The coefficient of variance amounted 2%. The inter-assay variance was determined on 7 different days and the coefficient of variance was 7,5 %.

Patients with localized disease showed median preoperative plasma concentrations of 16790 ng/L (6204-54834 ng/L) for latent TGF-ß1 and 455 ng/L (66-1610 ng/L) for active TGF-ß1. The control group had median concentrations of 20106 ng/L (2631-52285 ng/L) for latent TGF-ß1 and also 455 ng/L (56-1650 ng/L) for active TGF-ß1. The differences (nonparametric Kruskal-Wallis ANOVA) between the two groups were statistically insignificant (Figure 1). Patients with metastatic RCC showed median plasma concentrations of 34421 ng/L (6800-48960 ng/L) for latent TGF-ß1 and 720 ng/L (320-1120 ng/L) for active TGF-ß1. Comparing this TGF-ß1 plasma levels with the localized RCC group and the control group a statistically significant difference ($p<0,01$) was found (Figure 2). Stratifying the patients to the UICC TNM-system (2002) and nuclear grading we identified no significant differences between the pathological subgroups. Also no difference was found between the different locations of metastases. Comparing TGF-ß1 and latent TGF-ß1 plasma concentrations of the peripheral blood versus the renal vein blood no significant differences of TGF-ß1 levels were observed. Plasma levels after surgical therapy (days 1, 5 and 10) and during follow-up without evidence of disease (2-6 months) showed also no distinct differences (Figure 3).

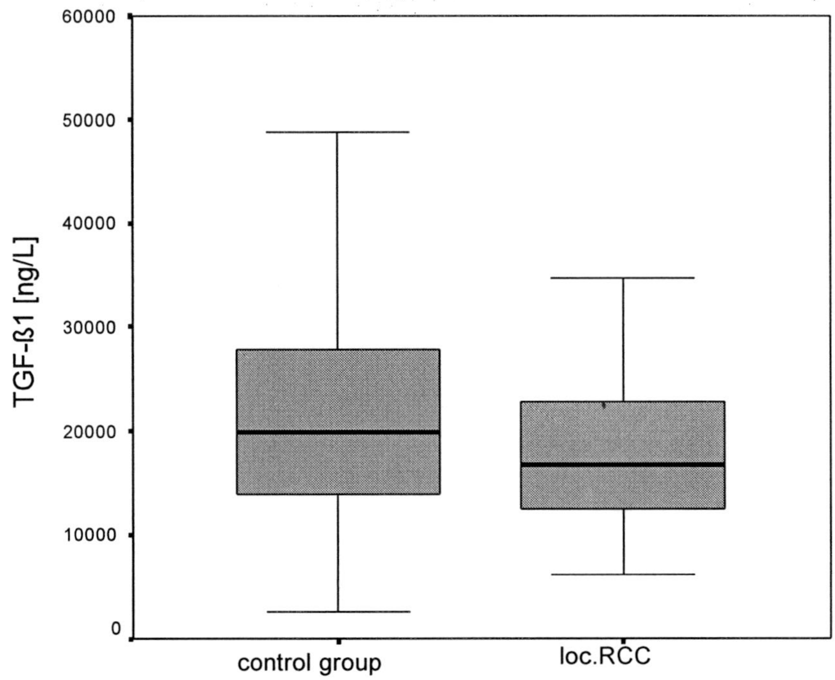

Figure 1. TGF-ß1 plasma levels in patients with localized RCC (n=39) and in patients with various benign urological disorders (n=100).

No significant difference (nonparametric Kruskal-Wallis ANOVA) was detectable.

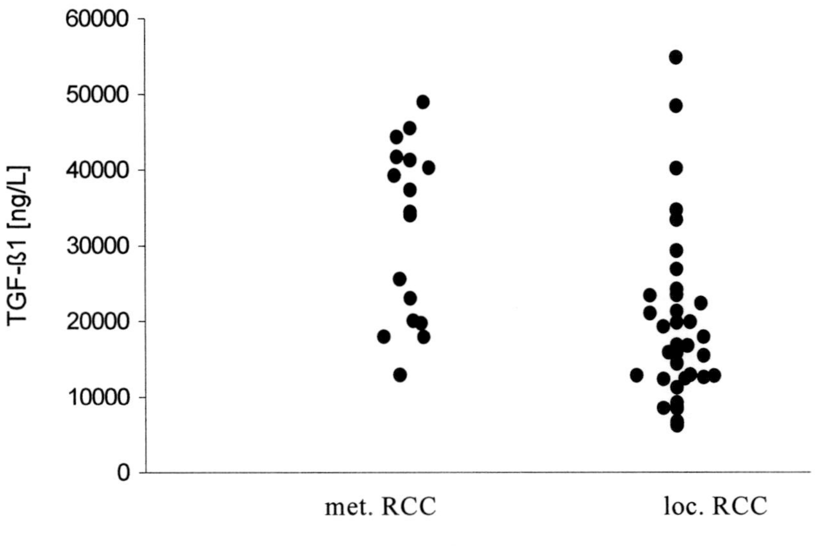

Figure 2. Concentration of TGF-ß1 in patients with localized (n=39) and metastatic RCC (n=17). Statistical analysis showed a significant difference ($p<0.01$).

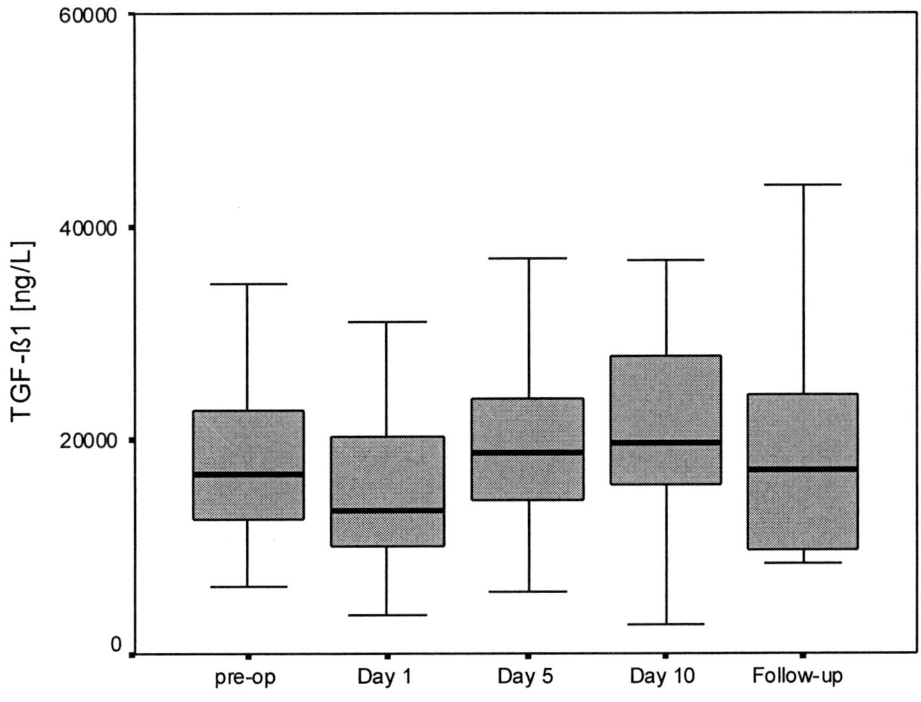

Figure 3. Plasma levels after surgical therapy (days 1, 5 and 10) and during follow-up without evidence of disease (2-6 months) showed no distinct differences.

DISCUSSION

The present study was performed to evaluate the clinical utility of TGF-ß1 plasma-levels in patients suffering from RCC in order to obtain prognostic reference and to facilitate postoperative monitoring. With several different functions like regulation of cell proliferation and differentiation, TGF-ß1 seems to play an important role in development and progression in RCC. We are aware that our results are in contrast to those reported by others (11,17,18). In contrast to our investigation, where TGF-ß1 was detected in plasma, Wunderlich and coworkers first measured TGF-ß1 levels in serum (11). In our opinion measuring serum-levels may produce false positive values as TGF-ß1 is released by platelets during the clotting process (19). This topic has been adressed extensively by Wakefield (20). In several cases of RCC a paraneoplastic, IL-6 induced, thrombocytosis occurs which can be quite responsible for higher, but not tumor specific, TGF-ß1 serum levels (21). However, measurement of TGF-ß1 in plasma have to be recommended (20). Wunderlich and coworkers described elevated TGF-ß1 plasma levels in 20 patients suffering from RCC by using an ELISA developed and published by Danielpour (18,22). In our opinion the different results can be caused by the different assays used. Especially with TGF-ß1 the problems of comparability between different analytical methods should be generally stressed (16). TGF-ß1 was also produced by renal cell carcinoma cell lines and expression TGF-ß1 mRNA in tumor samples was found (17). These results together with our findings underline the important but still unclear role of TGF-ß1 in different stages of RCC. We first describe significant higher plasma levels of TGF-ß1 in metastatic RCC compared to localized disease. This aspect seems to be of high interest for the follow-up after surgical therapy and respond of consecutive immunochemotherapy in case of metastases. Our results demonstrate that TGF-ß1 is not a suitable and reliable diagnostic tool to detect patients with localized RCC. Our data lead to conclusion that the tumor cells are not the predominant source of TGF-ß1 within the organism. Whether TGF-ß1 might be useful in early detection of RCC recurrence, to control success of immunochemotherapy in metastatic disease or as a prognostic parameter in the face of higher plasma levels in metastatic disease has to be proved in further investigations.

REFERENCES

[1] Russo P: Renal cell carcinoma: presentation, staging, and surgical treatment. *Semin Oncol* 2000;27:160-176.

[2] McLaughlin JK, Lipworth L: Epidemiologic aspects of renal cell cancer. *Semin Oncol* 2000;27:115-123.

[3] Gago-Dominguez M, Yuan JM, Castelao JE, Ross RK, Yu MC: Family history and risk of renal cell carcinoma. *Cancer Epidemiol Biomarkers Prev* 2001;10:1001-1004.

[4] Giberti C, Oneto F, Martorana G, Rovida S, Carmignani G: Radical nephrectomy for renal cell carcinoma: long-term results and prognostic factors on a series of 328 cases. *Eur Urol* 1997;31:40-48.

[5] Hegele A, Varga Z, Kosche B, Stief T, Heidenreich A, Hofmann R: Pyruvate kinase type tumor M2 in urological malignancies. *Urol Int* 2003;70:55-58.

[6] von Knobloch R, Hegele A, Brandt H, Varga Z, Wille S, Kalble T, Heidenreich A, Hofmann R: High frequency of serum DNA alterations in renal cell carcinoma detected by fluorescent microsatellite analysis. *Int J Cancer* 2002;98:889-894.

[7] Michael A, Pandha HS: Renal-cell carcinoma: tumour markers, T-cell epitopes, and potential for new therapies. *Lancet Oncol.* 2003; 4:215-223.

[8] Ozer G, Altinel M, Kocak B, Yazicioglu A, Gonenc F: Value of urinary NMP-22 in patients with renal cell carcinoma. *Urology.* 2002; 60:593-597.

[9] Phillips AO, Steadman R, Topley N, Williams JD: Elevated D-glucose concentrations modulate TGF-beta 1 synthesis by human cultured renal proximal tubular cells. The permissive role of platelet-derived growth factor. *Am J Pathol* 1995;147:362-374.

[10] Lawrence DA: Transforming growth factor-beta: an overview. *Kidney Int* 1995; 49:19-23.

[11] Wunderlich H, Steiner T, Junker U, Knofel B, Schlichter A, Schubert J: Serum transforming growth factor-beta1 in patients with renal cell carcinoma. *J Urol* 1997; 157:1602-1603.

[12] Reinhold D, Bank U, Buhling F, Lendeckel U, Ulmer AJ, Flad HD, Ansorge S: Transforming growth factor-beta 1 (TGF-beta 1) inhibits DNA synthesis of PWM-stimulated PBMC via suppression of IL-2 and IL-6 production. *Cytokine* 1994; 6:382-388.

[13] Roberts AB, Sporn MB: The transforming growth factor-beta. In: Sporn MB, Roberts AB, eds. Peptide growth factors and their receptors. *Handbook of experimental pharmacology*. Heidelberg 1990: Springer Verlag, p 419-472.

[14] Meager A: Assays for transforming growth factor beta. *J Immunol Methods* 1991; 141:1-14.

[15] Phillips AO, Steadman R, Donovan KD, Williams JD: A new antibody capture enzyme linked immunoassay specific for transforming growth factor beta. *Int J Biochem Cell Biol* 1995; 27:207-213.

[16] Kropf J, Schurek JO, Wollner A, Gressner AM: Immunological measurement of transforming growth factor-beta1 (TGF-beta1) in blood; assay development and comparison. *Clin Chem* 1997; 43:1965-1974.

[17] Junker U, Knoefel B, Nuske K, Rebstock K, Steiner T, Wunderlich H, Junker K, Reinhold D: Transforming growth factor beta 1 is significantly elevated in plasma of patients suffering from renal cell carcinoma. *Cytokine* 1996; 8:794-798.

[18] Wunderlich H, Steiner T, Kosmehl H, Junker U, Reinhold D, Reichelt O, Zermann DH, Schubert J: Increased Transforming Growth Factor ß1 Plasma Level in Patients with Renal Cell Carcinoma: A Tumor-Specific Marker? *Urol Int* 1998; 60:205-207.

[19] Assoian RK, Sporn MB: Type ß transforming growth factor in human platelets: release during platelet degranulation and action on vascular smooth muscle cells. *J Cell Biol* 1986; 102:1217-1223.

[20] Wakefield LM, Letterio JJ, Chen T, Danielpour D, Allison RS, Pai LH, Denicoff AM, Noone MH, Cowan KH, O'Shaughnessy JA, Sporn MB: Transforming growth factor-beta1 circulates in normal human plasma and is unchanged in advanced metastatic breast cancer. *Clin Cancer Res* 1995; 1:129-136.

[21] Blay JY, Favrot M, Rossi JF, Wijdenes J: Role of interleukin-6 in paraneoplastic thrombocytosis. *Blood* 1993; 82:2261-2262.

[22] Danielpour D: Improved sandwich enzyme-linked immunosorbent assays for transforming growth factor beta-1. *J Immunol Methods* 1993; 158:17.

In: Trends in Kidney Cancer Research
Editor: Kelvin R. Nunez, pp. 23-38
ISBN 1-59454-141-8

Chapter III

Prognostic and Predictive Implications of CD8highCD57+ Lymphocytes for Advanced Renal Cell Carcinoma Patients

Dainius Characiejus, [*] ***Vita Pašukonienė, Nijolė Kazlauskaitė, Tadas Petraitis and Konstantinas P. Valuckas***
Institute of Oncology, Vilnius University, Vilnius, Lithuania

Abstract

Before new agents for treatment of metastatic renal cell carcinoma (RCC) are developed, immunotherapy with cytokines (interferon-α or interleukin-2) remains a standard treatment option. The overall impact of immunotherapy on survival of metastatic RCC patients is small. However, long lasting remissions are achieved in some patients. Given the great variability in natural course of metastatic RCC, it is important to define patients with good or bad prognosis and those likely to benefit from immunotherapy with cytokines. Traditional clinical and laboratory prognostic factors (performance status, time from initial diagnosis, lactate dehydrogenase, hemoglobin level, etc.) are not sufficient for this purpose. Therefore, identification of new prognostic and predictive factors in advanced RCC is necessary. In the retrospective study, we analyzed the impact of pre-treatment levels of peripheral blood lymphocyte subsets (CD3+, CD19+, CD16&56+, CD4+, CD8+, CD4+CD45ROhigh and CD8highCD57+) on survival of advanced RCC patients treated and non-treated with interferon-α2b (IFN). Percentages and absolute levels of lymphocyte subsets in peripheral blood were determined in 85 consecutive advanced RCC patients using flow cytometry. Sixty patients with known IFN treatment status were selected for survival analysis. Thirty-two of these 60 patients were treated with IFN and 28 patients were non-treated. Survival of IFN-treated and non-treated

* Corresponding author: Dainius Characiejus, Institute of Oncology, Vilnius University, Santariškių 1, 08660 Vilnius, Lithuania. Telephone: +370 52786 816, Fax: +370 52720164, E-mail: dainius@banga.lt

patients was analyzed by testing gradually different cut-of levels of each lymphocyte subset. Of all lymphocyte subsets analyzed, only the CD8highCD57+ lymphocytes (‘cytotoxic/ regulatory’ CD8+ lymphocytes) were found to be significant in determining survival of IFN-treated and non-treated RCC patients. Non-treated patients with < 30% CD8highCD57+ lymphocytes in CD8+ subset survived significantly longer compared to patients with ≥ 30% CD8highCD57+ lymphocytes in CD8+ subset (median survival 23.5 months and 6 months, respectively; p = 0.01). Treatment with IFN increased overall survival only in the latter subgroup of advanced RCC patients (median survival increased from 6 to 18.5 months; p = 0.02), whereas in the former group, a trend towards decreased survival after treatment with IFN was observed (median survival 23.5 months and 13.6 months for non-treated and treated patients, respectively; p = 0.11). Thus, our results suggest that percentage of CD8highCD57+ lymphocytes in the CD8+ subset may have a prognostic significance for advanced RCC patients and may have a predictive value in patient selection for survival benefit due to treatment with IFN.

INTRODUCTION

Renal cell carcinoma (RCC) may have very different clinical outcomes in different patients and can be regarded as one of the most heterogeneous of adult malignancies. It is well known, that metastases of RCC may first appear 20 years or more after nephrectomy [6]. In about 1% to 7% of cases, spontaneous regression of pulmonary metastases after removal of the primary tumor may occur [22], [26]. This incidence is one of the highest reported incidences of spontaneous regression among all malignant tumors [10],[11]. In general, outcome of patients with metastatic RCC is poor with the median survival of approximately 1 year. However, some primary tumors and metastases of RCC, especially pulmonary parenchymal lesions, may have periods with little or no growth during many months [11]. A small subset (from 4.5% to 20%) of patients with metastatic RCC survive 5 or more years [11], [22], [25].

The above evidence clearly shows that the course of RCC is far from uniform and prognostic evaluation of metastatic RCC patients remains a major challenge. Several attempts have been made to divide metastatic RCC patients into different prognostic groups on the basis of clinical and laboratory risk factors. The risk factors for short survival usually include bad performance status, absence of nephrectomy, short disease to treatment interval, more than one metastatic site, location of metastases in liver, bone or brain, loss of weight, high erythrocite sedimentation rate, high lactate dehydrogenase, high neutrophil count and low hemoglobin [27],[35]. In a prognostic model developed in Memorial Sloan-Kettering Cancer Center, five variables were selected as the most significant risk factors for short survival: low Karnofsky performance status (< 80%), high lactate dehydrogenase (> 1.5 x upper limit of normal), low hemoglobin (< lower limit of normal), high “corrected” serum calcium (>10 mg/dl), and absence of nephrectomy. These prognostic factors were used to categorize patients into three groups of different risk. The median survival was 20 months for favorable risk patients (zero risk factors), 10 months for intermediate risk patients (one or two risk factors) and 4 months for poor risk patients (three or more risk factors) [27]. Thus, Memorial

Sloan-Kettering Cancer Center model proved suitable for stratification of metastatic RCC patients into three prognostic groups with substantially different survival.

Before new agents for treatment of metastatic RCC are developed, the standard treatment option remains immunotherapy with interferon-α or interleukin-2 [18], [35]. However, for both of these cytokines, the objective response rate is less than 15% [16],[32] and the overall impact on median survival of metastatic RCC patients is small [2],[7],[16],[26]. The individual response to treatment with cytokines is unpredictable, differing from patient to patient. Given considerable toxicity and varying responses to treatment, it is important to identify those metastatic RCC patients that benefit most from the cytokine therapy and to avoid overtreatment of the unresponsive subgroup of patients.

Predictive significance for cytokine therapy of various clinical prognostic factors and laboratory parameters have been studied by several investigators [7], [27], [35]. In general, prognostic risk factors for short survival were associated with lower responsiveness to cytokine therapy. On the contrary, a good performance status, a disease to treatment interval of more than 24 months and a single site of metastatic disease usually have been considered as factors associated with responsiveness of metastatic RCC patients to biological therapy [27],[33],[35]. In the retrospective analysis of the Memorial Sloan-Kettering Cancer Center prognostic model, there was a significant difference in survival between favorable-risk, intermediate-risk and poor-risk groups of patients, treated with interferon-α. When survival of the three risk groups of cytokine-treated patients was compared to survival of corresponding risk groups of patients treated with chemotherapy, the magnitude of difference in median survival was greater in favorable-risk and intermediate-risk groups. These and other observations suggest that favorable-risk and intermediate-risk patients benefit most from cytokine therapy in terms of survival. However, some survival benefit is obtained also in the poor-risk group [27],[35]. Therefore, although these prognostic models may be suitable for risk stratification in phase III trials with metastatic RCC using interferon-α as a comparative treatment arm [24], they hardly can help in deciding whether to treat or not to treat with cytokines an individual patient. For this purpose, new more precise prognostic and predictive factors, based on biology of tumor cells and on immune response of the patient are necessary.

It is generally believed that RCC is an immunogenic tumor and that immunotherapy with cytokines may act by supporting immune responses directed against RCC [31]. In spite of this, there is only a small amount of data on pre-treatment immunological parameters that would correlate with clinical response of RCC patients or their survival. In this context, the data by Göhring et al. [19] can be mentioned. These authors observed that pre-treatment numbers of T and B lymphocytes in peripheral blood were significantly higher in metastatic RCC patients with clinical response induced by treatment with interleukin-2/interferon-α in combination with 5-fluorouracil.

In our recent study [9], we analyzed in more detail the impact of pre-treatment levels of different lymphocyte subsets on survival of advanced RCC patients treated and non-treated with interferon-α2b (IFN henceforth). In addition to CD3+, CD19+ and CD16&56+ (T, B and NK lymphocytes, respectively), CD4+ (helper/inducer T lymphocytes), CD8+ (cytotoxic/suppressor T lymphocytes), we were especially interested in CD4+CD45ROhigh ('memory' CD4+ lymphocytes) and CD8highCD57+ ('cytotoxic/ regulatory' CD8+

lymphocytes). We considered the latter two lymphocyte subsets of major interest because they might indicate the exposure of the immune system to tumor-associated antigen [5], [13], [23].

Patients and Methods

Patients

Between February 1995 and May 1999, flow cytometric analysis of peripheral blood lymphocyte subsets was performed for 85 consecutive patients with advanced RCC, treated at Department of Oncological Urology, Institute of Oncology, Vilnius University. Sixty of these patients with histologically confirmed diagnosis of RCC, metastatic/inoperable disease and known IFN treatment status were selected for retrospective survival analysis. If administered, IFN therapy had to be started not later than 10 days after determination of lymphocyte subsets in peripheral blood. Patients who received radiation within three months prior to determination of lymphocyte subsets and patients who underwent radical surgery for RCC subsequently to determination of their lymphocyte subsets were not included in survival analysis.

Thirty-two of 60 patients selected for survival analysis were treated with recombinant IFN (Realdiron, Biotechna, Vilnius, Lithuania) and attended at least one visit at the Institute of Oncology after one month. These patients were known to have received treatment with IFN during one month and were administered IFN for at least one more month. IFN was administered intramuscularly at doses of 18 MU three times a week. Ten of 32 patients received IFN in combination with 5-fluorouracil. In the combination treatment regimen, patients received 750 mg/m^2 5-fluorouracil as an intravenous bolus infusion and 9 MU IFN intramuscularly daily during 5 consecutive days every 5 weeks. Between these cycles, IFN was administered intramuscularly at doses of 18 MU three times a week.

Twenty-eight of 60 patients selected for survival analysis were considered as non-treated with IFN. Four of these 28 patients refused or were not offered treatment with IFN, and the remaining 24 patients discontinued treatment with IFN within one month.

FACS Analysis of Peripheral Blood Lymphocyte Subsets

Peripheral venous blood samples from patients were collected using EDTA as anticoagulant. Whole blood was stained for 15 min at room temperature in the dark with saturating amounts of fluorochrome conjugated monoclonal antibodies. The following combinations of monoclonal antibodies were used: CD3-FITC/CD16&56-PE/CD19-PerCP, CD57-FITC/CD8-PE/CD4-PerCP and CD45RO-PE/CD4-PerCP (Becton Dickinson). After incubation with monoclonal antibodies, red blood cells were lysed by incubating the samples with 2 ml of FACS® Lysing Solution (Becton Dickinson) for 10 min at room temperature in the dark. Subsequently, the samples were centrifuged and the supernatant discarded. After washing with CellWash (Becton Dickinson) the cells were fixed with CellFix™ (Becton

Dickinson) and kept at 4°C until flow cytometric analysis. The samples were analyzed on a FACSort® (Becton Dickinson) flow cytometer with a laser tuned at 488 nm. Data were acquired and analyzed with LYSYS II software (Becton Dickinson). List mode files were collected for 10,000 cells from each sample. Forward and side scatter were used to gate lymphocytes and the absolute count of lymphocytes was calculated by multiplying the percentage of lymphocytes with the absolute number of white blood cells counted with a haemocytometer. The absolute counts of the following lymphocyte subsets were calculated: CD3+, CD19+, CD16&56+, CD4+, CD8+, CD4+CD45ROhigh, CD8highCD57+. The percentage of CD8highCD57+ lymphocytes in CD8+ subset, the percentage of CD4+CD45ROhigh lymphocytes in CD4+ subset and CD4+ / CD8+ ratio were determined.

Follow-Up and Statistics

Survival was calculated from the date of determination of lymphocyte subsets to the date of death or the last date the patient was known to be alive. All patients were followed-up with help of the Lithuanian Cancer Registry. The influence of lymphocyte subsets on survival of IFN-treated and non-treated patients was evaluated by placing patients in subgroups according to gradual cut-off levels in each lymphocyte subset. Survival of patient subgroups was analyzed using the Kaplan-Meier method. The difference between survival curves was determined using log-rank test.

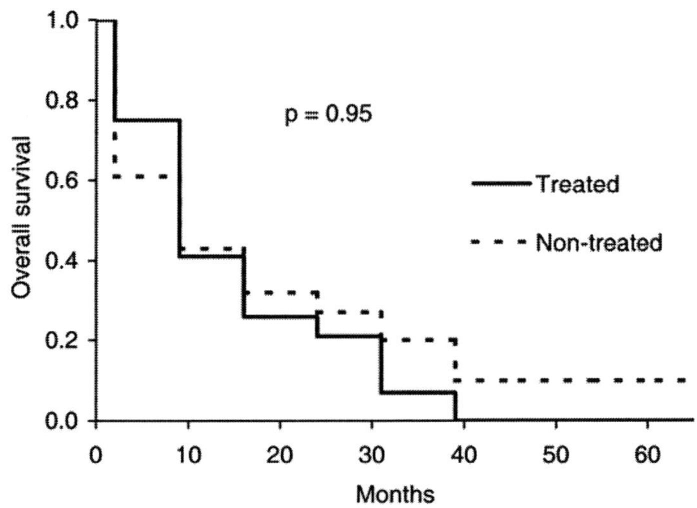

Figure 1. Kaplan-Meier overall survival curves for all IFN-treated (n = 32) and non-treated (n = 28) RCC patients (Anticancer Research 22: 3679-3684, 2002; reproduced with permission)

Results

The 60 patients with advanced RCC were analyzed. There were 39 men, 21 women, median age 62 years (range 34 – 81 years). Four patients had unresectable primary kidney tumor without evidence of distant metastases, but the majority of the patients (56) had metastatic disease. The median duration of follow-up was 15 months (range 2 – 69.3 months). Clinical characteristics of RCC patients treated with IFN and of IFN-non-treated patients are described in Table 1. The majority of the 32 patients treated with IFN continued treatment for 2 to 3 months (24 patients), 4 patients continued treatment for 3 to 12 months and another 4 patients for more than 12 months.

Overall survival data of 32 IFN-treated patients and 28 non-treated patients are given in Figure 1. Median survival time of these patient groups was 15 months and 15.5 months, respectively. There was no difference in overall survival between IFN-treated and non-treated patients in our analysis.

Table 1. Patients' Characteristics according to IFN Treatment Status

	IFN-treated (N = 32)	Non-treated (N = 28)
Age (years)		
Median	59	64
Range	34-72	40-81
Sex		
Male	21	18
Female	11	10
Prior nephrectomy	19	12
Duration of the disease (months)		
<12	20	20
>12	12	8
Metastatic disease	32	24
Sites of metastasis		
Lung	19	13
Liver	3	3
Bone	4	2
Lymph node	6	7
Other*	7	2
Prior therapy		
None	27	22
Radiation therapy	1	1
Chemotherapy	1	2
Embolization	3	3

* Includes: renal bed, soft tissue, spleen, peritoneum and contralateral kidney (Anticancer Research 22: 3679-3684, 2002; reproduced with permission).

Absolute counts and percentages of peripheral blood lymphocyte subsets were examined to find a cut-off that would categorize IFN-treated or non-treated patients into subgroups with significantly different survival. CD3+, CD19+, CD16&56+, CD4+, CD8+, CD4+CD45ROhigh lymphocytes and CD4+ / CD8+ ratio were not associated with survival of RCC patients (results not shown). The only lymphocyte subset that was significantly important in determining survival of IFN-treated and non-treated RCC patients was CD8highCD57+ lymphocytes (Figure 2) with the cut-off point of 30% in the CD8+ subset. In our study, CD8highCD57+ lymphocytes were determined for 66 of 85 patients (including 49 of 60 patients selected for survival analysis). Of these 66 patients, 32 patients (48%) had ≥ 30% of CD8highCD57+ lymphocytes in CD8+ subset.

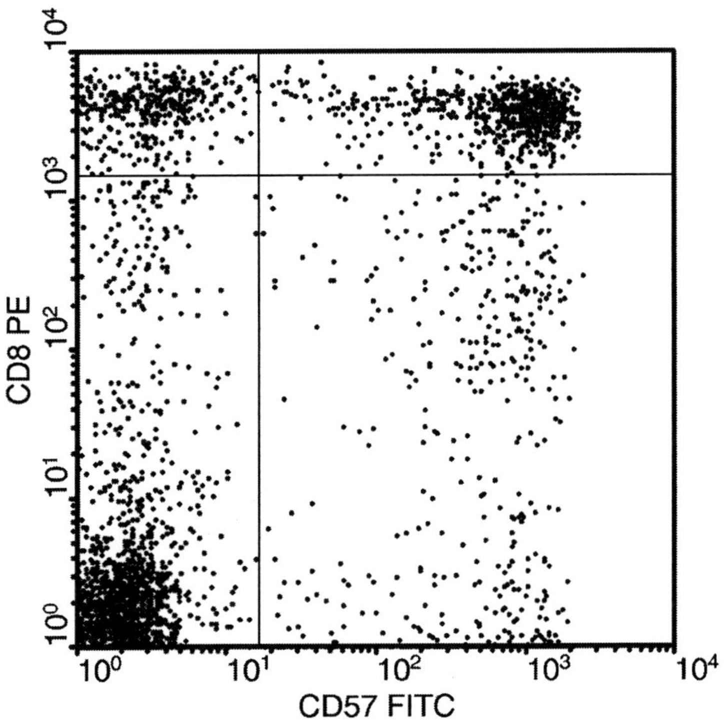

Figure 2. Two-parameter flow cytometric dot plot showing CD8highCD57+ lymphocytes (upper right quadrant) (Anticancer Research 22: 3679-3684, 2002; reproduced with permission)

Overall survival of IFN-non-treated RCC patients with ≥ 30% CD8highCD57+ lymphocytes in the CD8+ subset was significantly shorter compared to IFN-non-treated patients with < 30% CD8highCD57+ lymphocytes in the CD8+ subset (Figure 3). Median survival time of IFN-non-treated patients with ≥ 30% CD8highCD57+ and with < 30% CD8highCD57+ lymphocytes in the CD8+ subset was 6 months and 23.5 months, respectively.

Treatment with IFN significantly increased overall survival of RCC patients with ≥ 30% CD8highCD57+ lymphocytes in the CD8+ subset (Figure 4). Median survival time of IFN-treated patients with ≥ 30% CD8highCD57+ lymphocytes in the CD8+ subset was 18.5 months compared to 6 months of patients non-treated with IFN.

In contrast, treatment with IFN did not increase survival of RCC patients with < 30% CD8highCD57+ lymphocytes in the CD8+ subset. Moreover, a trend towards decreased overall survival of patients with < 30% of CD8highCD57+ lymphocytes in the CD8+ subset after treatment with IFN was observed (Figure 5). Median survival time of IFN-treated RCC patients with < 30% CD8highCD57+ lymphocytes in the CD8+ subset was 13.6 months compared to 23.5 months of patients non-treated with IFN.

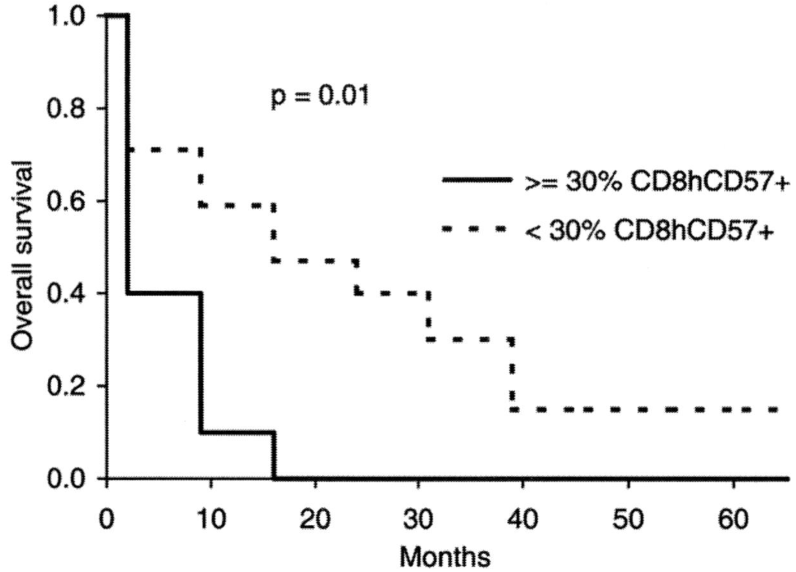

Figure 3. Kaplan-Meier overall survival curves for IFN–non-treated RCC patients with ≥ 30 % (n = 10) or < 30 % (n = 17) of CD8highCD57+ lymphocytes in CD8+ subset (Anticancer Research 22: 3679-3684, 2002; reproduced with permission).

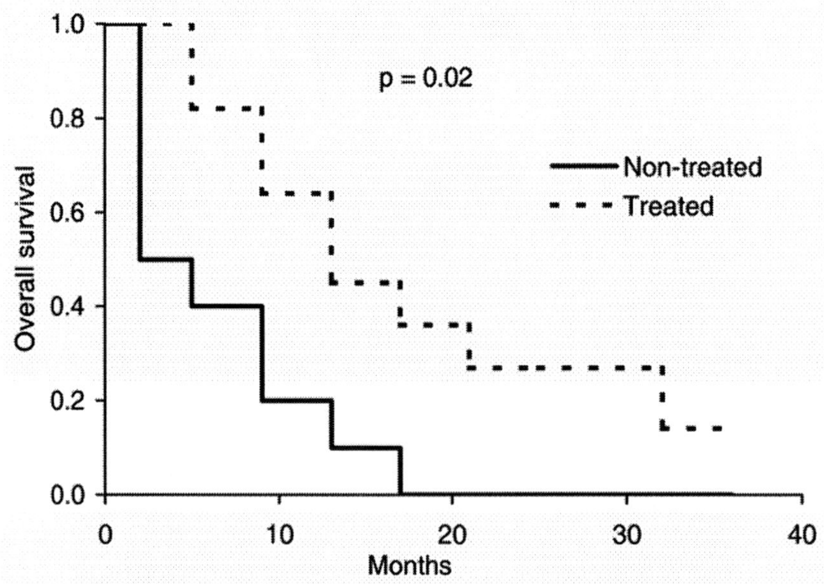

Figure 4. Kaplan-Meier overall survival curves for RCC patients with ≥ 30 % of CD8highCD57+ lymphocytes in CD8+ subset who were treated (n = 11) or non-treated (n = 10) with IFN (Anticancer Research 22: 3679-3684, 2002; reproduced with permission).

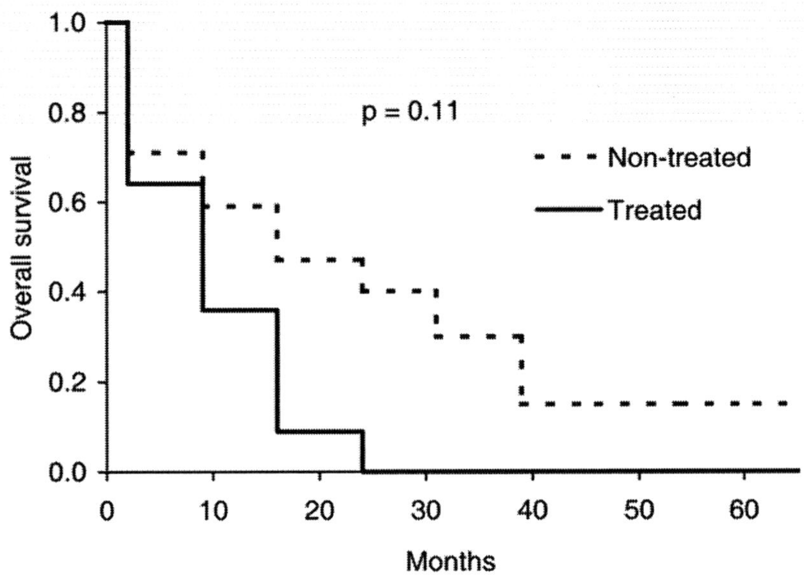

Figure 5. Kaplan-Meier overall survival curves for RCC patients with < 30 % of CD8highCD57+ lymphocytes in CD8+ subset who were treated (n = 11) or non-treated (n= 17) with IFN (Anticancer Research 22: 3679-3684, 2002; reproduced with permission).

Discussion

Non-selective treatment of all metastatic RCC patients with interferon-α can hardly be justified, because the overall impact on survival is low and the toxicity of this treatment is considerable. Given the well-know variability in natural course of RCC and in response to treatment, individualization of therapy is extremely important in this malignancy.

Many attempts have been made to find correlations between immunological changes and clinical response of RCC to cytokine therapy. The parameters studied include CD3+ CD25+/- HLADr+/-, CD45RA+ lymphocyte subsets, CD4+/CD8+ ratio, thyroid autoantibodies, T-lymphocyte signal transduction molecules and proliferation of T lymphocytes in the autologous mixed-lymphocyte reaction and allogeneic mixed-lymphocyte reaction [8],[17],[20],[34],[37]. The results of these studies are inconclusive and none of the above-mentioned immunological parameters can be used in making decision about treatment with cytokines of an individual patient.

The analysis of the predictive significance for treatment with cytokines of immunological parameters is not possible without a control group of non-treated patients. Such a control group nowadays would not be feasible for ethical reasons, because cytokines, in particular interferon-α, are considered a standard treatment in patients with metastatic RCC [2],[16], [33],[35].

During 1995-1999, interferon-α was just being introduced in Lithuania, and no strict guidelines towards its use for treatment of metastatic RCC were available. This was the reason for considerable variability in approach to treatment of metastatic RCC patients in Lithuania during that period. Therefore, we were able to select in our analysis a subgroup of advanced RCC patients who could be considered as non-treated with IFN [9]. Four of these 28 patients did not start treatment with IFN, and the remaining 24 patients discontinued the treatment within one month. It was unlikely that this short duration of treatment with IFN was sufficient to exert its antitumor effect, because, to our knowledge, at least two months of continuous treatment with interferon-α are necessary to achieve a clinical response in RCC patients [1], [15]. Therefore, although we are aware that these 28 patients are not a true control group, we think that the impact on survival of this very short treatment with IFN of 24 patients is negligible.

The remaining 32 patients were treated with IFN for at least two months. In our analysis, we combined patients treated with IFN monotherapy and patients treated with the combination of IFN and 5-fluorouracil, because the existing evidence did not support any advantage of the addition of 5-fluorouracil to interferon-α in treatment of RCC [14], [21], [28].

Both treated and non-treated patient subgroups had their lymphocyte subsets determined using flow-cytometry. Thus, we had a rather unique opportunity to analyze the prognostic / predictive significance of peripheral blood lymphocyte subsets in patients with advanced RCC.

Because of retrospective nature of our study, accurate data on objective response of treated patients are not available. However, the objective response may not always be related to survival of metastatic RCC patients and, therefore, should not be considered as the most important endpoint of the treatment outcome. This notion is substantiated by the results of Fosså SD et al. [15], who observed that addition of vinblastine to interferon in the treatment of metastatic RCC resulted in doubling of the response rate without prolongation of survival. Novel therapies such as immunotherapy or angiogenesis inhibition may produce prolonged stabilization of disease or slow tumor regression over many months without causing an objective response according to standard criteria [27].

In our retrospective analysis, we were not able to find any prognostic or predictive significance for treatment with IFN of CD3+, CD19+, CD16&56+, CD4+, CD8+, CD4+CD45ROhigh lymphocytes or CD4+ / CD8+ ratio in advanced RCC patients. In contrast with these negative results, the percentage of CD8highCD57+ lymphocytes in CD8+ subset was found to have a strong prognostic significance for advanced RCC patients and a strong predictive value for survival benefit for patients treated with IFN. Similarly to percentage of CD8highCD57+ lymphocytes in the CD8+ subset, the absolute count of CD8highCD57+ lymphocytes also has a prognostic and a predictive significance for advanced RCC patients (cut-off level 100 cells/μl; data not presented). At this time, however, we consider the percentage of CD8highCD57+ lymphocytes in the CD8+ subset as more reliable parameter because it is entirely flow-cytometric and avoids possible errors in manual/automatic counting of white blood cells.

CD57 is a 110-kDa glycoprotein, first identified on NK cells but also present on a subset of T cells. The density of CD8 antigen on T lymphocytes is higher than on NK cells. Therefore, CD8highCD57+ lymphocytes can be considered to be T cells, whereas CD8+CD57+ lymphocytes may contain NK cells as well [23], [36].

Clonal expansion of CD8highCD57+ or CD8+CD57+ lymphocytes has been described in a variety of clinical disorders associated with chronic antigenic stimulation: in patients with autoimmune diseases, in leukemia/lymphoma patients after allogeneic bone marrow transplantation, in patients with human cytomegalovirus or HIV infection [12],[13],[36]. It has been hypothesized that these expanded T cells represent antigen-specific effector cells directed against antigens to which the immune system is exposed [13]. On the other hand, regulatory or suppressive functions have been ascribed to CD8+CD57+ lymphocytes [23],[36].

Expanded CD8+CD57+ T-cell populations have been described in patients with multiple myeloma and associated with possible survival advantage [30]. Batliwalla et al. [4] have reported on the association between clonal expansion of CD8+CD57+ lymphocytes and improved outcome of AJCC stage III malignant melanoma patients treated with Newcastle disease virus oncolysate. To our knowledge, there are no studies on CD8highCD57+ or CD8+CD57+ lymphocytes in patients with other solid tumors.

Nearly half (48% according to our data) of advanced RCC patients have $\geq 30\%$ CD8highCD57+ lymphocytes in the CD8+ subset. These patients may benefit from IFN treatment in terms of survival. This proportion is considerably larger compared to the percentage of patients in whom the objective response is achieved (15%). On the other hand, RCC patients with $< 30\%$ CD8highCD57+ lymphocytes in the CD8+ subset do not benefit from IFN treatment at all. Obviously, this subset of patients experience considerable side effects of IFN therapy with likely deterioration of quality of life. Although not statistically significant, our results suggest that IFN treatment may even shorten survival of patients with low CD8highCD57+ lymphocyte counts. These our results may not seem entirely surprising, because a harmful effect of interferon-α therapy on event-free survival of RCC patients has already been demonstrated in the adjuvant setting [29].

Prognostic / predictive models based on clinical risk factors or their combinations [27],[35] have their value in designing phase III trials and in the risk-directed therapy of metastatic RCC patients with cytokines. The relationship of the prognostic / predictive potential of the CD8highCD57+ lymphocyte subset with that of clinical risk factors remains to be determined. It has to be emphasized, however, that none of the traditional clinical or laboratory risk factors or their combinations has been shown to be associated with complete unresponsiveness to interferon-α therapy. Stratification of metastatic RCC patients using clinical prognostic models is helpful in predicting the magnitude of treatment effect in different subsets of patients, but does not allow identifying patients, who are completely non-responsive to treatment with interferon-α. In contrast, CD8highCD57+ lymphocyte counts appear to be suitable for identifying patients, in whom treatment with interferon-α is entirely ineffective or even harmful. Thus, CD8highCD57+ lymphocyte counts apparently have higher "distinctive power" than traditional clinical factors and therefore might help to select patients who could be spared from ineffective treatment with interferon-α.

It is well known that cytokine therapy may induce prolonged remissions in a subset of metastatic RCC patients, whereas the net effect on survival of larger population of metastatic RCC patients is small or even negligible. This observation may lead to the hypothesis that cytokines may have the opposite effects on survival of different metastatic RCC patients, substantially prolonging survival in one subset of patients while actually shortening survival of the remaining subset of patients. Due to these opposite effects, non-selective treatment with cytokines has little influence on overall survival of metastatic RCC patients. Therefore, we hypothesize that the influence of interferon-α treatment on survival of the whole population of metastatic RCC patients would be considerably larger, if only patients selected according to CD8highCD57+ lymphocyte levels were treated.

We propose the following design for the prospective study to test the above hypothesis and to evaluate the effect on survival and quality of life of individualized treatment of metastatic RCC patients based on pre-treatment CD8highCD57+ lymphocyte counts. Metastatic RCC patients with high levels of CD8highCD57+ lymphocytes (≥30% in CD8+ subset) might be assigned to the interferon-α treatment arm, whereas patients with low levels of CD8highCD57+ lymphocytes (<30% in CD8+ subset) might be assigned to the observation arm. Watch-and-wait approach might be used for patients in the observation arm and changes in CD8highCD57+ lymphocyte levels as well as rate of growth of metastases assessed. Patients from the observation arm might be carried over to the interferon-α treatment arm if CD8highCD57+ lymphocyte levels increase or if the growth of metastases is rapid. Survival data of patients in both study arms could be combined and the median survival as well as the 5-year survival of the whole patient population evaluated.

According to our data, the median survival of both IFN-treated patients with high CD8highCD57+ lymphocyte levels and of IFN-non-treated patients with low CD8highCD57+ lymphocyte levels is close to 20 months. It has to be noted that none of the presently available cytokine-based therapies is able to reproducibly prolong median survival of metastatic RCC patients beyond 16 or 17 months [7]. Therefore, the increase in the median survival of the whole study population to 20 months or more would validate the approach of selecting interferon-α therapy for metastatic RCC patients according to CD8highCD57+ lymphocyte levels.

Although the response rate after treatment with cytokines of metastatic RCC is low and the long term survival is rare, the reproducibility of these treatment effects indicate the existence of pathogenetic relationship between tumor growth and the immune response of the patient. Our observation that higher levels of CD8highCD57+ lymphocytes in peripheral blood are associated with shorter survival of metastatic RCC patients suggests that suppressive functions of CD8highCD57+ lymphocytes may dominate in advanced RCC patients. The mechanisms of antitumor action of interferon-α have not been clarified, but are thought to be activation of macrophages, upregulation of MHC class I molecules and direct antitumor activities [7]. The relationship between the antitumor action of IFN and elevated levels of CD8highCD57+ lymphocytes suggest, that IFN may act by downregulating the suppressive functions or decreasing the numbers of these lymphocytes. The latter possibility is supported by our unpublished observations that elevated levels of CD8highCD57+ lymphocytes in peripheral blood decrease during therapy with IFN.

Thus, it seems likely that CD8highCD57+ lymphocytes are involved in the pathology of the immune response of the patient against RCC and, therefore, may play a role in other forms of immunotherapy for this disease. Apart from interferon-α, another cytokine used for immunotherapy of metastatic RCC is interleukin-2. The toxicity of interleukin-2 is higher than that of interferon-α [35]. Similarly to interferon-α, the median survival for all patients after treatment with interleukin-2 is not altered. However, the responses achieved with this cytokine seem to be more durable, with 10% to 20% patients estimated to be alive 5 to 10 years following treatment [7],[22],[27]. Studies of the predictive role of CD8highCD57+ lymphocytes for therapy of metastatic RCC with interleukin-2 would be interesting.

Another interesting area to study the role of CD8highCD57+ lymphocytes would be the treatment of metastatic RCC patients using non-myeloablative allogeneic stem cell transplantation. This type of treatment has shown very encouraging results in metastatic RCC patients. However, these promising results have been achieved at the cost of considerable transplant related mortality [3]. Therefore, predictive factors in patient selection for non-myeloablative allogeneic stem cell transplantation are necessary. Of interest, allogeneic bone marrow transplantation has been shown to be associated with clonal expansion of CD8+CD57+ lymphocytes in peripheral blood [12]. Thus, the involvement of CD8highCD57+ lymphocytes in non-myeloablative allogeneic stem cell transplantation in metastatic RCC patients cannot be ruled out.

In conclusion, our results suggest that the levels of CD8highCD57+ lymphocytes in peripheral blood might be of value in assessing the prognosis and in individualizing the interferon-α therapy of advanced RCC patients. Further investigations into the role of CD8highCD57+ lymphocytes during different modes of biological therapy of RCC seem warranted. It has to be emphasized, that the most important endpoints in kidney cancer research, as in clinical cancer research in general, are prolongation of survival and improvement in quality of life of patients. Probably, these endpoints can be achieved not only by developing new drugs, but also by investigating new ways to individualize treatment of patients with currently available drugs.

REFERENCES

[1] Abratt RP, Pontin AR, Ball HS: Activity of a short course of interferon alpha for metastatic renal cell carcinoma - a phase-2 study. *Cancer Immunol Immunother* 37:140-141, 1993.

[2] Anonymous: Interferon-α and survival in metastatic renal carcinoma: Early results of a randomised controlled trial. Medical Research Council Renal Cancer Collaborators. *Lancet* 353:14-17, 1999.

[3] Bahnson R, Hu HS, Vogelzang NJ: Non-myeloablative allogeneic stem cell transplantation for metastatic renal cell carcinoma. *Urol Oncol* 21: 79-81, 2003.

[4] Batliwalla FM, Bateman BA, Serrano D, et al: A 15-year follow-up of AJCC stage III malignant melanoma patients treated postsurgically with Newcastle disease virus oncolysate and determination of alterations in the CD8 T cell repertoire. *Mol Med* 4: 783-794, 1998.

[5] Bell EB, Sparshott SM, Bunce C: CD4+ T-cell memory, CD45R subsets and the persistence of antigen - a unifying concept. *Immunol Today* 19:60-64, 1998.

[6] Belldegrun A, Abi-Aad AS, Figlin RA, et al: Renal cell carcinoma: basic biology and current approaches to therapy. *Semin Oncol* 18: Suppl 7: 96-101, 1991.

[7] Bleumer I, Oosterwijk E, De Mulder P, et al: Immunotherapy for renal cell carcinoma. *Eur Urol* 44: 65-75, 2003.

[8] Bukowski RM, Olencki T, Wang Q, et al: Phase II trial of interleukin-2 and interferon-alpha in patients with renal cell carcinoma: Clinical results and immunologic correlates of response. *J Immunother* 20:301-311, 1997.

[9] Characiejus D, Pasukoniene V, Kazlauskaite N, et al: Predictive value of CD8highCD57+ lymphocyte subset in interferon therapy of patients with renal cell carcinoma. *Anticancer Res* 22: 3679-3684, 2002.

[10] Cole WH: Spontaneous regression of cancer: the metabolic triumph of the host? *Ann N Y Acad Sci* 230: 111-141, 1974.

[11] Dekernion JB, Ramming KP, Smith RB: The natural history of metastatic renal cell carcinoma: a computer analysis. *J Urol* 120: 148-152, 1978.

[12] Dolstra H, Preijers F, Van de Wiel-van Kemenade E, et al. Expansion of CD8+CD57+ T cells after allogeneic BMT is related with a low incidence of relapse and with cytomegalovirus infection. *Br J Haematol* 90: 300-307, 1995.

[13] Dolstra H, Van de Wiel-van Kemenade E, De Witte T, et al: Clonal predominance of cytomegalovirus-specific CD8+ cytotoxic T lymphocytes in bone marrow recipients. *Bone Marrow Transplant* 18:339-345, 1996.

[14] Elias L, Blumenstein BA, Kish J, et al: A phase II trial of interferon-α and 5-fluorouracil in patients with advanced renal cell carcinoma: A Southwest Oncology Group Study. *Cancer* 78:1085-1088, 1996.

[15] Fosså SD, Martinelli G, Otto U, et al: Recombinant interferon alfa-2a with or without vinblastine in metastatic renal cell carcinoma: Results of a European multi-center phase III study. *Ann Oncol* 3:301-305, 1992.

[16] Fosså SD: Interferon in metastatic renal cell carcinoma. *Semin Oncol* 27:187-193, 2000.

[17] Franzke A, Peest D, Probst-Kepper M, et al: Autoimmunity resulting from cytokine treatment predicts long-term survival in patients with metastatic renal cell cancer. *J Clin Oncol* 17:529-533, 1999.

[18] Goey SH, Verweij J, Stoter G: Immunotherapy of metastatic renal cell cancer. *Ann Oncol* 7:887-900, 1996.

[19] Göhring B, Riemann D, Rebmann U, et al: Prognostic value of the immunomonitoring of patients with renal cell carcinoma under therapy with IL-2/IFN-α-2 in combination with 5-FU. *Urol Res* 24:297-303, 1996.

[20] Hernberg M, Muhonen T, Pyrhönen S: Can the CD4+/CD8+ ratio predict the outcome of interferon-alpha therapy for renal cell carcinoma? *Ann Oncol* 8:71-77, 1997.

[21] Igarashi T, Marumo K, Onishi T, et al: Interferon-alpha and 5-fluorouracil therapy in patients with metastatic renal cell cancer: An open multicenter trial. The Japanese Study Group Against Renal Cancer. *Urology* 53:53-59, 1999.

[22] Martel CL, Lara PN: Renal cell carcinoma: current status and future directions. *Crit Rev Oncol Hematol* 45: 177-190, 2003.

[23] Morley JK, Batliwalla FM, Hingorani R, et al: Oligoclonal CD8+ T cells are preferentially expanded in the CD57+ subset. *J Immunol* 154:6182-6190, 1995.

[24] Motzer RJ, Bacik J, Murphy BA, et al: Interferon-alfa as a comparative treatment for clinical trials of new therapies against advanced renal cell carcinoma. *J Clin Oncol* 20: 289-296, 2002.

[25] Motzer RJ, Mazumdar M, Bacik J, et al: Effect of cytokine therapy on survival for patients with advanced renal cell carcinoma. *J Clin Oncol* 18: 1928-1935, 2000.

[26] Motzer RJ, Russo P. Systemic therapy for renal cell carcinoma. *J Urol* 163: 408-417, 2000.

[27] Motzer RJ: Prognostic factors and clinical trials of new agents in patients with metastatic renal cell carcinoma. *Crit Rev Oncol Hematol* 46: S33-S39, 2003.

[28] Négrier S, Caty A, Lesimple T, et al: Treatment of patients with metastatic renal carcinoma with a combination of subcutaneous interleukin-2 and interferon alfa with or without fluorouracil. *J Clin Oncol* 18:4009-4015, 2000.

[29] Pizzocaro G, Piva L, Colavita M, et al: Interferon adjuvant to radical nephrectomy in Robson stages II and III renal cell carcinoma: a multicentric randomized study. *J Clin Oncol* 19: 425-431, 2001.

[30] Raitakari M, Brown RD, Sze D, et al: T-cell expansions in patients with multiple myeloma have a phenotype of cytotoxic T cells. *Br J Haematol* 110:203-209, 2000.

[31] Schendel DJ, Oberneder R, Falk CS, et al: Cellular and molecular analyses of major histocompatibility complex (MHC) restricted and non-MHC-restricted effector cells recognizing renal cell carcinomas: problems and perspectives for immunotherapy. *J Mol Med* 75:400-413, 1997.

[32] Stadler WM, Vogelzang NJ: Low-dose interleukin-2 in the treatment of metastatic renal-cell carcinoma. *Semin Oncol* 22:67-73, 1995.

[33] Stebbing J, Gore M: The current status of interferon-α treatment in advanced renal cancer. *BJU Int* 87:599-601, 2001.

[34] Tsavaris N, Baxevanis C, Kosmidis P, et al: The prognostic significance of immune changes in patients with renal cancer, melanoma and colorectal cancer, treated with interferon alpha 2b. *Cancer Immunol Immunother* 43:94-102, 1996.

[35] van Herpen CM, De Mulder PH: Prognostic and predictive factors of immunotherapy in metastatic renal cell carcinoma. *Crit Rev Oncol Hematol* 41: 327-334, 2002.

[36] Wang ECY, Moss PAH, Frodsham P, et al: CD8highCD57+ lymphocytes in normal, healthy individuals are oligoclonal and respond to human cytomegalovirus. *J Immunol* 155:5046-5056, 1995.

[37] Wersäll P, Mellstedt H: Increased LAK and T cell activation in responding renal cell carcinoma patients after low dose cyclophosphamide, IL-2 and α-IFN. *Med Oncol* 12:69-77, 1995.

In: Trends in Kidney Cancer Research
Editor: Kelvin R. Nunez, pp. 39-54

ISBN 1-59454-141-8

Chapter IV

Thrombin Receptors in Renal Carcinoma Cells

Roland Kaufmann*
Medical Faculty, Friedrich Schiller University, Jena, Germany

Abstract

PAR(proteinase-activated receptor)-type thrombin receptors are members of a novel family of seven-transmembrane G-protein coupled receptors. The discovery of this receptor subclass has provided a framework for understanding how the coagulation proteinase thrombin communicates with cells. Recent studies provided evidence for the crucial role of PARs in tumor development and progression. Renal carcinomas belong to a coagulation type tumors where the tumor cells are associated with intact coagulation pathway that leads to thrombin formation. Therefore, investigation of PARs in this tumor entity is highly important on the definition of their significance in malignancy. In this chapter, the present knowledge of PAR-type thrombin receptors in renal carcinoma cells is summarized. After an overview including PAR structure and their effects in different tumor cell types; PAR characterization on RNA, protein, signaling and cellular level in renal carcinoma cells (permanent human renal carcinoma cell line A-498 and primary cultures obtained from surgically resected renal cell carcinomas) is described. A potential role of PAR-type thrombin receptors in renal cell carcinoma prognosis and therapy is discussed.

* Corresponding author: Medical Faculty, Friedrich Schiller University, Department of General and Visceral Surgery, Research Lab, Research Center Lobeda, Erlanger Allee 101, D-07747 Jena, Germany. Phone: +49-9325870; Fax: +49-9325872; e-mail: Roland.Kaufmann@med.uni-jena.de

Introduction

The role of the serine proteinase thrombin as a key player in the blood coagulation has been established for a number of decades. In addition, thrombin is known to have direct effects upon a number of cell types including tumor cells. These effects are mediated by thrombin receptors that belong to a new class of G protein coupled receptors, the proteinase activated receptors (PARs). During the last few years there is growing evidence for a crucial role of PAR-type thrombin receptors in cancer. Here, the present knowledge of PARs function in renal carcinoma is discussed.

PARs – A New Family of G-Protein Coupled Receptors (GPCR)

In recent years, it has become clear that seven transmembrane domain G-protein coupled receptors (GPCRs) mediate the actions of almost all types of chemical messengers from small transmitters, lipid messengers, neuropeptides, peptide hormones, to large biomolecules. These membrane receptors are activated by ligand binding inducing a conformational change in the receptor's structure. As a result, a signal transmitted across the cell membrane into the cell. The activation is reversible in that the ligand can dissociate from its receptor. Within this family of GPCRs, a different and unique mechanism of activation was discovered in 1991 with the cloning of a receptor signaling thrombin (Vu et al., 1991). This novel receptor was termed by the NC-UPHAR receptor nomenclature committee proteinase-activated receptor-1 (PAR_1; Hollenberg and Compton, 2002). PAR_1 is activated by proteolytic cleavage at a specific site within the extracellular amino-terminal domain, exposing a new amino terminus, which then interacts as a „tethered ligand" with a distal region of the receptor body, leading to receptor activation.

The discovery of this receptor has provided a basic concept for understanding how thrombin interacts with cells. Four PARs are currently known. PAR_1 (Rasmussen et al, 1991; Vu et al., 1991), PAR_3 (Ishihara et al, 1997), and PAR_4 (Xu et al. 1998) can be activated by the serine proteinase thrombin (EC 3.4.21.5), and thrombin is almost certainly a physiological activator of these receptors in vivo. However, several other proteases can cleave $PAR_{1/3}$ and or $_4$ productively and may also contribute to their function in vivo. PAR-2 (Nystedt et al., 1994) can be activated by multiple trypsin-like serine proteases including: trypsin itself, mast cell tryptase, neutrophil proteinase 3, tissue factor/factor VIIa/factor Xa, and membrane-tethered serine protease-1. However, PAR_2 is not cleaved by thrombin. PAR_1 is also the one that established the activation paradigm that in general terms applies to the other three PAR-family members. That paradigm includes the ability of PARs to respond not only to selected proteases as mentioned above, but also to peptides based upon the sequence of the tethered ligand (PAR activating peptides; PAR-APs). The one exception to the rule is PAR_3 for which no activating peptide agonist has been discovered thus far. Table 1 shows a number of potential useful selective peptide agonists for several PARs. Thus, the four PAR family

Table 1. Proteinase-Activated Receptors

IUPHAR recommended name	PAR_1	PAR_2	PAR_3	PAR_4
IUPHAR receptor code	2.1:PAR:1:PAR1:HUMAN:0 0	2.1:PAR:2:PAR2: HUMAN:00	2.1:PAR:3:PAR: 3:HUMAN:00	2.1:PAR:4:PAR:4: HUMAN:00
Alternate designators	Thrombin receptor	Trypsin receptor	Thrombin receptor	Thrombin receptor
Receptor variants		F240S mutation (h)		
Amino acid composition	425 aa (h)[a]	397 aa (h)	374 aa (h)	385 aa (h)
Agonist proteinases	Thrombin > trypsin	Trypsin, tryptase, trypsin 2, matriptase/MT- serine protease 1	Thrombin trypsin > factor X	Thrombin congrue nt Trypsin Cathepsin G; factors VIIa/X
Inactivating proteinases	Cathepsin G, proteinase 3, elastase, plasmin, chymase	Unknown	Unknown	Unknown
Tethered ligand sequences	SFLLR (h), SFFLR (m,r)	SLIGKV (h), SLIGRL (m,r)	TFRGAP (h), SFNGGP (m)	GYPGQV (h)[c], GYPGKF (m)
Subtype selective peptide agonists	TFRIFD[b]	SLIGKV-NH2, SLIGRL-NH2		GYPGKF-NH2
	TFLLR-NH2	Trans-cinnamoyl- *LIGRLO-NH2*		GYPGQV-NH2[c] AYPGKF-NH2
Antagonists	Trans-cinnamoyl-parafluoro- Phe-paraguanidino-Phe-Leu- Arg-Arg-NH2[d]			
	Mercaptopropionyl-Phe-Cha- Arg-Lys-Pro-Lys-Pro-Asn- Asp-Lys-NH2			TRANS- cinnamoyl- YPGKF-NH2[e]
	Non-peptide antagonists: RWJ56110 and RWJ58259			
Signal transduction mechanisms	Gq/11 (increased IP3/DAG); Gi; G12/13	---[g]	None known	---[g]
Gene/chromosome	F2R/5q13 (h) F2R/13D2 (m)	F2RL1/5q13 (h) F2RL1/13D2 (m)	F2RL2/5q13 (h) F2RL2/13D2 (m)	F2RL3/19p12 (h) F2RL3/8B3.3 (m)
NCBI accession no.	M62424 (h)	U34038 (h)	U92971 (h)	AF080214 AF055917 (h)
	L03529 (m) M81642 (r)	Z48043 (m) U61373 (r)	U92972 (m)	AF080215 (m)

[a] The IUPHAR receptor code is provided for each human (h) PAR, but not for murine (m), or rat (r) PARs.

[b] TFRIFD is the *Xenopus* thrombin receptor tethered ligand domain (the human PAR_1 tethered ligand domain sequence, SFLLRN, activates both PAR_1 and PAR_2 receptors).

[c] AYPGKF is 10 times more potent than the natural human (GYPGQV) or murine (GYPGKF) tethered ligand sequences, which are also PAR_4 selective.

[d] May also act at PAR_2 as agonist; also designated BMS 200261.

[e] Validated only in rat platelets.

[f] Antagonizes PAR_1; acts as an agonist at PAR_2.

[g] Stimulates phosphositide turnover through an uncharacterized G protein, probably $G_{q/11}$; G_i interactions with PAR_2 not evaluated; PAR_4 believed *not* to interact with G_i.

members share a number of similitaries, but some differences have emerged. As noted above, three of the receptors can be activated by thrombin. Two of these, PAR_1 and PAR_3, have similar dose/response curves when studied in expression systems. The third, PAR_4, requires 10-100-fold higher concentrations of thrombin, apparently because it lacks the hirudin-like sequences that can interact with thrombin′s anion-binding exosite and facilitate receptor cleavage (Kahn et al., 1998; Xu et al., 1998; Nakanishi-Matsui et al., 2000). Once activated by their tethered ligands, the PAR1 and PAR4 can cause an elevation of intracellular calcium via a presumed $G_{q/11}$-mediated process. For PAR_1, a role for intracellular loop 2 has been shown for G_q coupling (Verrall et al., 1997). PAR_1 (but not PAR_4; Faruqi et al., 2000) can couple not only to the G_q family, but also to the pertussis toxin-sensitive G_i (Hung et al., 1992; Swift et al., 2000) resulting in: 1) an inhibition of adenylyl cyclase and 2) presumably other processes, such as ion channel regulation and phospholipase Cβ and cSrc activation triggered by the $G_{i\alpha}$ units (reviewed by Macfarlane et al., 2001). The coupling of PAR_1 to G_q, G_i, or both very likely depends on the cell type and the relative abundance of the two G-proteins. Evidence also suggests that PAR_1 can couple to members of the $G_{12/13}$ family (Offermanns et al., 1994).

One difficulty in interpreting some of the data in the literature obtained before the discovery of PAR_4 is that thrombin, which can activate both PAR_1 and PAR_4, was often used as an agonist rather than the receptor-selective PAR-APs. Thus, although it is clear that both PAR_1 and PAR_4 can elevate intracellular calcium, the coupling of the different PARs to other specific members of the G-protein family remains to be established. It should be noted further that PAR_1 and PAR_4 can exhibit distinct signaling shut-off and internalization kinetics due to distinct potential phosphorylation sites in the C-terminal domains of the two receptors (Shapiro et al., 2000). Thus, the kinetics as well as the G-protein-coupling specificity among PAR_1 and PAR_4 will very likely be found to differ. Many of the downstream signal pathway targets that can be activated, including members of the extracellular signal-regulated kinase-type mitogen-activated protein kinases (ERK1/2; p42/44), stress-activated protein kinase, c-Jun NH_2-terminal kinase family, Src-family, other tyrosine kinases, and phosphatidylinositol-3 kinase, have been well summarized (Macfarlane et al., 2001).

The contribution of PAR_3 to signaling in primary cells has been examined especially in mouse platelets (Ishihara et al, 1997; Nakanishi-Matsui et al., 2000) and to a lesser extent in human endothelial cells. In neither case was it possible to demonstrate a signal triggered by mouse PAR_3 directly, despite the fact that human PAR_3 is expressed in fibroblasts clearly mediated phosholipase C activation (Ishihara et al., 1997) and ERK-type MAPK (our unpublished results). Following a new model PAR_3 seems to function as a cofactor to facilitate PAR_4 cleavage by thrombin but has lost the ability to signal independently. However, this remains to be determined in detail.

PAR-Type Thrombin Receptors in Cancer

Thrombin is generated from its precursor enzyme prothrombin in blood and has a critical function in blood coagulation Therefore, initially much of the available information about thrombin receptors relates to vascular biology, and their function in thrombosis, inflammation, vascular injury and remodelling and has been investigated intensively (for reviews see e.g. Coughlin, 2000; Mcfarlane et al., 2001). 1995 (Wojtukiewiz et al., 1995) demonstrated the expression of PAR_1 in carcinosarcoma and melanoma cells suggesting a role of thrombin receptors in carcinogenesis. During the following years, functional PAR_1-type thrombin receptors were characterized on the signaling and cellular level in cells from different tumor entities including the larynx (Kaufmann et al., 1997), pancreas (Rudroff et al., 1998), glioma (Kaufmann et al., 1996; Schafberg et al., 1997; Zieger et al., 2001), glioblastoma (Kaufmann et al., 1998) meningioma (Kaufmann et al., 1999), prostate (Chay et al., 2003; Liu et al., 2003) and colon (Darmaoul et al., 2003). In addition, increased tumor cell adhesion to endothelium, extracellular matrix and platelets, enhanced metastatic capacity of tumor cells, and activated cell growth and stimulation of angiogenesis in response to thrombin and PAR_1 agonist peptides was demonstrated (Nierodzik, et al., 1996; Klementsen and Jorgensen, 1997). In breast and pancreatic carcinoma cells, the level of PAR_1 expression has been correlated with the degree of invasiveness (Even-Ram et al, 1998; Rudroff et al., 2002). Furthermore, B16F10 melanoma cells transfected with PAR_1, enhanced thrombin-induced tumor cell adhesion to fibronectin 2.5-fold and pulmonary metastasis as high as 39-fold compared to untransfected thrombin-treated tumor cells (Nierodzik et al., 1998). In addition, PAR_1 seems not to be the only functional thrombin receptor in tumor cells as shown in a recently published report which demonstrated that PAR_1 and PAR_4 act as a dual receptor system in human astrocytoma cells (Kaufmann et al., 2000).

Thrombin/PAR-Type Thrombin Receptors in Renal Carcinoma Cells

Renal cell carcinomas (RCCs) belong to the coagulation-type tumors where the tumor cells are associated with an intact coagulation pathway that leads to thrombin formation (Zacharski et al., 1990; Zacharski et al., 1992; Zacharski and Constantini, 1995). Therefore, a role of thrombin and its receptors in RCCs under in vivo conditions is very likely and investigating this tumor entity seems to be obligatory for a definition of PAR/thrombin's significance in malignancy.

For studying the role of thrombin and PAR-type thrombin receptors in RCCs, different cellular models have been used.

A-498 Cells

In the human renal carcinoma cell line A-489, established from the kidney carcinoma of a 52-year-old male in 1973 (Giard et al., 1973) it was shown that thrombin activates different intracellular effector systems especially including $[Ca^{2+}]_i$, protein kinase C (PKC), protein kinase A (PKA), mitogen activated protein kinases (ERK1/2) and nuclear factor *k*B (NF*k*B; Kaufmann et al., 2002). These intracellular signaling molecules are well known to link G-protein coupled receptors to differentiation and growth pathways in various cell types (for a review see: van Biesen et al., 1996). On the cellular level, thrombin had no effect on cell proliferation but enhanced chemotactic cell migration. Migration was investigated by using a boyden chamber assay with a filter precoated with collagen. In this experimental setup, thrombin exhibit stimulatory effects on A-498 cell migration (Kaufmann et al. 2001). It is well known that cell movement is accompanied by morphological alterations where cellular extensions are prominent (Rorth, 2003). Fine filopodial extensions appear to form in a very dynamic way (Ribeiro et al., 2002; Sato and Kornberg), but more robust, long cellular extensions lead the way for migrating cells in a number of systems (for a review, see: Fulga and Rorth, 2002). In A-498 cells treated with thrombin (0.1- 1.0 NHI-U/ml) a drastically changed morphology with numerous filopodial extrusions in comparision with nontreated cells could be observed (Figure 1) for 4 hours.

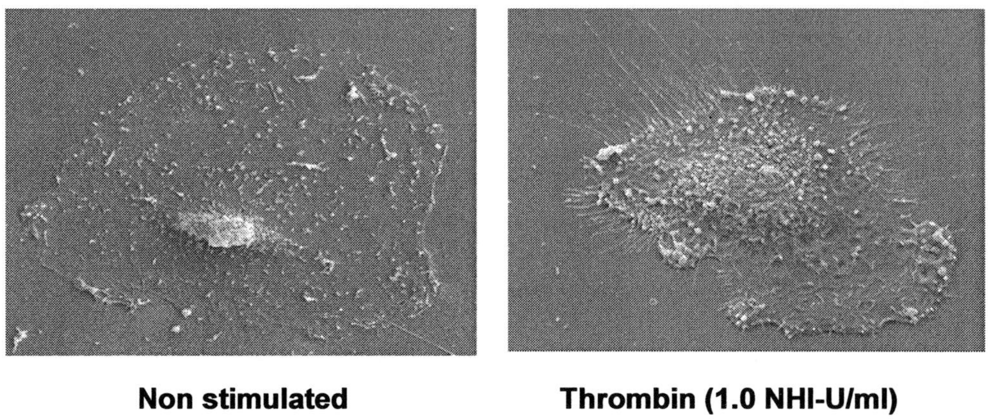

Figure 1. Thrombin-induced morphological changes on A-498 renal carcinoma cells. The cells grown on coverslips were fixed with glutaraldehyde. After critical point drying (Critical Point Dryer CPD-030; Bal-Tec, Liechtenstein) cells were coated with gold, using a sputter coating procces (Sputter Coater SCD-005; Bal-Tec, Liechtenstein) and investigated by scanning electron microscopy (LEO, Oberkochen, Germany).

The migratory effect of thrombin on A-498 cells could be blocked by pretreatment of cells with PKA inhibitor H-98 but not with PKC inhibitor BIM I, MAPK inhibitor PD98059 or NF-*k*B inhibitor SN50. In addition, the thrombin-induced effect on migration of A-498 cells was inhibited by the high affinity thrombin inhibitor hirudin. These results clearly indicate, that in renal A-498 renal carcinoma cells, thrombin prompted migration but was without effect on proliferation. Protein kinase A seems to be involved in thrombin´s migratory capacity in A-498 cells. PKA mediates the vast majority, but not all (Santorro et al, 1998; de Rooij et al., 1998; Kawasaki et al., 1998) of the cellular effects of cAMP, an intracellular second messenger, which is present in all cells and tissues. In eukaryotic cells, it is generated by an enzyme family designated adenylyl cyclases (Sunahara et al., 1996; Xia and Storm, 1997; Hanoune et al., 1997; Tang and Hurley, 1998). PKA, the first protein kinase to be discovered (Walsh et al., 1968), is comprised of two catalytic and two regulatory subunits (reviews: Krebs and Beavo, 1979, Walsh and Van Patten, 1994). Within the cell, a number of distinct isoforms are generated by assembly of the products of several regulatory and catalytic subunit genes (review: Dell'Aqua and Scott, 1997). In the absence of cAMP, the enzyme exists as an inactive tetrameric holoenzyme complex. Binding of cAMP to the holoenzyme leads to the dissociation into a regulatory dimer and two active C. It is the PKA catalytic (C-PKA) subunit that is the active form of the enzyme which may phosphorylate multiple target proteins in the cytosol, cytoskeleton, membrane or nucleus on serines in the consensus sequence X-Arg-Arg-X-Ser-X (review: McKnight et al., 1988). During activation of PKA, the catalytic subunit is released from the regulatory subunit, phosphorylates nearby proteins, and then translocates to the nucleus, where it regulates gene expression and other nuclear functions (Nigg et al., 1985; Riabowol et al., 1988; Bacskai et al., 1993). Our data suggest that PKA activation induced by thrombin rapidly altered the subcellular localization of C-PKA in A-498 cells leading to a translocation into the nucleus (Kaufmann et al. 2002).

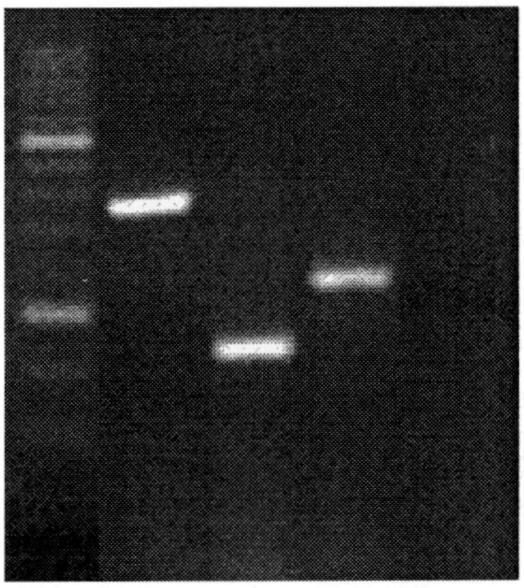

Figure 2. Detection of PAR-mRNA using RT-PCR and agarose gel electrophoresis. M Molecular weight Marker; A Actin; 1 PAR1; 3 PAR3 4 PAR4. Total mRNA was extracted and first-strand cDNA was synthesized by oligo (dt) primed reverse transcription using a commercial cDNA Cycle kit. For PAR_4 cDNA synthesis a specific primer (TGAGTAGCTGGGATTACAG) was used. Aliquots of A-498 cDNA were taken for PCR amplification using following primers: PAR_1: forward CTCGAATTCTGAAGGTCAAGAAGCCGG; reverse CTCGAATTCAGCTTTTTGTATATGCTG; PAR_3: forward TTCCTCACCTGCATCAG; reverse ACTGGGTCGAAGCAACTATT (Scase et al., 1997); PAR_4: forward AACCTCTATGGTGCCTACGTGC; reverse CCAAGCCCAGCTAATTTTTG (Kahn et al., 1999). PCR was performed as per the manufacturer's instruction (Perkin Elmer). PCR products were electrophoresed on a 1 % agarose gel containing ethidiumbromide and visualized under UV transillumination.

A number of extracellular factors utilize the cAMP/protein kinase A cascade to regulate a diverse array of physiological and cellular processes including mitogenesis and migration (Withers, 1997). In addition, protein kinase A has been shown to be an important intracellular signaling system in the signal transduction of thrombin in non-neoplastic cells (Walsh and van Patten, 1994). In cancer, it is suggested that PKA participates in the metastatic process and therefore has a function in cancer development and progression (Schwede et al, 1996; Krupitzka et al., 1996; Maier et al., 1996; Cho et al., 2000). In the study on Human A-498 renal carcinoma cells, has been shown for the first time that thrombin uses the PKA pathway to regulate migration of human tumor cells.

As stated above, thrombin exerts most of its cellular effects by catalytic interaction with proteinase-activated receptor (PAR)-type thrombin receptors. As shown in Figure 2, mRNA coding for PAR_1 and PAR_3 but not PAR_4 could be found in A-498 cells.

Therefore, the participation of thrombin receptors in thrombin-induced action in A-498 cells is highly indicated. However, the involvement of non-catalytic binding sites may not be excluded. This was suggested since thrombin is known from other cell types including endothelial cells to exert cellular effects via dual signaling pathways, with one of them being mediated by non-proteolytic actions (Herbert et al, 1994). Moreover, the specific thrombin inhibitor hirudin, which is known to bind very tightly not only to the catalytic site but also to the fibrinogen recognition site of thrombin (Rydel et al., 1990), blocked thrombin-mediated effect on migration in A-498 cells. Since cell migration is a crucial step in the highly-complicated sequence of tumor invasion, thrombin-induced PKA activation might be a signaling pathway promoting progression of human renal cell carcinoma.

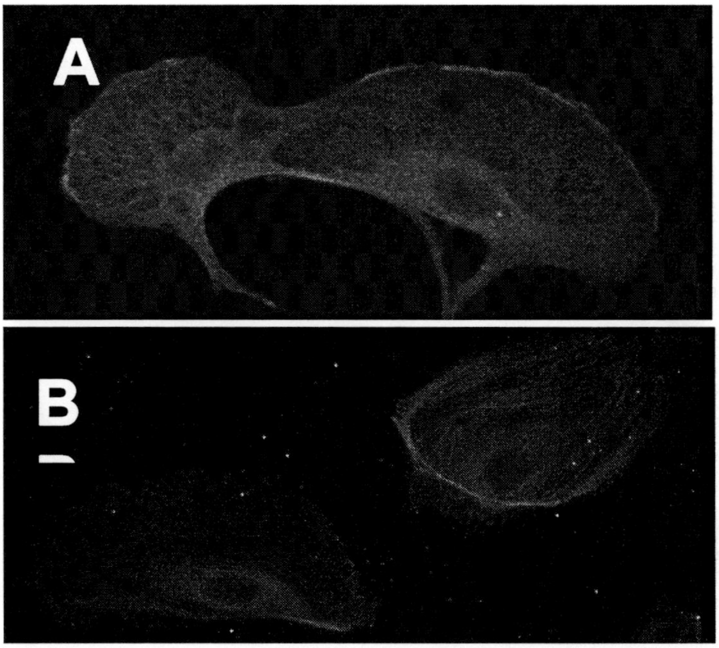

Figure 3. Immunofluorescence staining of PAR_1 (A) and PAR_3 (B) in human RCC cells. As a secondary antibody, a FITC-conjugated anti-mouse IgG or anti-rabbit IgG was used and fluorescence images were obtained with a confocal laser scanning microscope.

Primary Tumor Cell Cultures from Surgically Resected RCCs

Primary cultures were prepared by mechanical dissection and enzymatic digestion from surgically resected specimens of primary renal cell carcinomas classified histologically according to the UICC TNM classification (1997). Colonies of tumor cells were identified by phase contrast microscopy, removed and expanded individually. Individual cultures were tested for positivity for cytokeratin to exclude contamination by tumor stromal fibroblasts by standard immunocytochemistry using a PAN-cytokeratin antibody.

As seen for the permanent renal carcinoma cell line, A-498 primary cultures established from from RCCs express mRNA encoding PAR_1 and PAR_3 but not PAR_4. For PAR_1, first real time PCR data suggest a correlation between PAR1 expression and metastatic capacity of RCCs (R. Kaufmann, unpublished results). However, this has to be elucidated in detail. On the protein level, expression of PAR_1- and PAR_3-type thrombin receptors could be shown by confocal laser fluorescence microscopy (Figure 3) and freeze fracture electron microscopy (Figure 4).

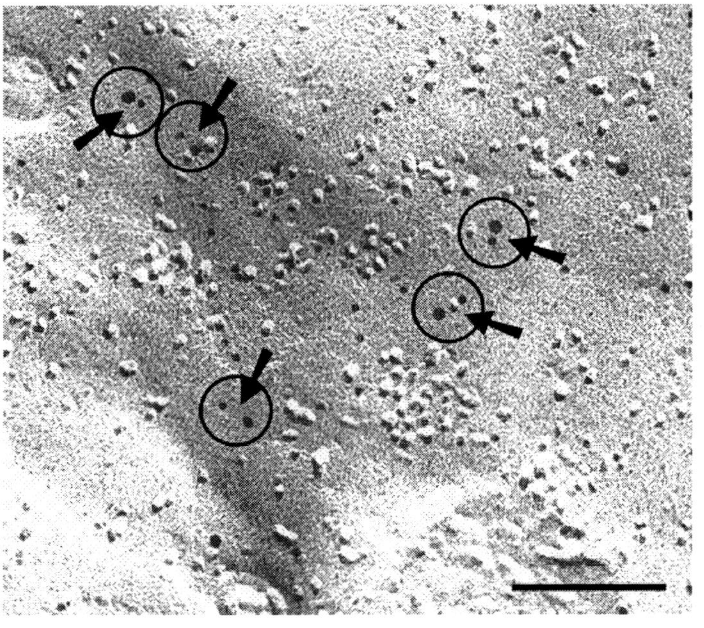

Figure 4. Transmission electron micrograph of a freeze-fractured RCC cell membrane immunolabeled with antibodies directed against PAR_1 and PAR_3, respectively.
PAR_1 (monoclonal anti-PAR_1 antibody Mab 61-1, secondary antibody conjugated with 5nm gold particles) and PAR_3 (polyclonal anti-PAR_3 antibody KAUF-17, secondary antibody conjugated with 10 nm gold particles). Bar 100 nm.

The fluorescence microscopic analysis revealed the presence of both receptors on cell membrane and intracellular compartments. PARs are well known to be membrane receptors. In addition, storage in intracellular pools has also been reported at least for PAR_1 (Hein et al., 1994; Shapiro and Coughlin, 1998). In RCC cells, a similar distribution pattern of PAR_1 and PAR_3 may be suggested. Their exact localization on intracellular compartments remains to be elucidated. In the past few years, a number of studies have demonstrated that oligomerization of G protein coupled receptors may play important roles in receptor trafficing and signaling, and heterodimerization has been proposed to lead to receptors with pharmacological and/or functional properties that are different from those of the individual receptors. The biological significance of this membrane receptor behaviour is undefined. However a modulatory role of receptor association/dissociation in cellular differentiation and growth including carcinogenesis is under discussion (for a review, see e.g. Angers et al., 2002). In renal cell carcinoma cells, $PAR_{1/3}$ colocalization could be partly noted. Therefore, it is very important to clearify whether PAR_1 and $_3$ are able to form mono- or/and heterodimer complexes and to evaluate their role in RCC.

PAR-Activating Peptide TFLLRN as a Helpful Tool in the Investigation of Thrombin Receptor Function in Renal Carcinoma Cells

Thrombin interacts with both PAR_1 and PAR_3. Therefore it is not possible to define the PAR-subtype responsible for effects measured after thrombin stimulation. For PAR_1, a highly selective peptide agonist exists that was derived from the sequence representing the first 6 amino acids of PAR_1 Neo-N-terminus after receptor cleavage. This peptide has been used to define PAR_1-mediated signaling in renal carcinoma cells.

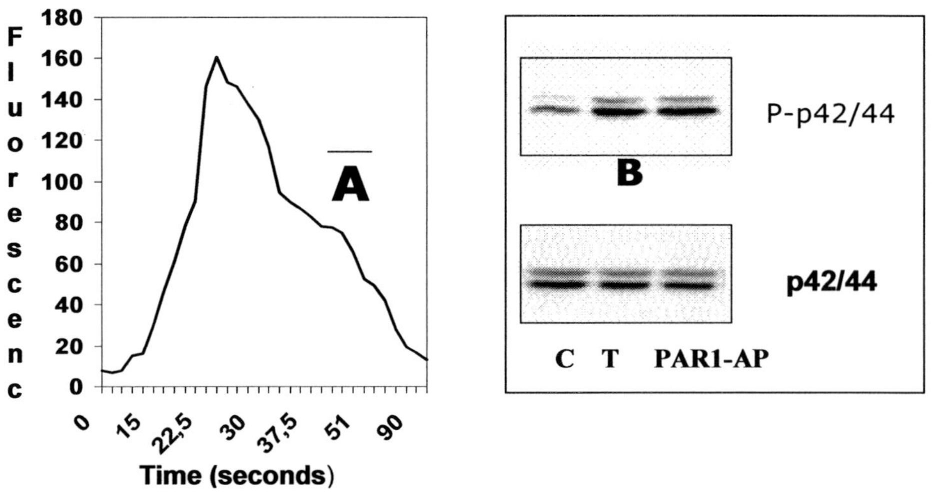

Figure 5. *(A)* TFLLRN (PAR_1-AP)-induced [Ca2+]i mobilization measured by laser fluorescence microscopy (final peptide concentration: 50 μM).
Cells were loaded with fluo-4 acetoxymethylester. For calcium measurement, an inverted confocal laser scanning microscope (LSM 510, Carl Zeiss, Göttingen, Germany) was used. Fluorescence images were collected by using the 488 nm argon ion laser line
(B) Effect of PAR1-AP(50 μM) and thrombin (1.0 NHI-U/ml) on activation of MAP kinases p42/44. Cell lysates were subjected to SDS-PAGE and Western blotting with an anti-P-p42/44 antibody. immunblot analysis with total p42/44 was performed as a control for constant protein loading in all lanes.

As shown in Figure 5, the PAR_1 selective agonist TFLLRN induced a transient calcium signal and p42/44 MAPK activation that indicated that PAR_1 signals both calcium and p42/44 MAP-Kinases in primary tumor cell cultures established from surgical resected RCCs. Since these intracellular effector systems are key elements in the regulation of cell processes as growth and differentiation (for review see Pearson et al., 2001) a role of PAR_1 in RCC development and progression is undoubted. The participation of PAR_3 in thrombin´s effects in renal carcinoma cells remains an open question up to now and has to be defined in the future.

Perspectives - PARs as Prognostic and Therapeutic Targets in RCCs

Renal cell carcinoma is characterized by an unpredictable clinical course. Therefore, prognostic factors are urgently needed. So far, clinical staging is the most powerful predictor of the progression of RCC. In principle, a better understanding of cell biological and molecular changes associated with the development of this disease is highly necessary. In recent years it has become evident that molecular targets including membrane receptors are suitable targets for both tumor prognosis and therapy (Ullrich, 2002). Following this strategy, studies on PAR-type thrombin receptors on tumor cells may provide novel insights into the complex mechanisms of carcinogenesis.

On kidney cancer, knowledge about thrombin receptors function is still in its infancy. Since preliminary results demonstrated a relationship between receptor expression and metastatic capacity, PAR expression might be suitable as a tool in the estimation of RCC prognosis. Since PAR_1 has been shown to be functional in both permanent cell lines and primary tumor cell cultures obtained from surgical resected RCCs, receptor inhibition studies are needed, especially including PAR1 antagonists. With the development of small-molecule antagonists (Zhang et al., 2001), it is now clear that intervening in processes mediated by PAR_1 presents a new approach to treating a variety of disorders dependent on thrombin generation (Derian et al., 2003). The full potential of PAR-1 antagonists has yet to be realized, but the promise of novel therapeutics that modulate receptor function rather than thrombin's proteolytic activity, provides an alternative means to dampen the pathological effects of thrombin. In this context, application of PAR antagonsts might contribute to development of novel basic approaches in cancer therapy including RCC.

The development of cancer is thought of as a progressive multi-step process during which a cell accumulates multiple and consecutive genetic alterations ultimately resulting in the phenotypic changes that lead to malignant tumor growth. This tumor cell-centered view of cancer development has lead to numerous useful discoveries and greatly furthered our understanding of the molecular mechanisms lying at the base of cellular transformation. At present, studies on PAR function in cancer are focused on the tumor cell itself including investigation on permanent tumor cell lines, primary tumor cell cultures and tissue sections. However, the characteristic phenotypic changes which enable a cancer cell to grow to a tumor are still less apparent. This is mainly a consequence of their analysis being restricted to the tissue level, a much more complicated situation than conventional cell-culture models. Over the past decade, it has become increasingly apparent that the complex interplay between different cell types, e.g. epithelial cells, fibroblasts, mast cells, macrophages, smooth muscle cells and endothelial cells, is critical for maintaining normal balanced tissue homeostasis. As a consequence, in tumor tissue the microenvironment will also profoundly influence many steps of tumor development and progression. It is known that all of the above - mentioned cell types in the tumor microenvironment are able to express PAR1-type thrombin receptors. The presence of PAR_1 in these cell types in the tumor microenvironment suggests a role of thrombin and its receptors in the highly complicated cell-cell conversation during tumor development and has to be taken into consideration in future research of PAR-type thrombin receptors in kidney cancer.

Experimental data represented are the result of collaborative work of the author´s Laboratory with Dr. Kerstin Junker, Department of Urology, and Dr. Martin Westermann, Centre for Electron Microscopy, Medical Faculty of the Friedrich Schiller University Jena, and Dr. Peter Henklein, Institute of Biochemistry, Charité, Humboldt University of Berlin.

References

Angers S, Salahpour A, Bouvier M (2002). Dimerization: an emerging concept for G protein-coupled receptor ontogeny and function. *Annu Rev Pharmacol Toxicol* 42: 409-435.

Bacskai BJ, Hochner B, Mahaut-Smith M, Adams SR, Kaang BK, Kandel ER, Tsien RY (1993). Spatially resolved dynamics of cAMP and protein kinase A subunits in Aplysia sensory neurons. *Science* 260: 222-226.

Chay CH, Cooper CR, Gendernalik JD, Dhanasekaran SM, Chinnaiyan AM, Rubin MA, Schmaier AH, Pienta KJ (2002). A functional thrombin receptor (PAR1) is expressed on bone-derived prostate cancer cell lines. *Urology* 60: 760-5.

Cho YS, Lee YN, Cho-Chung YS (2000). Biochemical characterization of extracellular cAMP-dependent protein kinase as a tumor marker. *Biochem Biophys Res Commun* 278: 679-684.

Coughlin SR (2000). Thrombin signalling and protease-activated receptors. *Nature* 407: 258-264.

Darmoul D, Gratio V, Devaud H, Lehy T, Laburthe M (2003). Aberrant expression and activation of the thrombin receptor protease-activated receptor-1 induces cell proliferation and motility in human colon cancer cells. *Am J Pathol* 162: 1503-1513.

Dell`Acqua ML, Scott JD (1997). Protein kinase A anchoring. *J Biol Chem* 272: 12881-12884.

Derian CK, Maryanoff BE, Zhang HC, Andrade-Gordon P (2003). Therapeutic potential of protease-activated receptor-1 antagonists. *Expert Opin Investig Drugs* 12: 209-21.

De Rooij J, Zwartkruis FJ., Verheijen MHG, Cool RH, Nijman S.B, Wittinghofer A, Bos JL (1998). Epac is a Rap1 guanine-nucleotide-exchange factor directly activated by cyclic AMP. *Nature* 396: 474-477.

Even-Ram S, Uziely B, Cohen P, Grisaru-Granovsky S, Maoz M, Ginzburg Y, Reich R, Vlodavsky I and Bar-Shavit R (1998). Thrombin receptor overexpression in malignant and physiological invasion processes. *Nat Med* 4: 909-914.

Faruqi TR, Weiss EJ, Shapiro MJ, Huang W, Coughlin SR (2000). Structure-function analysis of protease-activated receptor 4 tethered ligand peptides. Determinants of specificity and utility in assays of receptor function. *J Biol Chem* 275: 19728-19734.

Fulga TA, Rorth P (2002). Invasive cell migration is initiated by guided growth of long cellular extensions. *Nat Cell Biol* 4: 715-719.

Giard DJ, Aaronson SA, Todara GJ, Arnstein P, Kersey JH, Dosik H, Parks WP (1973). In vitro cultivation of human tumors: establishment of cell lines derived from a series of solid tumors. *J Natl Cancer Inst* 51: 1417-23.

Hanoune J, Pouille Y, Tzavara E, Shen TS, Lipskaya L, Miyamoto N, Suzuki Y, Defer N (1997). Adenylyl cyclases - structure, regulation and function in an enzyme superfamily. *Mol Cell Endocrinol* 128: 179-194.

Herbert JM, Dupuy E, Laplace MC, Zini JM, Bar Shavit R, Tobelem G. (1994). Thrombin induces endothelial cell growth via both a proteolytic and a non-proteolytic pathway. *Biochem J* 303: 227-31.

Hein L, Ishii K, Coughlin SR, Kobilka BK (1994). Intracellular targeting and trafficking of thrombin receptors. A novel mechanism for resensitization of a G protein-coupled receptor. *J Biol Chem* 269: 27719-27726.

Hollenberg MD, Compton SJ (2002). International Union of Pharmacology. XVIII. Proteinase-activated receptors. *Pharmacol Rev* 54: 203-217.

Hung DT, Wong YH, Vu TK, Coughlin SR (1992). The cloned platelet thrombin receptor couples to at least two distinct effectors to stimulate phosphoinositide hydrolysis and inhibit. adenylyl cyclase. *J Biol Chem* 267: 20831-20834.

Ishihara H, Connolly AJ, Zeng D, Kahn ML, Zheng YW, Timmons C, Tram T and Coughlin SR (1997). Protease-activated receptor 3 is a second thrombin receptor in humans. *Nature* 386: 502-506.

Kahn ML, Zheng YW, Huang W, Bigornia V, Zeng D, Moff S, Farese RV Jr, Tam C, Coughlin SR (1998). A dual thrombin receptor system for platelet activation. *Nature* 394: 690-694.

Kahn ML, Nakanishi-Matsui, Shapiro MJ, Ishihara I, Coughlin SH (1999). Protease-activated receptors 1 and 4 mediate activation of human platelets by thrombin. *J Clin Invest* 103: 879-887.

Kaufmann R, Lindschau C, Höer A, Henklein P, Adomeit A, Haller H, Liebmann C, Oberdisse E, Henklein P, Nowak G (1996). Signaling effects of alpha-Thrombin and SFLLRN in rat glioma C_6 cells. *J Neurosci Res* 46: 641-651.

Kaufmann, Schafberg H, Rudroff C, Nowak G (1997). Thrombin receptor activation results in calcium signalling and PKC-dependent Stimulation of DNA Synthesis in Hep-2 laryngeal carcinoma cells. *Cancer* 80: 2068-2074.

Kaufmann R, Patt S, Schafberg H, Kalff R, Neupert G, Nowak G (1998). Functional thrombin receptor PAR1 in primary cultures of human glioblastoma cells. *NeuroReport* 9: 709-712.

Kaufmann R, Patt S, Zieger M, Kraft R, Neupert G, Nowak G (1999). PAR1-type thrombin receptors are involved in thrombin-induced calcium signaling in human meningioma cells. *J Neuro-Oncol* 42: 131-136.

Kaufmann R, Patt S, Zieger M, Kraft R, Tausch S, Henklein P, Nowak G (2000). The two-receptor system PAR-1/PAR-4 mediates alpha-thrombin-induced [Ca2+]i mobilization in human astrocytoma cells. *J Cancer Res Clin Oncol* 126: 91-94.

Kawasaki H, Springett GM, Mochizuki N, Toki S, Nakaya M, Matsuda M, Housman DE, Graybiel AM (1998). A family of cAMP-binding proteins that directly activate Rap1. *Science* 282: 2275-2279.

Krebs EG, Beavo JA (1979). Phosphorylation-dephosphorylation of enzymes. *Annu Rev Bioch* 48: 923-959.

Krupitza G, Grill S, Harant H, Hulla W, Szekeres T, Huber H, Dittrich C (1996). Genes related to growth and invasiveness are repressed by sodium butyrate in ovarian carcinoma cells. *Brit J Cancer* 73: 433-438.

Liu J, Bastian M, Kohlschein P, Schuff-Werner P, Steiner M (2003).Expression of functional protease-activated receptor 1 in human prostate cancer cell lines. *Urol Res*. 31:163-8.

Macfarlane SR, Seatter MJ, Kanke T, Hunter GD and Plevin R (2001). Proteinase-activated receptors. *Pharmacol Rev* 53: 245-282.

Maier GD, Vellody K, Meisinger J, Djordjevic A, Lozano Y, Young MR (1996). Protein kinase A regulates Lewis lung carcinoma adherence to extracellular matrix components and spontaneous metastasis. *Clin Exp Metastas* 14: 314-322.

McKnight GS, Clegg CH, Uhler MD, Chrivia JC, Cadd GG, Correll LA, Otten AD (1988). Analysis of the cAMP-dependent protein kinase system using molecular genetic approaches. *Rec Progr Hormone Res* 44: 307-335.

Nierodzik ML, Bain RM, Liu L-X, Shivji M, Takeshita K, Karpatkin S (1996). Presence of the seven transmembrane thrombin receptor on human tumour cells: effect of activation on tumour adhesion to platelets and tumor tyrosine phosphorylation. *Br J Haematol* 92: 452-457.

Klementsen B, Jorgensen L (1997). Mechanisms involved in the early interaction between HeLa cells, platelets and endothelial cells in vitro under the influence of thrombin. Effects of acetylsalicylic acid and Na-salicylate. *APMIS* 105: 546-558.

Nakanishi-Matsui M, Zheng YW, Sulciner DJ, Weiss EJ, Ludeman MJ, Coughlin SR (2000). PAR3 is a cofactor for PAR4 activation by thrombin. *Nature* 404: 609-613.

Nierodzik M L, Chen K, Takeshita K, Li J-J, Huang Y-Q, Feng X-S, D'Andrea M R, Andrade-Gordon P, Karpatkin S. (1998). Protease-activated receptor 1 (PAR-1) is required and rate-limiting for thrombin-enhanced experimental pulmonary metastasis. *Blood* 92: 3694-3700.

Nigg EA, Hilz H, Eppenberger HM, Dutly F (1985). Rapid and reversible translocation of the catalytic subunit of cAMP-dependent protein kinase type II from the Golgi complex to the nucleus. *EMBO Journal* 4: 2801-2806.

Nystedt S, Emilsson K, Wahlestedt C and Sundelin J (1994). Molecular cloning of a potential proteinase activated receptor. *Proc Natl Acad Sci USA* 91: 9208-9212.

Offermanns S, Laugwitz KL, Spicher K, Schultz G (1994). G proteins of the G12 family are activated via thromboxane A2 and thrombin receptors in human platelets. *Proc Natl Acad Sci. USA* 91: 504-508.

Pearson G, Robinson F, Beers Gibson T, Xu B-E, Karandikar M, Berman K, Cobb MH.

Mitogen-Activated Protein (MAP) Kinase Pathways. Regulation and Physiological (2001). *Endocrine Rev* 22: 153-183.

Rasmussen UB, Vouret-Craviari V, Jallat S, Schlesinger Y, Pages G, Pavirani A, Lecocq JP, Pouyssegur J, VanObberghen-Schilling E (1991). cDNA cloning and expression of a hamster alpha-thrombin receptor coupled to Ca2+ mobilization. *FEBS Lett* 288: 123-128.

Riabowol KT, Fink JS, Gilman MZ, Walsh DA, Goodman RH, Feramisco JR (1988). The catalytic subunit of cAMP-dependent protein kinase induces expression of genes containing cAMP-responsive enhancer elements. *Nature* 336: 83-86.

Ribeiro, C., Ebner, A., and Affolter, M. (2002). In vivo imaging reveals different cellular functions for FGF and Dpp signaling in tracheal branching morphogenesis. *Dev Cell 2*, 677-683.

Rorth P (2003). Communication by touch: role of cellular extensions in complex animals.*Cell* 112: 595-8.

Rudroff C, Schafberg H, Nowak G, Weinel R, Scheele J, Kaufmann R (1998). Characterization of functional thrombin receptors in human pancreatic tumor cells (MIA PaCa-2. *Pancreas* 16: 189-194.

Rudroff C, Seibold S, Kaufmann R, Cu Zetina C, Reise K, Schafer U, Schneider A, Brockmann M, Scheele J, Neugebauer, EAM (2002). Expression of the thrombin receptor PAR-1 correlates with tumour cell differentiation of pancreatic adenocarcinoma in vitro. *Clin Exp Metastasis* 19: 181-189.

Rydel TJ, Ravichandran KG, Tulinsky A, Bode W, Huber R, Roitch C, Fenton II JW (1990). The structure of a complex of recombinant hirudin and human alpha-thrombin. *Science*, 249, 277-280.

Santoro B, Liu DT, Yao H, Bartsch D, Kandel ER, Siegelbaum SA, Tibbs GR (1998). Identification of a gene encoding a hyperpolarization-activated pacemaker channel of brain. *Cell* 93: 717-729.

Sato M, Kornberg TB (2002). FGF is an essential mitogen and chemoattractant for the air sacs of the drosophila tracheal system. *Dev Cell* 3: 195-207.

Scase TJ, Heath MF, Evans RJ (1997). Cloning of PAR3 from human platelets, and human erythroleukemic and human promonocytic cell lines. *Blood* 90: 2113-2114.

Schafberg H, Nowak G, Kaufmann R (1997). Thrombin has a bimodal effect on glioma cell growth. *Brit J Cancer* 76: 1592-1596.

Schwede F, Maronde E, Genieser H, Jastorff B (2000). Cyclic nucleotide analogs as biochemical tools and prospective drugs. *Pharmacol Therapeut* 87: 199-226.

Shapiro MJ, Coughlin SR (1998). Separate signals for agonist-independent and agonist-triggered trafficking of protease-activated receptor 1. *J Biol Chem* 273: 29009-29014.

Sunahara, RK, Dessauer CW, Gilman AG (1996). Complexity and diversity of mammalian adenylyl cyclases. *Annu Rev Pharm Toxicol* 36: 461-480.

Swift S, Sheridan PJ, Covic L, Kuliopulos A (2000). PAR1 thrombin receptor-G protein interactions. Separation of binding and coupling determinants in the galpha subunit. *J Biol Chem* 275: 2627-2635.

Tang WJ, Hurley, JH (1998). Catalytic mechanism and regulation of mammalian adenylyl cyclases. *Mol Pharmacol* 54: 231-240.

Ullrich A (2002). Molecular targets in cancer therapy and their impact on cancer management. *Oncology.* 63(Suppl 1): 1-5.

Van Biesen T, Luttrell LM, Hawes BE, Lefkowitz RJ (1996). Mitogenic signaling via G protein coupled receptors. *Endocrine Rev* 17: 698-714.

Verrall S, Ishii M, Chen M, Wang L, Tram T, Coughlin SR (1997). The thrombin receptor second cytoplasmic loop confers coupling to Gq-like G proteins in chimeric receptors. Additional evidence for a common transmembrane signaling and G protein coupling mechanism in G protein-coupled receptors. *J Biol Chem* 272: 6898-6902.

Vu TK, Hung DT, Wheaton VI and Coughlin SR (1991). Molecular cloning of a functional thrombin receptor reveals a novel proteolytic mechanism of receptor activation. *Cell* 64: 1057-1068.

Walsh DA, Perkins JP, Krebs, EG (1968). An adenosine 3',5'-monophosphate-dependant protein kinase from rabbit skeletal muscle. *J Biol Chem* 243: 3763-3765.

Walsh DA, van Patten SM (1994). Multiple pathway signal transduction by the cAMP-dependent protein kinase. *FASEB J* 8: 1227-1236.

Withers DJ (1997). Signaling pathways involved in the mitogenic effects of cAMP. *Clin Sci* 92: 445-451.

Xia ZG, Storm DR (1997). Calmodulin-regulated adenylyl cyclases and neuromodulation. *Curr Opin Neurobiol* 7: 391-396.

Xu WF, Andersen H, Whitmore TE, Presnell SR, Yee DP, Ching A, Gilbert T, Davie EW and Foster DC (1998). Cloning and characterization of human protease-activated receptor 4. *Proc Natl Acad Sci USA* 95: 6642-6646.

Zhang HC, McComsey DF, White KB, Addo MF, Andrade-Gordon P, Derian CK, Oksenberg D, Maryanoff BE (2001). Thrombin receptor (PAR-1) antagonists. Solid-phase synthesis of indole-based peptide mimetics by anchoring to a secondary amide. *Bioorg Med Chem Lett* 11: 2105-9.

Zacharski LR, Memoli VA, Costantini V, Wojtukiewicz MZ, Ornstein DL (1990). Clotting factors in tumour tissue: implications for cancer therapy. *Blood Coagul Fibrinol* 1: 71-78

Zacharski LR, Wojtukiewicz MZ, Costantini V, Ornstein DL, Memoli VA (1992). Pathways of coagulation/fibrinolysis activation in malignancy. *Sem Thromb Hemostas* 18: 104-116.

Zacharski LR, Constantini V (1995). Blood Coagulation activation in cancer: challenges for cancer treatment. *Hämostaseol* 15: 14-20.

Zieger M, Tausch S, Henklein P, Nowak G, Kaufmann R (2001). A novel PAR-I-type thrombin receptor signaling pathway: Cyclic AMP-independent activation of PKA in SNB-19 glioblastoma cells. *Biochem Biophys Res Commun* 282: 952-957.

In: Trends in Kidney Cancer Research
Editor: Kelvin R. Nunez, pp. 55-76
ISBN 1-59454-141-8

Chapter V

Von Hippel-Lindau Gene and Protein Alterations in Carcinogen-Induced Rat Kidney Tumors: Implications for Renal Tumorigenesis in Humans

Yih-Horng Shiao *
National Cancer Institute-Frederick, Frederick, MD

Abstract

N-nitroso compounds act as alkylating agents, and several such compounds are present in tobacco smoke and are detectable in patients treated with diuretics for hypertension and after long-term dialysis treatment for end-stage kidney disease. Rat kidney tumors of various histological types, morphologically resembling their human counterparts, are inducible by *N*-nitroso compounds, thus providing direct evidence to link tobacco smoking and renal dialysis to kidney tumors in humans. These carcinogen-induced rat kidney tumors are also useful for identification of molecular mechanisms of renal tumorigenesis. As seen in humans, alterations in the *von Hippel-Lindau* (*VHL*) gene have been frequently detected in rat kidney tumors of the clear cell phenotype and are rare in eosinophilic renal epithelial tumors, mesenchymal tumors, and nephroblastomas in rats. When rat non-clear cell kidney tumors are examined for VHL protein, almost all tumors show down-regulation of the protein in comparison with adjacent non-neoplastic tissues. This finding suggests that reduction of wild-type VHL protein can also contribute to kidney tumor development regardless of histology. Further analysis of human renal cell carcinomas confirms that down-regulation of VHL protein occurs more frequently than *VHL* gene mutations. Differential localization of VHL protein has been also observed using various antibodies against different VHL epitopes and has been associated with tumor characteristics and patients' survival. In contrast to the significance of protein alteration, clinical utility of *VHL* gene mutational status has not been consistently demonstrated, even though many tumorigenic and angiogenic factors are up-regulated in kidney tumors or cancer cells carrying *VHL* gene alterations. The broad implications of VHL protein for renal tumorigenesis are further highlighted by the discovery of differential expression of VHL protein variants in different organs in rats.

Kidney Tumor Statistic

Kidney tumors are still a major cancer burden in several continents, especially in developed countries [1]. These tumors affected 189,077 patients and caused 91,137 deaths worldwide in year 2000. In the United States, a total of 31,900 new cancer cases and 11,900 deaths have been estimated for the year 2003 [2]. Although kidney tumor incidence ranks 10th among human neoplasms, the average annual increase of 2.2% since 1950 makes kidney tumors the 6th fast-rising tumor type among all organ sites. Males are more frequently diagnosed with kidney tumors than females. The rate of increase is higher in black than in white populations. Peoples of Asian/Pacific origin are half as likely to develop kidney malignancies than other ethnic groups. Kidney tumors respond poorly to radiotherapy and chemotherapy [3,4]. Therefore, understanding of the etiology and elucidation of molecular mechanism(s) contributing to tumor development are crucial to formulation of plans for early prevention, diagnosis, and treatment intervention.

The Risk Factors for Kidney Tumors

Tobacco smoking, obesity, hypertension, and chronic renal failure have been consistently demonstrated to be major risk factors for kidney tumors [5-8]. Except obesity, which may relate to reactive oxygen species production [9], the other three risk factors all may involve N-nitroso compounds. An increase of N-nitroso compounds is observed in patients exposed to tobacco smoking, diuretic treatment for hypertension, and long-term dialysis for end-stage renal failure [10-15]. Tobacco smoke contains thousands of chemicals with known carcinogenic potential, including several N-nitroso compounds [10,11]. Diuretics, such as hydrochlorothiazide, a secondary amine, can be converted to N-nitroso compounds via nitrosation reaction in the stomach [12, 13]. Endogenous formation of N-nitrosodimethylamine has been also detected in patients with chronic renal failure [14,15]. Many N-nitroso compounds require metabolic activation to become alkylating carcinogens, which form DNA adducts through their alkyl functional group [10,16-18]. The common DNA adducts include O^6-alkylguanine and O^4-alkylthymine, which are promutagenic for GC

* Corresponding author: Yih-Horng Shiao, Ph.D., Laboratory of Comparative Carcinogenesis, Building 538, Room 205, National Cancer Institute-Frederick, National Institutes of Health, Frederick, MD 21702; Tel: 301-846-1246; Fax: 301-846-5946; E-mail: shiao@mail.ncifcrf.gov

to AT and TA to CG transitions, respectively [19,20]. Consumption of fruits and vegetables has been associated with reduced risk for kidney tumors [7,8]. These diets contain many anti-alkylating agents, such as vitamins D and E [21,22], supporting the idea that alkylation is one mechanism leading to kidney tumor formation. Some N-nitroso compounds can also generate reactive oxygen species to damage DNA through oxidation [23-25]. The risks of suspected chemicals are usually assessed and validated in animals (see the "Animal models for renal tumorigenesis" below).

CANCER PHENOTYPE AND GENETICS

The majority of kidney tumors (>80%) are derived from renal parenchyma [26,27]. A small fraction of kidney tumors is of renal pelvic origin. Of kidney parenchymal tumors in humans, about 90% are renal cell carcinomas, originating from mature epithelium [26,28]. Wilms' tumors, also called nephroblastomas and arising from embryonic metanephric blastema, comprise about 6% while tumors of mesenchymal origin make up approximately 4% of the total [26,28]. Renal cell carcinomas can be grouped into various tumor types based on cytology and growth pattern [29,30]. The cytology may be clear, chromophilic (basophilic or eosinophilic), chromophobic, oncocytic, or spindle-shaped/pleomorphic. The growth pattern can be compact, acinar, tubulopapillary, or cystic. According to recent international consensus, combining morphological and genetic criteria, renal cell tumors are classified into benign and malignant neoplasms [31,32]. Benign neoplasms include Wilms' tumor-like metanephric adenoma and adenofibroma, papillary adenoma, and oncocytoma. Malignant neoplasms consist of conventional clear cell (70-80%, characterized primarily by alteration in the *VHL* gene), papillary (10-15%, with basophilic and/or eosinophilic cytology and often carrying trisomy of chromosomes 3q, 7, 12, 16, and 17, and loss of Y chromosome), chromophobic (about 5%, with monosomy of chromosomes 1, 2, 6, 10, 13, 17, and 21, and hypodiploidy), collecting duct (1%), and unclassified tumors (3-5%). With this classification, the 5-year survival for each tumor type are 78-100% for chromophobic, 56-86% for papillary, 50-76% for clear cell, and about 24% for unclassified kidney tumors [33,34].

Studies of hereditary diseases predisposing to renal cell carcinomas have identified several cancer-causing genes, which are also altered in sporadic kidney tumors [35]. The *VHL* gene, originally isolated from the von Hippel-Lindau disease and located in the chromosome 3p25-26, is commonly lost (90%), mutated (30-60%), or hypermethylated in the promoter region (20%) in renal cell carcinomas of clear cell phenotype [36]. Mutations in the *MET* oncogene, which plays a key role in familial papillary renal cell carcinomas and resides in 7q31.3, are also detectable in sporadic counterparts [37]. The *BHD* gene is linked to the Birt-Hogg-Dube syndrome and is mapped to chromosome 17p11.2 [35]. Alterations in the *BHD* gene are observed in different histological types of renal cell carcinomas and appear to have no association with a specific phenotype [38,39]. Other genes, such as the *TSC1* (9q34) and the *TSC2* (16p13) from tuberous sclerosis syndrome, and the *FH*, fumarate hydratase (1q42-43) from familial leiomyoma renal cell carcinoma, have been also implicated in a small fraction of kidney tumors [35]. The role of VHL in renal tumorigenesis has been extensively examined in *in vitro* and *in vivo* systems and is discussed in detail here.

Animal Models for Renal Tumorigenesis

Animal studies have an advantage for examination of cause-effect relationships with strictly controlled experimental conditions, which are impossible for research using human subjects. Although humans and other animals are different entities, information from animal studies can be later extrapolated carefully for human use. Overall, animal studies provide alternative *in vivo* systems useful for 1) validation of descriptive observations from humans and 2) providing less variable and more accessible materials for new discoveries.

Validation of Risk Factors and *VHL* Mutations

Rats have a very low incidence of spontaneous kidney tumors [40,41], and their kidneys are sensitive to tumor induction by chemicals [42,43]. In addition to N-nitroso compounds commonly detected in patients with high kidney tumor risk, some synthetic N-nitroso compounds, acting as direct carcinogens with no need of bioactivation, have been used as alkylating agents in animal carcinogenesis studies [40,44,45]. These compounds have been proven to induce kidney tumors of various histological types in different rat strains through specific routes of exposure (see the reference 46 for comprehensive review). The resulted tumor types resemble human counterparts. With dietary manipulation, kidney tumor incidence can be enhanced by shifting bioactivation of N-nitroso compounds from the liver to the kidney in rats fed exclusively glucose/sucrose diet during carcinogen treatment [47,48]. This particular model may have implications for obesity-related kidney tumor risk in humans, because a change in dietary pattern to a diet with a high carbohydrate to fat ratio in the United States has been associated with an increase in obesity [49,50].

N-nitrosodimethylamine (NDMA) and N-nitrosomorpholine induce a small percentage of kidney tumors with the clear cell phenotype, which is the most common histological type in humans but is rare in rats [45,51,52]. In these animal models, the clear cell phenotype has been confirmed by periodic acid-Schiff staining for glycogen accumulation [45,52]. The predominant tumor type of epithelial origin arising from these treatments is a basophilic tumor with solid, cystic, tubular, or papillary growth pattern. Eosinophilic tumors, having similar growth spectra as basophilic tumors, are also observed and often overtake co-existing clear cells to become the major cell type inside tumor areas. N-nitroso-ethyl(2-hydroxyethyl)amine (EHEN) induces mainly eosinophilic kidney tumors in adult male Fischer 344 rats [46]. Chromophobic tumors are incidental findings in rats and have been reported in chemical carcinogenesis studies using various N-nitroso compounds and in Eker rats with inherited *TSC2* gene alteration [46]. Oncocytomas are also inducible with several N-nitroso compounds and can develop spontaneously in aged animals [46]. An oncocyte-like tumor has been also described in the Eker rat model. N-nitroso-N-ethylurea (NEU), a synthetic direct-acting alkylating agent, has been used to induce nephroblastomas in the offspring of Noble rats with transplacental exposure [46]. N-nitrosomethyl(methoxymethyl)amine (DMN-OMe), also a synthetic chemical, which is an activated compound similar to that resulting from NDMA metabolism. It induces renal tumors of mesenchymal cell origin in neonatal Fischer 344/NCr rats [46]. Induction of nephroblastoma and mesenchymal tumors are also reported with other N-nitroso compounds [46].

VHL mutations are frequently observed in human renal cell carcinomas, especially of clear cell phenotype [36]. Detection of *VHL* mutations in rat kidney tumors can provide direct evidence linking genetic alterations to a specific exposure. To pursue this, mutation analysis has been carried out for chemically-induced clear cell and non-clear cell kidney tumors in many laboratories. Early screening for *VHL* mutations was disappointing because no mutations were detected in about 40 rat kidney tumors, including 10 EHEN-induced eosinophilic tumors, 10 NEU-induced nephroblastomas, 7 DMN-OMe-induced mesenchymal tumors and 23 rat kidney tumors from other exposures [53-55]. However, none of these tumors show conventional clear cell phenotype. After examination of a collection of NDMA-induced rat kidney tumors, a total of 4 mutations in the coding region of *VHL* were demonstrated in 3 of 8 clear or mixed clear/eosinophilic cell tumors [47]. The mutations consist of three G to A and one A to G transitions, consistent with known mutagenic properties of NDMA involving formation of O^6-methylguanine and O^4-methylthymine [19,20]. This mutation spectrum has been also observed in 30%-70% of *VHL* base substitutions in human sporadic renal cell carcinomas, confirming a possible role of NDMA in the induction of *VHL* mutations and causation of renal tumors in humans. Among three tumors carrying *VHL* mutations, two yielded no wild-type *VHL* sequence, suggestive of allele loss, as is often seen in the corresponding human disease [56]. Since NDMA has been shown to have a clastogenic effect on DNA [57,58], it is possible that allele loss was also ascribable to the carcinogen. The other finding was that the tumors having *VHL* mutations tended to have abundant swollen cells in which the nuclei are located against the cytoplasmic membrane, giving a ring-like appearance. In human clear cell renal carcinomas, cells contain glycogen, lipid, and/or vacuoles of unknown type in variable proportion [59]. This suggests that the swollen cells are a subset of clear cells and *VHL* mutation may be involved in formation of this phenotype.

The above EHEN-induced eosinophilic tumors and/or NEU-induced nephroblastomas have been further examined for mutation in the non-coding region of the *VHL* exon 1 and for possible DNA hypermethylation in 14 CpG sites of this putative promoter region. In humans, DNA hypermethylation in the equivalent region is seen and suppresses *VHL* gene expression in clear cell tumors without detectable intragenic mutations [60,61]. Still, no mutation or hypermethylation has been observed in those animal non-clear cell tumors [62]. These results confirm findings in humans that intragenic *VHL* mutations and promoter hypermethylation in non-clear cell kidney tumors are uncommon [63].

Discovery of New Types of VHL Changes

To examine possible VHL alterations other than mutation, the protein level has been examined by immunohistochemistry in EHEN-induced eosinophilic tumors originating from mature renal tubule and NEU-induced nephroblastomas arising from the metanephric blastema, the precursor of renal tubules. Expression of VHL in the tubules and in the blastema has been reported in normal kidneys previously [64-67]. Down-regulation of VHL protein was observed in 6 of 8 eosinophilic tumors and in all 10 nephroblastomas when compared with adjacent non-neoplastic tissues [62]. The immunostaining signal was located in the cytoplasm and was more intense in the tubules of normal cortex than in those of the normal medullary area. The glomeruli and stromal tissues were not stained. This is the first demonstration of VHL down-regulation as a novel mechanism leading to kidney tumor formation, although the gene is not mutated. Down-regulation of VHL protein in non-clear cell kidney tumors may also provide an explanation for the hypervascular phenotype commonly observed in these tumors.

Another new discovery from examination of VHL protein was differential expression of 2 VHL protein isoforms (20 and 22 kilodalton) between fetal and adult tissues in untreated rats [36]. All examined tissues, including kidney, cerebrum, cerebellum, adrenal, liver, lung, and pancreas known to be target organs for the human VHL disease, expressed both isoforms except adult kidney. Fetal tissues appeared to have higher protein level than adult counterparts. Higher level of the 22-kilodalton variant was observed in adult adrenal gland, adult cerebrum, adult cerebellum, fetal lung, and fetal liver. No difference of the two protein variants is seen in adult pancreas, adult lung, adult liver, and fetal kidney. In kidneys, the two VHL isoforms of 20 and 22 kilodalton have been detected in 16-day fetal rats but only the 20-kilodalton VHL protein has been seen in adult kidneys [36,62]. This differential expression of VHL isoforms had not been reported before, although expression of 2 VHL isoforms in human and mouse cell lines has been known for sometime [68-70]. The finding is very exciting because it may have implications for the development of eosinophilic tumors (adult renal tubule origin) and that of nephroblastomas (embryonic metanephric blastema origin). Further, functional difference between two human VHL isoforms (30 and 19 kilodalton) has been reported in *in vitro* studies, although both isoforms can bind elongin B/C and down-regulate vascular endothelial growth factor [68,69,71]. The 30-kilodalton variant has a stronger tumor suppressor activity than the 19-kilodalton protein [72], and the latter protein loses capability to bind fibronectin [69]. In light of possible functional difference, analysis of two isoforms in sporadic tumors is certainly needed in the future.

Further analysis of a putative promoter region in the *VHL* in rat kidney tumors induced by $KBrO_3$, an environmental agent used in cosmetics manufacture and food processes, and detected in drinking water, revealed another new mechanism. Mutations of C to T in a putative *VHL* promoter region, containing three 5'-CCGCCC(A/C)(C/G/T)-3', a Sp1 transcription factor binding motif known to regulate gene expression [73], were detected in some clear cell tumors and also in an aged control [74]. The same C to T mutation at the fourth position of the conserved core region (5'-CGCC-3') was seen in 2 of 9 clear cell tumors. Two other C to T mutations outside the Sp1 core region were also detected, one in a clear cell tumor and the other in 1 of 3 untreated 2-year old rats. These C to T mutations were located at non-CpG sites and are consistent with the hypothesis that the base change arises from promutagenic 5'-OH-cytosine [75], an oxidative lesion resulting from $KBrO_3$-initiated oxidative stress [76]. Although mutation frequency is low in this series of clear cell tumors, the repeated mutation in the Sp-1 sites suggests that this region may be sensitive to either $KBrO_3$-induced oxidative or age-related DNA damage.

THE VON HIPPEL-LINDAU GENE

The *VHL* gene, containing 3 exons, was first cloned in 1993 in humans with the VHL disease, a familial syndrome with predisposition to various tumors [77,78]. These tumors, including retinal angioma, hemangioblastoma in the central nervous system, renal cell carcinoma, and pheochromocytoma, also have a common hypervascular phenotype, linking *VHL* alteration to tumorigenesis and angiogenesis. Beside tumors arising from germline *VHL* abnormalities, sporadic tumors with a highly vascular phenotype, such as clear cell renal carcinomas and hemangioblastomas, also carry frequent *VHL* gene alterations [79-81]. The *VHL* genes of other species were subsequently cloned and the predicted protein sequences share a high percentage of similarity among species [70,82-84]. The known chromosomal locations for the *VHL* are 3p25-26 for humans [77], 4q41 for rats [85], and 6 (at 49.45 cM region) for mice [70]. Two *VHL* mRNA transcripts (long and short) are detectable using sensitive techniques in almost all normal adult tissues and tissues during embryogenesis in humans and mice [64,77,86-88]. These include tissues commonly affected in the VHL disease, such as kidney, brain, adrenal gland, and retina. It appears that the long transcript is more abundant than the short transcript in most adult and fetal tissues [70,86,87]. Expression of long transcript only has been observed in some renal cancer cell lines, such as the 786-O [86], frequently used in functional assays. VHL protein is also ubiquitously detected in normal adult tissues by immunohistochemistry [65-67]. The level of protein is highly variable among tissues. VHL protein is either poorly expressed or undetectable in smooth muscle and endothelial cells. Up-regulation of VHL protein in endothelial cells is observed in several pathological lesions, including lung metastasis of pancreatic adenocarcinoma, inflammatory areas of esophageal ulcer, sprouting microvessels in atherosclerotic areas, and proliferating endothelial cells in placenta [67,89]. This suggests that VHL protein is overexpressed in response to the change of cellular environments. Two VHL protein isoforms have been frequently observed in humans and rodents [62,68,70,71,90]. In addition to tumorigenesis and angiogenesis, VHL has been also linked to morphogenesis of different histological types of renal tumors [46], and normal tissue development, including placental vasculogenesis, trachea, neuronal cells, and spermatogenesis [83,91-94]. The accumulated evidence that VHL alterations contribute to angiogenesis and tumorigenesis from *in vitro* and *in vivo* experiments are summarized in the following section.

Molecular Mechanisms Revealed in *in vitro* Experiments

Molecular pathways involving VHL protein have been extensively examined using cell culture systems. *VHL*-deficient cell lines are often used to generate daughter lines bearing different *VHL* transfectants, including wild-type *VHL*, and the daughter lines are then compared with *VHL*-deficient parental lines to determine the specificity of protein-protein interaction and downstream effectors. The yeast two-hybrid system is also used to isolate many VHL partners [95]. The angiogenic and tumorigenic pathways are discussed separately.

VHL-related Angiogenesis

It has been well established that VHL suppresses angiogenesis via down-regulation of hypoxia-inducible factor-alpha (HIF-alpha). Under normoxia conditions, hydroxylation of the proline at the 564 or 402 residue of HIF-alpha oxygen-dependent degradation domain (ODDD) inside the amino-terminal transactivation region is catalyzed by prolyl hydroxylases in the presence of molecular oxygen, Fe(2+), and 2-oxoglutarate [96-98]. Supplementation of ascorbate enhances the hydroxylase activity [99]. Cobalt(2+) blocks the binding of VHL to hydroxylated HIF-alpha by occupying the ODDD domain [100]. The proline-564 hydroxylated HIF-alpha is recognized by a hydrophobic pocket of VHL [101,102], which is a part of the VHL-elongin B/C-Cul2 (VBC) complex also known to function as an ubiquitin ligase [103-105]. The VBC complex initiates polyubiquitination of the HIF-alpha and subsequently degradation of the HIF-alpha by the 26S proteasome [106-108]. Since HIF-alpha can form a heterodimer with HIF-beta (also called aryl hydrocarbon receptor nuclear translocator) and p300/CBP coactivators to mediate transcription of many angiogenic molecules, including vascular endothelial growth factor (VEGF) and plasminogen activator inhibitor 1 [109,110], removal of HIF-alpha plays an important role in suppression of angiogenesis. *VHL* mutations in both elongin C- and HIF-binding domains abolish the VBC ubiquitin ligase-mediated HIF-alpha polyubiquitination and result in HIF-alpha accumulation [109,110]. This inverse relationship of VHL to HIF-alpha or to VEGF has been validated in primary human renal carcinomas and hemangioblastomas [111-113]. Under hypoxic conditions, HIF-alpha may escape from VHL-regulated degradation by lack of prolyl hydroxylation or nuclear translocation [114]. Hypoxia also prevents hydroxylation of asparagines in the HIF-alpha carboxyl-terminal transactivation domain by the FIH-1 hydroxylase [115,116]. This allows p300 and cAMP-response-element-binding protein coactivators to bind to the transactivation domain of HIF-alpha and initiates downstream gene transcription [117-119]. Inability to control HIF-alpha protein level and transcription activity by VHL under hypoxia may explain in part why some sporadic tumors with a hypervascular phenotype do not have detectable *VHL* mutations.

A HIF-independent pathway has been also observed for VHL anti-angiogenic function. VHL is able to down-regulate VEGF by sequestering the Sp1 transcription factor/protein kinase C zeta complex from activating VEGF transcription [120-123]. VHL can also down-regulate TGF-beta1, a potent angiogenic factor in renal tumors [124].

VHL-Related Tumorigenesis

VHL protein is capable of regulating the cell cycle, cell signaling, cellular environment, and metabolism. VHL alterations may contribute to tumor growth, invasiveness, and metastasis. Wild-type VHL raises the level of p27, a cell cyclin-dependent kinase (CDK) inhibitor, and results in G1 cell cycle arrest [125,126]. VHL-dependent up-regulation of p27 is also observed in cells grown at high density and in cells after neutralizing TGF-alpha activity [90,125,127]. In contrast to p27, cyclin D1 mRNA and protein are down-regulated by wild-type VHL [128-130]. This reduction prevents the Rb tumor suppressor from cyclin D1/CDK4-elicited phosphorylation [130]. Up-regulation of cyclin D1 is commonly detected in cancer cells regardless of *VHL* genetic status [128,129]. Cyclin D1 is a cyclin-dependent kinase cofactor for CDK4 and the cyclin D1/CDK4 complex can bind to p27 [129], which may in turn sequester p27 from cell cycle control. Recently, the tumor suppressing function of VHL has been also linked to increase of p53 protein [131], a well known multifunctional tumor suppressor [132].

VHL and TGF-alpha, a mitogen initiating the Ras-Raf-Map kinase signaling cascade, appears to be antagonistic, with higher VHL level in favor of growth suppression but higher TGF-alpha leading to cell growth [36]. Another mitogenic factor, platelet-derived growth factor-B (PDGF-B) and its signaling effectors can be also down-regulated by VHL, possibly by inhibiting Sp1-mediated PDGF-B transcription [133]. In addition, TGF-alpha and PDGF may stimulate HIF-alpha expression via MAP kinase signaling [134,135], and induce angiogenesis under non-hypoxic conditions [136]. Loss of functional VHL can also trigger tumorigenesis via up-regulation of protein the kinase C (PKC) family. Wild-type VHL has been shown to bind and to prevent PKC zeta and delta from activating the MAP kinase signaling pathway [120]. Wild-type VHL can also sequester PKC delta from interaction with insulin-like growth factor 1 (IGF1) receptor, and subsequently inhibits IGF1-mediated signaling pathway and reduces the invasiveness of renal cancer cells [137]. IGF1 can also stimulate the expression of HIF-alpha to produce an angiogenic phenotype in *VHL*-deficient cells [134]. The down-regulation of PKC lambda is controlled by VHL-dependent ubiquitination [138].

Inactivation of VHL may also alter the cellular environment and facilitates tumor progression at normoxia. Up-regulation of HIF-alpha is the major mediator to induce many downstream effectors contributing to tumor aggressiveness [139,140]. A HIF-dependent response element is identified in the *CA9* promoter region and therefore the HIF is able to regulate *CA9* gene expression [141]. Overproduction of CA9 and CA12, which are carbonic anhydrases and catalyze hydration of CO_2, creates an acidic extracellular environment and is frequently detected in tumors [142]. Increase of acidity has been associated with tumor invasiveness [143]. HIF-alpha is also involved in metastasis through two known mechanisms. Angiogenesis has been described above. The other mechanism is the expression of CXCR4, a chemokine receptor commonly detected in metastatic tumors, which is up-regulated by HIF-alpha [144]. Hypoxia (low oxygen tension), another cellular environmental change in tumors, is known to counteract VHL-dependent down-regulation of TGF-alpha [145], cyclin D1 [129,130], HIF-alpha [100], and carbonic anhydrases 9 and 12 [141,142]. The HIF-alpha can in turn up-regulate TGF-alpha, cyclin D1, and CA9. 130,141,146]. It appears that oxygen is needed for VHL-mediated tumor suppression. Other VHL effectors include Jade1 [147], STRA13 [148], matrix metalloproteinases and their inhibitors [149], and hepatocyte nuclear factor 1-alpha [150]. These are mediators of VHL-induced cell differentiation and suppression of invasiveness.

Involvement of VHL in carbohydrate metabolism comes from two lines of evidence. First, HIF-alpha, escaped from VHL-dependent ubiquitination because of VHL alteration or hypoxia, has been shown to increase transport of glucose into cancer cells and to induce expression of many glycolytic enzymes [134]. Second, wild-type VHL localizes to the mitochondria, and altered VHL changes the mitochondrial phenotype to resemble that in human clear cell renal carcinomas [151]. These two observations are consistent with the Warburg effect [152,153], that accumulation of lactic acid in tumor cells is a result of increase of glycolysis and reduction of cell respiration by the mitochondria. It is noteworthy that the same molecular mechanisms leading to the Warburg effect may also increase environmental acidity and angiogenesis [134,154]. Further, localization of VHL to the mitochondria has many implications for renal tumorigenesis in general and for the morphogenesis of clear cell renal tumors, because mitochondria play an essential role in apoptosis [155,156] and in glucose/lipid metabolism [157]. Cells resistant to apoptosis, a programmed cell death, are prone to cell transformation and tumor development [158]. Accumulation of glycogen and/or lipid, as seen in clear cell tumors, can occur if the catabolism of pyruvate, the aerobic glycolytic end product, and fatty acid from lipolysis through the mitochondria is reduced.

Mechanisms Revealed in in Vivo Experiments

Although VHL-related angiogenic and tumorigenic pathways have been extensively characterized *in vitro*, use of cancer-derived cells cannot exclude the possibility of contributions other than VHL. Knockout animals provide the opportunity to alter selected genes specifically and to determine whether the resulting phenotypic changes are consistent with findings in humans. An initial experiment demonstrated that mice with a homozygous knockout of *VHL* were lethal at 10.5 to 12.5 days of gestation, while heterozygous $VHL^{+/-}$ animals at 15 months of age did not have any detectable abnormality [91]. The main defect in those $VHL^{-/-}$ embryos was the failure of vasculogenesis in the placenta, which may associate with lack of VEGF expression. Expression of VEGF was observed in age-matched normal $VHL^{+/+}$ embryos. Defective extracellular fibronectin matrix assembly was detected in other $VHL^{-/-}$ mice [159]. To examine the susceptibility of the $VHL^{+/-}$ mice to carcinogen exposure, streptozotocin, a renal carcinogen, has been used in a tumor end-point study [160]. Although carcinogen-induced kidney tumor incidence in $VHL^{+/-}$ mice was similar to treated $VHL^{+/+}$ mice, treatment induced a higher frequency of hepatic vascular lesions in $VHL^{-/-}$ mice than in $VHL^{+/+}$ mice and incidental vascular lesions in the uterus, spleen, ovary, and heart were exclusively detected in treated $VHL^{+/-}$ mice. This and other $VHL^{+/-}$ mouse systems show various degrees of susceptibility to develop spontaneous hepatic vascular lesions. BALB/c mouse strain was most susceptible, C57BL/6 strain least susceptible, and A/J strain intermediate [94]. These experiments suggest that loss of VHL tends to induce abnormal angiogenesis. To avoid embryonic lethality, mice with a conditional *VHL* allele have been created and subjected to recombinase-initiated homozygous *VHL* deletion in selected organs to determine the phenotypic changes as the result of complete VHL inactivation. Liver is still the major target organ for vascular lesions with a high frequency [94, 161]. Vascular lesions are also seen in heart, kidney, pancreas, lung, and testis [94]. The loss of VHL is accompanied with increase of HIF-alpha, VEGF, and erythropoietin in those vascular lesions [94,161]. Although an abnormality of angiogenesis and a diversity of affected organs are demonstrated, no tumors of parenchymal cell origin or related to human VHL disease have been detected in those conditional mice. Species difference between human and mouse and/or requirement of other gene alterations may account for this discrepancy.

EXTENSION OF VHL FINDINGS FROM ANIMAL STUDIES TO HUMANS

Alteration in the *VHL* intragenic region has been widely examined in human kidney tumors [36]. Although loss of the chromosome 3p25 region is observed in more than 90% of sporadic clear cell renal cell carcinomas, mutations in the *VHL* coding sequence are only seen in about 30-60% of those tumors from various populations. Also, *VHL* mutations are not commonly detected in non-clear cell kidney tumors. This discrepancy is often interpreted as possible involvement of VHL-independent pathways in tumors without *VHL* intragenic mutations. However, another view is that *VHL* mutation alone is not sufficient to account for contributions of VHL to tumor development. This view is further supported by no clear association of *VHL* mutations to tumor characteristics, including tumor stage, tumor grade, microvessel density, and metastasis [162-164]. A recent population-based study in fact shows that *VHL* mutation is associated with better cancer-free survival in clear cell renal carcinoma patients compared to those with wild-type *VHL* allele after radical nephrectomy treatment [165]. The finding of VHL protein down-regulation in N-nitroso-compound-induced non-clear cell kidney tumors in rats, described above, is provocative. This study showed that alkylating agents still target VHL for alteration in tumors without *VHL* intragenic mutations. It also signifies the role of protein level in general renal tumorigenesis and emphasizes the importance of VHL protein analysis for all kidney tumor types in humans. Further, the differential expression of VHL isoforms, observed in embryonic and adult rat kidneys, needs to be explored in humans.

Following these studies in animals, VHL protein has been examined in human kidney tumors and the results support that down-regulation of VHL protein is more frequent than *VHL* intragenic mutations, and that differential localization of VHL protein is a better prognostic factor for kidney tumors. In one study, an apparent decline of VHL level (positive in <50% of tumor cells) was observed in 49 (65%) tumors when tumor and adjacent non-neoplastic tissues were compared directly [166]. In contrast to the presence of VHL signal in all non-neoplastic tubular cells, lack of VHL expression was always seen in patchy areas of all 75 tumors. This change in protein level was more frequent than *VHL* mutations (28/75, 37%). While VHL signal in adjacent non-neoplastic tubules was detected in the cytoplasm, VHL was localized to the cytoplasm and/or the cell membrane in tumors. The occurrence of a predominantly membranous signal was significantly associated with missense mutations (9 of 14 tumors with missense mutations versus 14 of 61 tumors with either no or non-missense mutations, $p=0.0025$) and tumor stage (23 of 60 tumors with stage TI versus 0 of 15 tumors with TII and TIII, $p=0.0034$). VHL protein has been also examined in another patient population with renal cell carcinomas using different antibodies. No detectable VHL expression in either the nuclei or the cytoplasm was seen in 123 of 398 (31%) clear cell, 20 of 62 (32%) papillary, and 6 of 25 (24%) chromophobe renal carcinomas, and 1 of 6 (6%) oncocytoma [167]. Expression of nuclear and/or cytoplasmic VHL is associated with better tumor-specific survival. Combined nuclear and cytoplasmic VHL expression is associated with low histological grade (Grade 1: 31/46; Grade 2: 110/225; Grade 3: 33/127, $p<0.0001$) and early tumor stage (Stage TI and TII: 83/173; TIII: 92/225, $p<0.05$).

Conclusion

Distinct VHL alterations have been identified in chemically-induced rat kidney tumors. These animal models validate the carcinogenic effects of compounds associated with kidney tumor risk in humans and provide a resource for new discoveries. N-nitroso compounds alter the *VHL* gene and/or VHL protein expression, similar to VHL alteration spectra in human kidney tumors, supporting the proposal that alkylating agents present in or derived from tobacco smoke, diuretics, and long-term dialysis are responsible for renal tumorigenesis. Down-regulation of VHL protein was first detected in rat kidney tumors. The subsequent VHL protein analysis in human kidney tumors not only confirmed the observation, but also discovered differential cellular localization of VHL protein. In addition to these important findings, animal models continue to yield new observations for future testing in human tumor counterparts. Two parameters, differential expression of VHL isoforms and oxidative damage at the core region of Sp-1 transcription factor binding motif, deserve further investigation.

Acknowledgments

I sincerely thank Ms. Kathy Breeze for help in manuscript preparation, and Drs. Lucy M. Anderson and Richard J. Calvert for critical review of this manuscript.

References

[1] Ferlay J, Bray F, Pisani P, et al. GLOBOCAN 2000: Cancer Incidence, Mortality and Prevalence Worldwide, Version 1.0, IARC CancerBase No. 5, Lyon, IARC Press; 2001. http://www-dep.iarc.fr/globocan/globocan.htm

[2] Ries LAG, Eisner MP, Kosary CL, et al., eds. *SEER Cancer Statistics Review*, 1975-2000, Bethesda, MD: National Cancer Institute; 2003. http://seer.cancer.gov/csr/1975_2000.

[3] Bukowski RM, Novick AC. Clinical practice guidelines: renal cell carcinoma. *Cleve Clin J Med.* 1997;64:SI1-44.

[4] Godley PA, Taylor M. Renal cell carcinoma. *Curr Opin Oncol.* 2001;13:199-203.

[5] Dhote R, Pellicer-Coeuret M, Thiounn N, et al. Risk factors for adult renal cell carcinoma: a systematic review and implications for prevention. *BJU Int.* 2000;86:20-27.

[6] McLaughlin JK, Lipworth L. Epidemiologic aspects of renal cell cancer. *Semin Oncol.* 2000;27:115-123.

[7] Martel CL, Lara PN. Renal cell carcinoma: current status and future directions. *Crit Rev Oncol Hematol.* 2003;45:177-190.

[8] Whang YE, Godley PA. Renal cell carcinoma. *Curr Opin Oncol.* 2003;15:213-216.

[9] Gago-Dominguez M, Castelao JE, Yuan JM, et al. Lipid peroxidation: a novel and unifying concept of the etiology of renal cell carcinoma (United States). *Cancer Causes Control.* 2002;13:287-293.

[10] Hecht SS. Biochemistry, biology, and carcinogenicity of tobacco-specific N-nitrosamines. *Chem Res Toxicol.* 1998;11:559-603.

[11] Hoffmann D, Wynder EL. Chemical constituents and bioactivity of tobacco smoke. *IARC Sci Publ.* 1986;74:145-165.

[12] Messerli FH, Grossman E. Beta-blockers and diuretics: to use or not to use. *Am J Hypertens.* 1999;12:157S-163S.

[13] Gold B, Mirvish SS. N-Nitroso derivatives of hydrochlorothiazide, niridazole, and tolbutamide. *Toxicol Appl Pharmacol.* 1977;40:131-136.

[14] Dunn SR, Simenhoff ML, Lele PS, et al. N-nitrosodimethylamine blood levels in patients with chronic renal failure: modulation of levels by ethanol and ascorbic acid. *J Natl Cancer Inst.* 1990;82:783-787.

[15] Simenhoff ML, Dunn SR, Lele PS. Analysis for and intestinal metabolism of precursor nitroso compounds in normal subjects and in patients with chronic renal failure. *IARC Sci Publ.* 1984;57:161-170.

[16] Magee PN. Nitrosamines and human cancer: introduction and overview. *Eur J Cancer Prev.* 1996;5 Suppl 1:7-10.

[17] Yang CS, Smith TJ. Mechanisms of nitrosamine bioactivation and carcinogenesis. *Adv Exp Med Biol.* 1996;387:385-394.

[18] Singer B. N-nitroso alkylating agents: formation and persistence of alkyl derivatives in mammalian nucleic acids as contributing factors in carcinogenesis. *J Natl Cancer Inst.* 1979;62:1329-1339.

[19] Swann PF. Why do O6-alkylguanine and O4-alkylthymine miscode? The relationship between the structure of DNA containing O6-alkylguanine and O4-alkylthymine and the mutagenic properties of these bases. *Mutat Res.* 1990;233:81-94.

[20] Singer B. DNA damage: chemistry, repair and mutagenic potential. *Regul Toxicol Pharmacol.* 1996;23:2-13.

[21] Fujioka T, Suzuki Y, Okamoto T, et al. Prevention of renal cell carcinoma by active vitamin D3. *World J Surg.* 2000;24:1205-1210.

[22] Ricciarelli R, Zingg JM, Azzi A. Vitamin E 80th anniversary: a double life, not only fighting radicals. *IUBMB Life.* 2001;52:71-76.

[23] Wells PG, Kim PM, Laposa RR, et al. Oxidative damage in chemical teratogenesis. *Mutat Res.* 1997;396:65-78.

[24] Lin H, Hollenberg PF. N-nitrosodimethylamine-mediated formation of oxidized and methylated DNA bases in a cytochrome P450 2E1 expressing cell line. *Chem Res Toxicol.* 2001;14:562-566.

[25] Weisburger JH, Chung FL. Mechanisms of chronic disease causation by nutritional factors and tobacco products and their prevention by tea polypenols. *Food Chem Toxicol.* 2002;40:1145-1154.

[26] Lucké B, Schumberger HG. *Tumors of the Kidney, Renal Pelvis and Ureter.* Washington, DC: Armed Forces Institute of Pathology; 1957.

[27] Devesa SS, Silverman DT, McLaughlin JK, et al. Comparison of the descriptive epidemiology of urinary tract cancers. *Cancer Causes Control.* 1990;1:133-141.

[28] Murphy WM, Beckwith JB, Farrow GM. *Tumors of the Kidney, Bladder, and Related Urinary Structures.* Washington, DC: Armed Forces Institute of Pathology; 1994.

[29] Thoenes W, Storkel S, Rumpelt HJ. Histopathology and classification of renal cell tumors (adenomas, oncocytomas and carcinomas). The basic cytological and histopathological elements and their use for diagnostics. *Pathol Res Pract.* 1986;181:125-143.

[30] Thoenes W, Storkel S, Rumpelt HJ, et al. Cytomorphological typing of renal cell carcinoma–a new approach. *Eur Urol.* 1990;18 Suppl 2:6-9.

[31] Kovacs G, Akhtar M, Beckwith BJ, et al. The Heidelberg classification of renal cell tumours. *J Pathol.* 1997;183:131-133.

[32] Storkel S, Eble JN, Adlakha K, et al. Classification of renal cell carcinoma: Workgroup No. 1. Union Internationale Contrele Cancer (UICC) and the American Joint Committee on Cancer (AJCC). *Cancer.* 1997;80:987-989.

[33] Moch H, Gasser T, Amin MB, et al. Prognostic utility of the recently recommended histologic classification and revised TNM staging system of renal cell carcinoma: a Swiss experience with 588 tumors. *Cancer.* 2000;89:604-614.

[34] Amin MB, Amin MB, Tamboli P, et al. Prognostic impact of histologic subtyping of adult renal epithelial neoplasms; an experience of 405 cases. *Am J Surg Pathol.* 2002;26:281-291.

[35] Choyke PL, Glenn GM, Walther MM, et al. Hereditary renal cancers. *Radiology.* 2003;226:33-46.

[36] Shiao YH. The von Hippel-Lindau gene and protein in tumorigenesis and angiogenesis: a potential target for therapeutic designs. *Curr Med Chem.* 2003;10:2461-2470.

[37] Schmidt L, Duh FM, Chen F, et al. Germline and somatic mutations in the tyrosine kinase domain of the MET proto-oncogene in papillary renal carcinomas. *Nat Genet.* 1997;16:68-73.

[38] Nickerson ML, Warren MB, Toro JR, et al. Mutations in a novel gene lead to kidney tumors, lung wall defects, and benign tumors of the hair follicle in patients with the Birt-Hogg-Dube syndrome. *Cancer Cell.* 2002;2:157-164.

[39] Khoo SK, Kahnoski K, Sugimura J, et al. Inactivation of BHD in sporadic renal tumors. *Cancer Res.* 2003;63:4583-4587.

[40] Hard GC. Comparative kidney carcinogenesis in laboratory rodents and humans. In: *Carcinogenicity, Testing, Predicting, and Interpreting Chemical effects.* Kitchin KT, ed. New York: Marcel Dekker; 1999:439-466.

[41] Chandra M, Riley MG, Johnson DE. Spontaneous renal neoplasms in rats. *J Appl Toxicol.* 1993;13:109-116.

[42] Huff J, Cirvello J, Haseman J, et al. Chemicals associated with site-specific neoplasia in 1394 long-term carcinogenesis experiments in laboratory rodents. *Environ Health Perspect.* 1991;93:247-270.

[43] Haseman JK, Crawford DD, Huff JE, et al. Results from 86 two-year carcinogenicity studies conducted by the National Toxicology Program. *J Toxicol Environ Health.* 1984;14:621-639.

[44] Hiasa Y, Ito N. Experimental induction of renal tumors. *Crit Rev Toxicol.* 1987;17:279-343.

[45] Bannasch P, Zerban H. Pathology of tumours in laboratory animals. Tumours of the rat. Tumours of the liver. *IARC Sci Publ.* 1990;99:199-240.

[46] Shiao YH. Role of the von Hippel-Lindau gene and protein in kidney tumor phenotypes: animal models. *Recent Res Devel Histopathol.* 2002;1:21-37. www.researchsignpost.com

[47] Shiao YH, Rice JM, Anderson LM, et al. von Hippel-Lindau gene mutations in N-nitrosodimethylamine-induced rat renal epithelial tumors. *J Natl Cancer Inst.* 1998;18:1720-1723.

[48] Swann PF, McLean AE. Cellular injury and carcinogenesis. The effect of a portein-free high-carbohydrate diet on the metabolism of dimethylnitrosamine in the rat. *Biochem J.* 1971;124:283-288.

[49] Drewnowski A. Fat and sugar: an economic analysis. *J Nutr.* 2003;133:838S-840S.

[50] Centers for Disease Control and Prevention (CDC). *Trends in Intake of Energy and Macronutrients-United States, 1971-2000. MMWR Morb Mortal Wkly Rep.* 2004;53:80-82.

[51] Hard GC. High frequency, single-dose model of renal adenoma/carcinoma induction using dimethylnitrosamine in Crl:(W)BR rats. *Carcinogenesis.* 1984;5:1047-1050.

[52] Brummer C, Rabes HM. Morphology and proliferation kinetics of early tumor stages induced by dimethylnitrosamine in rat kidneys. *Virchows Arch B Cell Pathol Incl Mol Pathol.* 1992;62:133-142.

[53] Shiao YH, Diwan BA, Perantoni AO, et al. Polymerase chain reaction-single-strand conformation polymorphism analysis for the VHL gene in chemically induced kidney tumors of rats using intron-derived primers. *Mol Carcinog.* 1997;19:230-235.

[54] Kikuchi Y, Kobayashi E, Nishizawa M, et al. Cloning of the rat homologue of the von Hippel-Lindau tumor suppressor gene and its non-somatic mutation in rat renal cell carcinomas. *Jpn J Cancer Res.* 1995;86:905-909.

[55] Walker C, Ahn YT, Everitt J, et al. Renal cell carcinoma development in the rat independent of alterations at the VHL gene locus. *Mol Carcinog.* 1996;15:154-161.

[56] Gnarra JR, Duan DR, Weng Y, et al. Molecular cloning of the von Hippel-Lindau tumor suppressor gene and its role in renal carcinoma. *Biochim Biophys Acta.* 1996;1242:201-210.

[57] Sivikova K, Dianovsky J. Induction of chromosomal aberrations, sister-chromatid exchanges and cell-cycle delay in cow peripheral blood lymphocytes treatment with two N-nitroso compounds in vitro. *Mutat Res.* 1993;290:311-315.

[58] Robbiano L, Mereto E, Migliazzi-Morando A, et al. An in vivo micronucleus assay for detecting the clastogenic effect in rat kidney cells. *Mutat Res.* 1997;390:51-57.

[59] Ericsson JL, Seljelid R, Orrenius S. Comparative light and electron microscopic observations of the cytoplasmic matrix in renal carcinomas. *Virchows Arch Pathol Anat Physiol Klin Med.* 1966;341:204-223.

[60] Herman JG, Latif F, Weng Y, et al. Silencing of the VHL tumor-suppressor gene by DNA methylation in renal carcinoma. *Proc Natl Acad Sci USA*. 1994;91:9700-9704.

[61] Herman JG, Graff JR, Myohanen S, et al. Methylation-specific PCR: a novel PCR assay for methylation status of CpG islands. *Proc Natl Acad Sci USA*. 1996;93:9821-9826.

[62] Shiao YH, Ramakrishna G, Anderson LM, et al. Down-regulation of von Hippel-Lindau protein in N-nitroso compound-induced rat non-clear cell renal tumors. *Cancer Lett*. 2002;179:33-38.

[63] Decker HJ, Weidt EJ, Brieger J. The von Hippel-Lindau tumor suppressor gene. A rare and intriguing disease opening new insight into basic mechanisms of carcinogenesis. *Cancer Genet Cytogenet*. 1997;93:74-83.

[64] Kessler PM, Vasavada SP, Rackley RR, et al. Expression of the von Hippel-Lindau tumor suppressor gene, VHL, in human fetal kidney and during mouse embryogenesis. *Mol Med*. 1995;1:457-466.

[65] Los M, Jansen GH, Kaelin WG, et al. Expression pattern of the von Hippel-Lindau protein in human tissues. *Lab Invest*. 1996;75:231-238.

[66] Corless CL, Kibel AS, Iliopoulos O, et al. Immunostaining of the von Hippel-Lindau gene product in normal and neoplastic human tissues. *Hum Pathol*. 1997;28:459-464.

[67] Sakashita N, Takeya M, Kishida T, et al. Expression of von Hippel-Lindau protein in normal and pathological human tissues. *Histochem J*. 1999;31:133-144.

[68] Schoenfeld A, Davidowitz EJ, Burk RD. A second major native von Hippel-Lindau gene product, initiated from an internal translation start site, functions as a tumor suppressor. *Proc Natl Acad Sci USA*. 1998;95:8817-8822.

[69] Iliopoulos O, Ohh M, Kaelin WG, Jr. pVHL19 is a biologically active product of the von Hippel-Lindau gene arising from internal translation initiation. *Proc Natl Acad Sci USA*. 1998;95:11661-11666.

[70] Gao J, Naglich JG, Laidlaw J, et al. Cloning and characterization of a mouse gene with homology to the human von Hippel-Lindau disease tumor suppressor gene: implications for the potential organization of the human von Hippel-Lindau disease gene. *Cancer Res*. 1995;55:743-747.

[71] Blankenship C, Naglich JG, Whaley JM, et al. Alternate choice of initiation codon produces a biologically active product of the von Hippel-Lindau gene with tumor suppressor activity. *Oncogene*. 1999;18:1529-1535.

[72] Chen F, Kishida T, Duh FM, et al. Suppression of growth of renal carcinoma cells by the von Hipppel-Lindau tumor suppressor gene. *Cancer Res*. 1995;55:4804-4807.

[73] Cook T, Gebelein B, Urrutia R. Sp1 and its likes: biochemical and functional predictions for a growing family of zinc finger transcription factors. *Ann NY Acad Sci*. 1999;880:94-102.

[74] Shiao YH, Kamata SI, Li LM, et al. Mutations in the VHL gene from potassium bromate-induced rat clear cell renal tumors. *Cancer Lett*. 2002;187:207-214.

[75] Suen W, Spiro TG, Sowers LC, et al. Identification by UV resonance Raman spectroscopy of an imino tautomer of 5-hydroxy-2'-deoxycytidine, a powerful base analog transition mutagen with a much higher unfavored tautomer frequency than that of the natural residue 2'-deoxycytidine. *Proc Natl Acad Sci USA*. 1999;96:4500-4505.

[76] Umemura T, Takagi A, Sai K, et al. Oxidative DNA damage and cell proliferation in kidneys of male and female rats during 13-weeks exposure to potassium bromate (KBrO3). *Arch Toxicol.* 1998;72:264-269.

[77] Latif F, Tory K, Gnarra J, et al. Identification of the von Hippel-Lindau disease tumor suppressor gene. *Science.* 1993;260;1317-1320.

[78] Neumann HP, Lips CJ, Hsia YE, et al. Von Hippel-Lindau syndrome. *Brain Pathol.* 1995;5:181-193.

[79] Fishman M, Seigne J, Antonia S. Novel therapies for renal cell carcinoma. *Expert Opin Investig Drugs.* 2001;10:1033-1044.

[80] Kanno H, Kondo K, Ito S, et al. Somatic mutations of the von Hippel-Lindau tumor suppressor gene in sporadic central nervous system hemangioblastomas. *Cancer Res.* 1994;54:4845-4847.

[81] Oberstrass J, Reifenberger G, Reifenberger J, et al. Mutation of the von Hippel-Lindau tumour suppressor gene in capillary haemangioblastomas of the central nervous system. *J Pathol.* 1996;179:151-156.

[82] Woodward ER, Buchberger A, Clifford SC, et al. Comparative sequence analysis of the VHL tumor suppressor gene. *Genomics.* 2000;65:253-265.

[83] Adryan B, Decker HJ, Papas TS, et al. Trachael development and the von Hippel-Lindau tumor suppressor homolog in Drosophila. *Oncogene.* 2000;19:2803-2811.

[84] Duan DR, Humphrey JS, Chen DY, et al. Characterization of the VHL tumor suppressor gene product: localization, complex formation, and the effect of natural inactivating mutations. *Proc Natl Acad Sci USA.* 1995;92:6459-6463.

[85] Aldaz CM, Yeung RS, Latif F, et al. Colocalization of the rat homolog of the von Hippel-Lindau (Vhl) gene and the plasma membrane Ca++ transporting ATPase isoform 2 (Atp2b2) gene to rat chromosome bands 4q41.3-42.1. *Cytogenet Cell Genet.* 1995;71:253-256.

[86] Whaley JM, Naglich J. Gelbert L, et al. Germ-line mutations in the von Hippel-Lindau tumor-suppressor gene are similar to somatic von Hippel-Lindau aberrations in sporadic renal cell carcinoma. *Am J Hum Genet.* 1994; 55:1092-1102.

[87] Richards FM, Schofield PN, Fleming S, et al. Expression of the von Hippel-Lindau disease tumour suppressor gene during human embryogenesis. *Hum Mol Genet.* 1996;5:639-644.

[88] Nagashima Y, Miyagi Y, Udagawa K, et al. Von Hippel-Lindau tumour suppresor gene. Localization of expression by in situ hybridization. *J Pathol.* 1996;180:271-274.

[89] Los M, Kerckhaert OA, Zewald R, et al. Mutational analysis of endothelial cells derived from von Hippel-Lindau-related renal cancer. *J Natl Cancer Inst.* 2000;92:1688-1689.

[90] Baba M, Hirai S, Kawakami S, et al. Tumor suppressor protein VHL is induced at high cell density and mediates contact inhibition of cell growth. *Oncogene.* 2001;20:2727-2736.

[91] Gnarra JR, Ward JM, Porter FD, et al. Defective placental vasculogenesis causes embryonic lethality in VHL-deficient mice. *Proc Natl Acad Sci USA.* 1997;94:9102-9107.

[92] Kanno H, Saljooque F, Yamamoto I, et al. Role of the von Hippel-Lindau tumor suppressor protein during neuronal differentiation. *Cancer Res*. 2000;60:2820-2824.

[93] Genbacev O, Krtolica A, Kaelin W, et al. Human cytotrophoblast expression of the von Hippel-Lindau protein is downregulated during uterine invasion in situ and upregulated by hypoxia in vitro. *Dev Biol*. 2001;233:526-536.

[94] Ma W, Tessarollo L, Hong SB, et al. Hepatic vascular tumors, angiectasis in multiple organs, and impaired spermatogenesis in mice with conditional inactivation of the VHL gene. *Cancer Res*. 2003;63:5320-5328.

[95] Galban S, Fan J, Martindale JL, et al. von Hippel-Lindau protein-mediated repression of tumor necrosis factor alpha translation revealed through use of cDNA arrays. *Mol Cell Biol*. 2003;23:2316-2328.

[96] Jaakkola P, Mole DR, Tian YM, et al. Targeting HIF-alpha to the von Hippel-Lindau ubiquitylation complex by O2-regulated prolyl hydroxylation. *Science*. 2001;292:468-472.

[97] Ivan M, Kondo K, Yang H, et al. HIF-alpha targeted for VHL-mediated destruction by proline hydroxylation: implications for O2 sensing. *Science*. 2001;292:464-468.

[98] Masson N, William C, Maxwell PH, et al. Independent function of two destruction domains in hypoxia-inducible factor-alpha chains activated by prolyl hydroxylation. *EMBO J*. 2001;20:5197-5206.

[99] Knowles HJ, Raval RR, Harris AL, et al. Effect of ascorbate on the activity of hypoxia-inducible factor in cancer cells. *Cancer Res*. 2003;63:1764-1768.

[100] Yuan Y, Hilliard G, Ferguson T, et al. Cobalt inhibits the interaction between hypoxia-inducible factor-alpha and von Hippel-Lindau protein by direct binding to hypoxia-inducible factor-alpha. *J Biol Chem*. 2003;278:15911-15916.

[101] Hon WC, Wilson MI, Harlos K, et al. Structural basis for the recognition of hydroxyproline in HIF-1 alpha by pVHL. *Nature*. 2002;417:975-978.

[102] Min JH, Yang H, Ivan M, et al. Structure of an HIF-1 alpha-pVHL complex: hydroxyproline recognition in signaling. *Science*. 2002:296:1886-1889.

[103] Stebbins CE, Kaelin WG, Jr., Pavletich NP. Structure of the VHL-ElonginC-ElonginB complex: implications of VHL tumor suppressor function. *Science*. 1999;284;455-461.

[104] Lisztwan J, Imbert G, Wirbelauer C, et al. The von Hippel-Lindau tumor suppressor protein is a component of an E3 ubiquitin-protein ligase activity. *Genes Dev*. 1999;13:1822-1823.

[105] Iwai K, Yamanaka K, Kamura T, et al. Identification of the von Hippel-Lindau tumor-suppressor protein as part of an active E3 ubiquitin ligase complex. *Proc Natl Acad Sci USA*. 1999;96:12436-12441.

[106] Kamura T, Sato S, Iwai K, et al. Activation of HIF1alpha ubiquitination by a reconstituted von Hippel-Lindau (VHL) tumor suppressor complex. *Proc Natl Acad Sci USA*. 2000;97:10430-10435.

[107] Cockman ME, Masson N, Mole DR, et al. Hypoxia inducible factor-alpha binding and ubiquitylation by the von Hippel-Lindau tumor suppressor protein. *J Biol Chem*. 2000;275:25733-25741.

[108] Tanaka K. Proteasomes: structure and biology. *J Biochem*. 1998;123:195-204.

[109] Maxwell PH, Ratcliffe PJ. Oxygen sensors and angiogenesis. *Semin Cell Dev Biol.* 2002;13:29-37.

[110] Kaelin WG, Jr. Molecular basis of the VHL hereditary cancer syndrome. *Nat Rev Cancer.* 2002;2:673-682.

[111] Krieg M, Marti HH, Plate KH. Coexpression of erythropoietin and vascular endothelial growth factor in nervous system tumors associated with von Hippel-Lindau tumor suppressor gene loss of function. *Blood.* 1998;92:3388-3393.

[112] Brieger J, Weidt EJ, Schirmacher P, et al. Inverse regulation of vascular endothelial growth factor and VHL tumor suppressor gene in sporadic renal cell carcinomas is correlated with vascular growth: an in vivo study on 29 tumors. *J Mol Med.* 1999;77:505-510.

[113] Turner KJ, Moore JW, Jones A, et al. Expression of hypoxia-inducible factors in human renal cancer: relationship to angiogenesis and to the von Hippel-Lindau gene mutation. *Cancer Res.* 2002;62:2957-2961.

[114] Tanimoto K, Makino Y, Pereira T, et al. Mechanism of regulation of the hypoxia-inducible factor-1 alpha by the von Hippel-Lindau tumor suppressor protein. *EMBO J.* 2000;19:4298-4309.

[115] Mahon PC, Hirota K, Semenza GL. FIH-1: a novel protein that interacts with HIF-1alpha and VHL to mediate repression of HIF-1 transcriptional activity. *Genes Dev.* 2001;15:2675-2686.

[116] Hewitson KS, McNeill LA, Riordan MV, et al. Hypoxia-inducible factor (HIF) asparagine hydroxylase is identical to factor inhibiting HIF (FIH) and is related to the cupin structural family. *J Biol Chem.* 2002;277:26351-26355.

[117] Lando D, Peet DJ, Whelan DA, et al. Asparagine hydroxylation of the HIF transactivation domain a hypoxic switch. *Science.* 2002;295:858-861.

[118] Sang N, Fang J, Srinivas V, et al. Carboxyl-terminal transactivation activity of hypoxia-inducible factor 1 alpha is governed by a von Hippel-Lindau protein-independent, hydroxylation-regulated association with p300/CBP. *Mol Cell Biol.* 2002;22:2984-2992.

[119] Freedman SJ, Sun ZY, Poy F, et al. Structural basis for recruitment of CBP/p300 by hypoxia-inducible factor-1 alpha. *Proc Natl Acad Sci USA.* 2002;99:5367-5372.

[120] Pal S, Claffey KP, Dvorak HF, et al. The von Hippel-Lindau gene product inhibits vascular permeability factor/vascular endothelial growth factor expression in renal cell carcinoma by blocking protein kinase C pathways. *J Biol Chem.* 1997;272:27509-27512.

[121] Mukhopadhyay D, Knebelmann B, Cohen HT, et al. The von Hippel-Lindau tumor suppressor gene product interacts with Sp1 to repress vascular endothelial growth factor promoter activity. *Mol Cell Biol.* 1997;17:5629-5639.

[122] Cohen HT, Zhou M, Welsh AM, et al. An important von Hippel-Lindau tumor suppressor domain mediates Sp1-binding and self-association. *Biochem Biophys Res Commun.* 1999;266:43-50.

[123] Pal S, Claffey KP, Cohen HT, et al. Activation of Sp1-mediated vascular permeability factor/vascular endothelial growth factor transcription requires specific interaction with protein kinase C zeta. *J Biol Chem.* 1998;273:26277-26280.

[124] Ananth S, Knebelmann B, Gruning W, et al. Transforming growth factor beta1 is a target for the von Hippel-Lindau tumor suppressor and a critical growth factor for clear cell renal carcinoma. *Cancer Res*. 1999;59:2210-2216.

[125] Pause A, Lee S, Lonergan KM, et al. The von Hippel-Lindau tumor suppressor gene is required for cell cycle exit upon serum withdrawal. *Proc Natl Acad Sci USA*. 1998;95:993-998.

[126] Kim M, Katayose Y, Li Q, et al. Recombinant adenovirus expressing von Hippel-Lindau-mediated cell cycle arrest is associated with the induction of cyclin-dependent kinase inhibitor p27Kip1. *Biochem Biophys Res Commun*. 1998;253:672-677.

[127] Perera AD, Kleymenova EV, Walker CL. Requirement for the von Hippel-Lindau tumor suppressor gene for functional epidermal growth factor receptor blockade by monoclonal antibody C225 in renal cell carcinoma. *Clin Cancer Res*. 2000;6:1518-1523.

[128] Zatyka M, da Silva NF, Clifford SC, et al. Identification of cyclin D1 and other novel targets for the von Hippel-Lindau tumor suppressor gene by expression array analysis and investigation of cyclin D1 genotype as a modifier in von Hippel-Lindau disease. *Cancer Res*. 2002;62:3803-3811.

[129] Bindra RS, Vasselli JR, Stearman R, et al. VHL-mediated hypoxia regulation of cyclin D1 in renal carcinoma cells. *Cancer Res*. 2002;62:3014-3019.

[130] Baba M, Hirai S, Yamada-Okabe H, et al. Loss of von Hippel-Lindau protein causes cell density dependent deregulation of CyclinD1 expression through hypoxia-inducible factor. *Oncogene*. 2003;22:2728-2738.

[131] Galban S, Martindale JL, Mazan-Mamczarz K, et al. Influence of the RNA-binding protein HuR in pVHL-regulated p53 expression in renal carcinoma cells. *Mol Cell Biol*. 2003;23:7083-7095.

[132] Vogelstein B, Lane D, Levine AJ. Surfing the p53 network. *Nature*. 2000;408:307-310.

[133] Rafty LA, Khachigian LM. von Hippel-Lindau tumor suppressor protein represses platelet-derived growth factor B-chain gene expression via the Sp1 binding element in the proximal PDGF-B promoter. *J Cell Biochem*. 2002;85:490-495.

[134] Semenza GL, Artemov D, Bedi A, et al. 'The metabolism of tumours': 70 years later. *Novartis Found Symp*. 2001;240:251-260.

[135] Richard DE, Berra E, Gothie E, et al. p42/p44 mitogen-activated protein kinases phosphorylate hypoxia-inducible factor 1alpha (HIF-1alpha) and enhance the transcriptional activity of HIF-1. *J Biol Chem*. 1999;274:32631-32637.

[136] Richard DE, Berra E, Pouyssegur J. Nonhypoxic pathway mediates the induction of hypoxia-inducible factor 1alpha in vascular smooth muscle cells. *J Biol Chem*. 2000;275:26765-26771.

[137] Datta K, Nambudripad R, Pal S, et al. Inhibition of insulin-like growth factor-I-mediated cell signaling by the von Hippel-Lindau gene product in renal cancer. *J Biol Chem*. 2000;275:20700-20706.

[138] Okuda H, Saitoh K, Hirai S, et al. The von Hippel-Lindau tumor suppressor protein mediates ubiquitination of activated atypical protein kinase C. *J Biol Chem*. 2001;276;43611-43617.

[139] Kondo K, Klco J, Nakamura E, et al. Inhibition of HIF is necessary for tumor suppression by the von Hippel-Lindau protein. *Cancer Cell.* 2002;1:237-246.

[140] Maranchie JK, Vasselli JR, Riss J, et al. The contribution of VHL substrate binding and HIF-1-alpha to the phenotype of VHL loss in renal cell carcinoma. *Cancer Cell.* 2002;1:247-255.

[141] Wykoff CC, Beasley NJ, Watson PH, et al. Hypoxia-inducible expression of tumor-associated carbonic anhydrases. *Cancer Res.* 2000;60:7075-7083.

[142] Ivanov S, Liao SY, Ivanova A, et al. Expression of hypoxia-inducible cell-surface transmembrane carbonic anhydrases in human cancer. *Am J Pathol.* 2001;158:905-919.

[143] Gatenby RA, Gawlinski ET. Mathematical models of tumour invasion mediated by transformation-induced alteration of microenvironmental pH. *Novartis Found Symp.* 2001;240:85-96.

[144] Staller P, Sulitkova J, Lisztwan J, et al. Chemokine receptor CXCR4 downregulated by von Hippel-Lindau tumour suppressor pVHL. *Nature.* 2003;425:307-311.

[145] de Paulsen N, Brychzy A, Fournier MC, et al. Role of transforming growth factor-alpha in von Hippel-Lindau (VHL)(-/-) clear cell renal carcinoma cell proliferation: a possible mechanism coupling VHL tumor suppressor inactivation and tumorigenesis. *Proc Natl Acad Sci USA.* 2001;98:1387-1392.

[146] Gunaratnam L, Morley M, Franovic A, et al. Hypoxia inducible factor activates the transforming growth factor-alpha/epidermal growth factor receptor growth stimulatory pathway in VHL(-/-) renal cell carcinoma cells. *J Biol Chem.* 2003;278:44966-44974.

[147] Zhou MI, Wang H, Ross JJ, et al. The von Hippel-Lindau tumor suppressor stabilizes novel plant homeodomain protein Jade-1. *J Biol Chem.* 2002;277:39887-39898.

[148] Ivanova AV, Ivanov SV, Danilkovitch-Miagkova A, et al. Regulation of STRA13 by the von Hippel-Lindau tumor suppressor protein, hypoxia, and the UBC9/ubiquitin proteasome degradation pathway. *J Biol Chem.* 2001;276:15306-15315.

[149] Koochekpour S, Jeffers M, Wang PH, et al. The von Hippel-Lindau tumor suppressor gene inhibits hepatocyte growth factor/scatter factor-induced invasion and branching morphogenesis in renal carcinoma cells. *Mol Cell Biol.* 1999;19:5902-5912.

[150] Davidowitz EJ, Schoenfeld AR, Burk RD. VHL induces renal cell differentiation and growth arrest through integration of cell-cell and cell-extracellular matrix signaling. *Mol Cell Biol.* 2001;21:865-874.

[151] Shiao YH, Resau JH, Nagashima K, et al. The von Hippel-Lindau tumor suppressor targets to mitochondria. *Cancer Res.* 2000;60:2816-2819.

[152] Warburg O. On the origin of cancer cells. *Science.* 1956;123:309-314.

[153] Warburg O. On respiratory impairment in cancer cells. *Science.* 1956;124:269-270.

[154] Dang CV, Semenza GL. Oncogenic alterations of metabolism. *Trends Biochem Sci.* 1999;24:68-72.

[155] Parone PA, James D, Martinou JC. Mitochondria: regulating the inevitable. *Biochimie.* 2002;84:105-111.

[156] Plas DR, Thompson CB. Cell metabolism in the regulation of programmed cell death. *Trends Endocrinol Metab.* 2002;13:75-78.

[157] Lodish H, Baltimore D, Berk A, et al. Molecular Cell Biology, Ed. 3. New York: Scientific American Books; 1995:745-759.

[158] Thompson CB. Apoptosis in the pathogenesis and treatment of disease. *Science.* 1995;267:1456-1462.

[159] Ohh M, Yauch RL, Lonergan KM, et al. The von Hippel-Lindau tumor suppressor protein is required for proper assembly of an extracellular fibronectin matrix. *Mol Cell.* 1998;1:959-968.

[160] Kleymenova E, Everitt JI, Pluta L, et al. Susceptibility to vascular neoplasms but no increased susceptibility to renal carcinogenesis in VHL knockout mice. *Carcinogenesis.* 2003;25:309-315.

[161] Haase VH, Glickman JN, Socolovsky M, et al. Vascular tumors in livers with targeted inactivation of the von Hippel-Lindau tumor suppressor. *Proc Natl Acad Sci USA.* 2001;98:1583-1588.

[162] Schraml P, Struckmann K, Hatz F, et al. VHL mutations and their correlation with tumour cell proliferation, microvessel density, and patient prognosis in clear cell renal cell carcinoma. *J Pathol.* 2002;196:186-193.

[163] Kondo K, Yao M, Yoshida M, et al. Comprehensive mutational analysis of the VHL gene in sporadic renal cell carcinoma: relationship to clinicopathological parameters. *Genes Chromosomes Cancer.* 2002;34:58-68.

[164] Brauch H, Weirich G, Brieger J, et al. VHL alterations in human clear cell renal cell carcinoma: association with advanced tumor stage and a novel hot spot mutation. *Cancer Res.* 2000;60:1942-1948.

[165] Yao M, Yoshida M, Kishida T, et al. VHL tumor suppressor gene alterations associated with good prognosis in sporadic clear-cell renal carcinoma. *J Natl Cancer Inst.* 2002;94:1569-1575.

[166] Shiao YH, Forsti A, Egevad L, et al. VHL down-regulation and differential localization as mechanisms in tumorigenesis. *Kidney Int.* 2003;64:1671-1674.

[167] Schraml P, Hergovich A, Hatz F, et al. Relevance of nuclear and cytoplasmic von Hippel-Lindau protein expression for renal carcinoma progression. *Am J Pathol.* 2003;163:1013-1020.

In: Trends in Kidney Cancer Research
Editor: Kelvin R. Nunez, pp. 77-88

ISBN 1-59454-141-8

Chapter VI

UPPER URINARY TRACT CARCINOMA AFTER INTAKE OF *ARISTOLOCHIA FANGCHI*: VALUE OF URINARY CYTOLOGY IN END-STAGE "CHINESE-HERB NEPHROPATHY"

J.L. Nortier,* A. Zlotta, M. Petein, M. Depierreux, M.C. Muniz-Martinez and J.L. Vanherweghem
Erasme Hospital, Université Libre de Bruxelles, B-1070 Brussels, Belgium

ABSTRACT

Chinese-herb nephropathy (CHN) is a progressive interstitial fibrosis associated with the use of *Aristolochia* species, a Chinese herb regularly replacing *Stephania tetrandra, Akebia, Asarum, Clematis* and *Cocculus* species in herbal remedies and containing nephrotoxic and carcinogenic aristolochic acids (AA). Moderate to end-stage renal disease (ESRD) may develop, requiring renal replacement therapy by dialysis or transplantation. Experimental models reproducing the clinical entity are available in rabbits and rats.

Aristolochic acids are powerful carcinogens in animal experiments. Removal of the native kidneys and ureters in CHN patients with ESRD has confirmed a high prevalence of upper urinary tract carcinoma (46 %). Tissue samples contained AA-related DNA adducts, which are not only specific markers of prior exposure to AA but are also involved in the tumorigenesis.

We took the opportunity of planned nephroureterectomies in our 41 end-stage CHN patients treated by dialysis (N=10) or renal transplantation (N=31) to assess the diagnostic value of urinary cytologic tests prior to surgery. Fresh voided urine samples

* Corresponding author: J.L. Nortier, MD, PhD, Dept of Nephrology, Erasme Hospital, 808, route de Lennik, B-1070 Brussels, Belgium. jnortier@ulb.ac.be

were available in 37 cases (4 hemodialysed patients were anuric). Cystoscopy with bilateral ureteral brushings and random bladder biopsies (if no bladder lesions were visible) were performed. Cytologic data were compared to histologic findings in the surgical specimens. All preoperative bladder biopsies were normal, except in 5 patients with mild-to-moderate dysplasia and one with superficial pTa bladder cancer. Neoplastic lesions were almost equally distributed between the renal pelvis and ureters. Of the 37 voided urine samples, 3 only showed atypia in relation with upper urinary tract carcinoma, whereas 18 patients had cancer diagnosed histologically. By contrast, bilateral ureteral brushings enabled to detect 14 out of 26 malignant lesions (in those 18 patients) by cytologic examinations. According to these results, specificity of cytologic analyses on voided urine and brushing samples were 100% and 96%, respectively and sensitivity 17% and 54%, respectively. In this specific population where the urinary output from native kidneys was impaired by terminal renal failure, the sensitivity of cytologic analysis of voided urine was much less helpful as compared to what could be expected in the general population.

In summary, exposure to *Aristolochia* species is associated with the development of renal interstitial fibrosis (CHN) and urothelial cancer in humans. Cystoscopy with ureteral brushings should be considered as a first-line screening procedure in patients with renal failure at risk of developing upper urinary tract carcinoma.

Key words: Aristolochia species; Aristolochic acids; Herbal remedies; Renal fibrosis; Urothelial carcinoma

INTRODUCTION

In 1993, cases of renal failure rapidly progressing to end-stage renal disease (ESRD) were reported in Belgium in relation with daily intake of slimming pills including root extracts of Chinese herbs (*Stephania Tetrandra* and *Magnolia officinalis*) [1]. Very soon, the inadvertent replacement of *Stephania Tetrandra* by *Aristolochia Fangchi* was suspected, as in traditional Chinese medicine, *Stephania Tetrandra* (Pin Yin name: Han fang ji) and *Aristolochia Fangchi* (Pin Yin name: Guang fan ji) are classified within the same therapeutic "Fang-chi" family. This initial hypothesis was confirmed in 1994 by phytochemical analyses of the so-called *Stephania* batches which actually detected the presence of aristolochic acids (AA), the main compounds of *Aristolochia* species [2]. Moreover, renal tissue samples from patients exposed to the so-called *Stephania Tetrandra* contained specific AA-DNA adducts [3,4]. This new renal disease called "Chinese-herb nephropathy" (CHN) or even "Aristolochic acid nephropathy" has been experimentally reproduced by AA administration to rabbits (intraperitoneal injections during 17 months) [5] and to rats (subcutaneous injections during 35 days) [6].

From a clinical point of view, CHN is characterized by a paucisymptomatic chronic renal failure without proteinuria or alteration of the urinary sediment [7,8]. Some cases presented with a Fanconi syndrome [reviewed in 9 and 10]. Histologically, an extensive interstitial fibrosis is observed in the superficial cortex, mainly composed of proximal tubules, progressing towards the deep cortex [11]. This destructive process led to a severe atrophy of the proximal tubular population, remaining intact the glomeruli at least in the beginning of the disease. The measurement of urinary levels of neutral endopeptidase- an ectoenzyme of the proximal tubule brush border- and microproteins- such as Clara cell protein- in CHN patients with different degrees of renal failure, confirmed the progressive structural and functional impairment of this part of the nephron, further correlated with the severity of the disease [12].

UROTHELIAL CARCINOMA IN CHINESE-HERB NEPHROPATHY

Moderate atypia and atypical hyperplasia of the urothelium were first described in 4 pieces of nephroureterectomies performed in 3 CHN patients prior or at time of transplantation [13]. Three cases of urinary tract cancer were further reported: in the first one, bladder involvement (papillary tumors) was described in a renal transplanted patient for CHN [14]; the second case presented with hematuria secondary to a papillary transitional cell carcinoma of the right pelvis [15]; the third case developed a hydronephrosis of her left native kidney after a successful transplantation for terminal CHN diagnosed in UK. The piece of nephroureterectomy showed a multifocal transitional cell carcinoma of the ureter [16]. Therefore, at the end of 1997, we informed our CHN patients in ESRD treated by dialysis or transplantation about the risk of developing urothelial carcinoma and suggested the prophylactic removal of their native kidneys and ureters. Among 39 patients who agreed to undergo surgery, a dramatically high prevalence of upper urinary tract cancer (46%) was reported: 17 cases of carcinoma of the ureter, renal pelvis, or both and 1 papillary bladder tumor [4]. Cosyns et al had also reported a prevalence of 40% (4 positive cases out of 10 patients) [17]. Nineteen of our remaining patients had mild-to-moderate urothelial dysplasia, and two had normal urothelium. All tissue samples analysed contained AA-related DNA adducts. No statistically significant differences were observed in the mean levels of the major DNA adduct, 7-(deoxyadenosine-N^6-yl)-aristolactam I DNA adduct, in renal tissue samples between patients in whom urothelial carcinoma had developed and those in whom it had not developed. The cumulative dose of *Stephania* (in fact, *Aristolochia*) was a significant risk factor for urothelial carcinoma, with total doses of more than 200 grams associated with a higher risk of urothelial carcinoma. Finally, only 4 of the 25 tissue samples analyzed for ochratoxin A-related DNA adducts were weakly positive - in fact, close to the background level of the assay-, indicating that ochratoxin A did not have a key role in CHN [4].

Urothelial cancer seemed to be a late complication of CHN since all the cases had been detected in ESRD patients. However, we reported a case presented with cervical adenopathy secondary to metastatic carcinoma of the left pelvic cavity, in a woman after intake of Chinese herbal medicine containing AA but with only mild renal failure, suggesting a possible dissociation between carcinogenicity and nephrotoxicity [18].

Pathomorphological Changes

In case of invasive urothelial carcinoma, solid neoplastic tissue may be seen in the pelvis and/or within the ureteral wall, as typically seen on Figure 1.

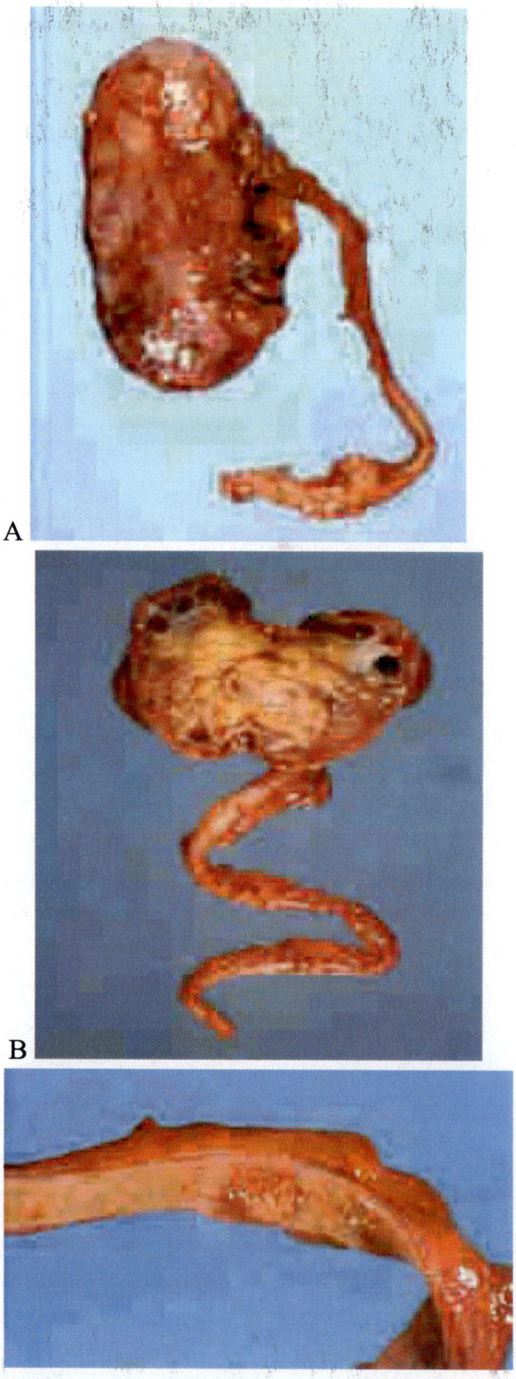

A

B

C

Figure 1. Macroscopic appearance of an invasive urothelial carcinoma (T2) involving the lower third of the right ureter in a patient with end-stage Chinese-herb nephropathy (CHN) (A); severe cortical atrophy of the kidney typically seen in end-stage CHN patients (B); section of the left ureter from another end-stage CHN patient showing a thickened wall of tumoral origin (T1 grade III) (C).

Surgical samples from nephroureterectomies were very informative to the pathologist. Serial samples were taken, including lower extremity and intermediate part of each ureter, renal pelvis and kidney. Specimens were fixed in formalin, dehydrated and embedded in paraffin. Sections were stained with hematoxylin-eosin, periodic acid-Shiff and Masson's trichrome. The urothelial epithelium was classified as normal, dysplastic, or neoplastic [19]. The stage of the tumors was defined according to the tumor-node-metastasis classification [20]. We used the histologic grading system of the World Health Organization for invasive urothelial carcinoma, which has three histologic grades: mild, moderate, and severe dysplasia [21]. Severe dysplasia was considered to indicate carcinoma in situ [22,23].

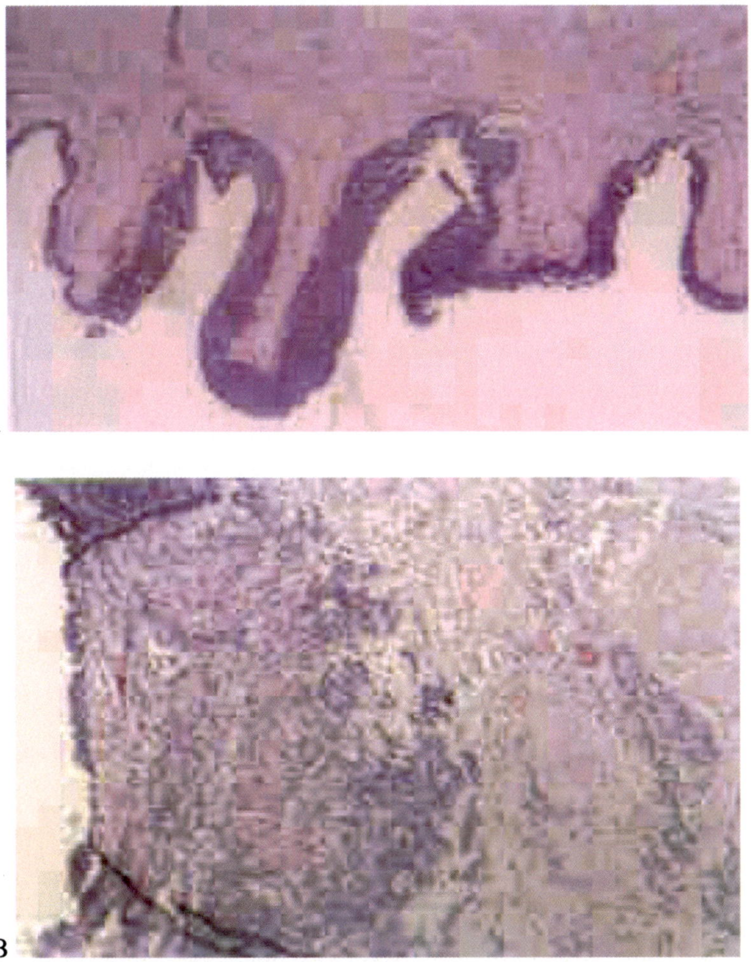

A

B

Figure 2. Urothelial carcinoma of the pelvic cavities from an end-stage CHN patient with different co-existing stages: in situ carcinoma of the left pelvis (A) and invasive tumor of the right pelvis with lymphatic permeation by neoplastic cells (B). *H & E* staining, orig. magnif. X 200.

As described earlier, multifocal urothelial lesions ranging from moderate dysplasia to in situ or even invasive carcinoma were located in the upper urinary tract and almost equally distributed between the renal pelvis and ureters [4]. Histologic findings were then classified according to the highest stage and grade identified. Indeed, as illustrated on Figure 2, multiple tumors of the renal pelvis and ureters usually co-existed in the upper urinary tract of the same patient. All preoperative bladder biopsies were normal, except in 5 patients with mild-to-moderate dysplasia and one with superficial pTa bladder cancer.

Screening Procedures of Upper Urinary Tract Carcinoma

We took the opportunity of planned surgical removal of native kidneys and ureters in 41 CHN patients treated by dialysis (N=10) or renal transplantation (N=31) to assess the diagnostic value of urinary cytologic tests prior to surgery.

Fresh voided urine samples were available in 37 cases (since 4 hemodialysed patients were anuric). After informed consent, cystoscopy with bilateral ureteral brushings and random bladder biopsies (if no bladder lesions were visible) were performed prior to surgery. No technical complications consecutive to these endourological procedures were observed. Fresh voided urine samples as well as samples obtained from washing and brushing of right and left urinary tract, were collected on Carbowax and microscopically studied after classical Papanicolaou staining.

Cytologic data compared to histologic findings in the surgical specimens are summarized in Table 1. Of the 37 voided urine samples, 3 only showed atypia in relation with upper urinary tract carcinoma, whereas 18 patients had cancer diagnosed histologically. A positive finding in such a urinary cytologic study was thus highly predictive only of the presence of an invasive neoplasm of the upper urinary tract. Cellular abnormalities detected in these situations were characterized by giant multinucleated cells and/or nucleolar atypias (Figure 3). By contrast, bilateral ureteral brushings enabled to detect 14 out of 26 malignant lesions (in those 18 patients) by cytologic examinations. According to these results, specificity of cytologic analyses on voided urine and brushing samples were 100% and 96%, respectively and sensitivity 17% and 54%, respectively.

Table 1. Histologic Findings and Cytologic Studies prior Surgical Removal of Native Kidney and Ureter from 41 Patients with End-Stage Chinese-Herb Nephropathy

Histologic Findings* (N=41)	Cytology of Voided Urine (N=37)	Cytology of Brushing Samples (N=41)
Normal urothelium (N=2)	Normal (2)	Normal (2)
Mild-to-moderate Dysplasia (N=21)	Normal (16)	Normal (18)
	Atypia (1)	Atypia (3)
pTa / pTis (N=15)	Normal (15)	Normal (8)
		Atypia (5)
		Malignant (2)
≥T1 (N=3)	Atypia (3)	Atypia (1)
		Malignant (2)

* Histologic findings were classified according to the highest stage and grade identified; the stage of the tumors was defined according to the tumor-node-metastasis classification; pTa denotes nononvasive papillary carcinoma, and pTis noninvasive (flat) carcinoma in situ.

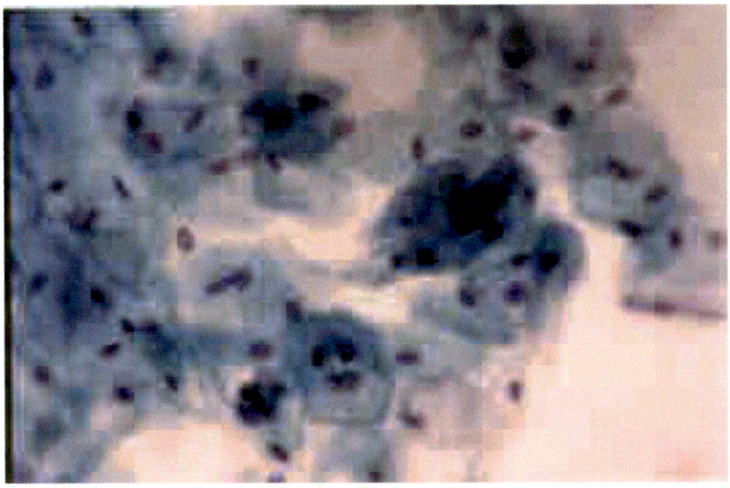

Figure 3. Representative cytological abnormalities found in a sample from ureteral washing and brushing of the right upper urinary tract of an end-stage CHN patient (same case as depicted in Figure 2): increased cellular size, giant nucleoli and multinuclear cells are typical signs of malignancy. *Papanicolaou staining*.

Carcinogenicity of Aristolochia sp

Aristolochic acids, the main compounds of *Aristolochia* sp, are nitrophenanthrene derivatives known for their potent carcinogenic action in rodents [24] as well as for their mutagenic properties in bacterial [25] and mammalian models [26]. Aristolactams, activated metabolites formed by AA nitroreduction, are able to form DNA adducts through covalent binding sites with adenosine and guanosine. The formation of these adducts was studied in vitro: cytochrome P4501A1 and 1A2 [27] as well as prostaglandin H synthetase [28] were shown to be involved in the metabolic activation of AA. These observations could explain inter-individual variations in the susceptibility to AA toxicity and also the preferential localization in the kidney and urinary tract. Carcinogenicity of AA DNA adducts has also been related to the mutation in the codon 61 of the protooncogen Has-ras [29] as well as in a mutation of p53 [17]. Specific AA-DNA adducts are then not only recognized as markers of prior exposure to AA, but also involved in the tumorigenesis process as recently detailed in a comprehensive pathophysiological review by molecular toxicologists [30]. It shoud be added that in our experimental model of AA induced renal fibrosis, urothelial dysplasia as well as carcinoma of the pelvic cavities were observed during the 35-day protocol [6]. Moreover, several rats developed malignant fibrohistiocytic sarcoma of the skin at the sites of AA injections two months after the end of injections (upper back) [6].

Regarding these experimental data and additional clinical observations in humans, herbal remedies containing plant species of the genus *Aristolochia* were evaluated by the International Agency for Research on Cancer (IARC) and considered as carcinogenic to humans with the first evidence level [31].

DISCUSSION

Urologic neoplasms are frequent in uremic patients and greatly contribute to the reported increased incidence of cancer in patients on maintenance dialysis (standardized incidence ratio for kidney and bladder cancers of 3.6 and 1.5, respectively [32]). In addition to the uremic environment, carcinogenic factors such as analgesic abuse, ochratoxin A (mycotoxin possibly involved in the etiology of Balkan endemic nephropathy [33]) and now aristolochic acids are recognized as strong promoting factors of urologic malignancy development.

At the time of the present study, we hypothesized that our specific CHN population was running at least a similar risk to patients with end-stage analgesic nephropathy. We then attempted to design screening procedures on the basis of existing recommendations for this patient group. Consensus was found in the literature about combined radiological imaging and cystoscopy with retrograde ureteric catheterisation [34,35]. However, ultrasonography and CT scanning were rapidly found ineffective in our end-stage CHN patients, considering the extreme atrophy of the native kidneys due to the extensive fibrotic process and the insufficiency of contrast-medium excretion in these terminal kidneys. Magnetic resonance imaging also proved to be disappointing in this matter (personal data). By contrast, well-documented studies from Germany and Australia discussed the efficacy of regular endourological procedures before and after renal transplantation of patients with end-stage analgesic nephropathy. Annual cystoscopy and ureteral washings and brushings were advocated by the ones [35], while prophylactic nephroureterectomy was considered as an alternative solution before transplantation by the others [36]. In the present case of our end-stage CHN patients, the sensitivity of cytologic analysis of voided urine proved to be much less helpful as compared to what could be expected in the general population (66 and 79% in two large series) [37]. This could be explained by the fact that voided urine mainly originated from the kidney transplant and not from the native kidneys and ureters. As a consequence, invasive cytological studies of material from ureteral brushings gave better results then voided urine examinations.

CONCLUSIONS

Chronic exposure to *Aristolochia* toxins (AA but also possibly other derivatives) is associated with the development of renal interstitial fibrosis (CHN) and upper urinary tract carcinoma. Cases of CHN have been reported in France, Spain, Japan, United Kingdom and Taiwan [9,10,30]. Health professionals should be aware that in traditional herbal medicine, traditional Chinese medicine, Japanese kampo and Ayurvedic medicine, *Aristolochia* sp are still in use and regularly replace *Stephania tetrandra*, *Akebia*, *Asarum*, *Clematis* sp and *Cocculus* sp in herbal remedies. Despite strong warnings from the Food and Drug Administration (FDA) in 2001 [38] and the classification of *Aristolochia* sp containing products as human carcinogens in 2002 by IARC [31], a lot of products containing AA or suspected to contain AA are currently sold on US Web sites, as recently reported [39]. These observations support the evidence that extracts of herbal preparations often considered without any risk by the public should be submitted to quality controls as strict as for any conventional drug [40]. Faced with a renal disease or a urothelial carcinoma of "unknown origin", nephrologists and urologists should extend their anamnestic inquiry to the most frequent use of "non western" medicine. More accurate diagnostic tests are urgently needed to improve the early detection of upper urinary tract cancer. From our point of view, cystoscopy with ureteral brushings should be considered as a first-line screening procedure in patients with renal failure at risk of developing urinary tract carcinoma.

REFERENCES

[1] Vanherweghem J.L., Depierreux M., Tielemans C., et al. Rapidly progressive interstitial renal fibrosis in young women: Association with slimming regimen including Chinese herbs. *Lancet* 341: 387-391, 1993.

[2] Vanhaelen M., Vanhaelen-FASTRE R., But P., Vanherweghem J.L. Identification of aristolochic acid in Chinese herbs. *Lancet* 343: 174, 1994.

[3] Schmeiser H.H., Bieler C.., Wiessler M., van Ypersele de Strihou C., Cosyns JP. Detection of DNA adducts formed by aristolochic acid in renal tissue from patients with Chinese herbs nephropathy. *Cancer Res* 56: 2025-2028, 1996.

[4] Nortier J.L., Muniz Martinez M-C., Schmeiser H.H., et al. Urothelial carcinoma associated with the use of a Chinese herb (*Aristolochia Fangchi*). *N Engl J Med* 342: 1686-92, 2000.

[5] Cosyns J-P., Dehoux JP., Guiot Y., et al. Chronic aristolochic acid toxicity in rabbits: a model of Chinese herb nephropathy? *Kidney Int* 59: 2164-73, 2001.

[6] Debelle F., Nortier J., Deprez E., et al. Aristolochic acids induce chronic renal failure with interstitial fibrosis in salt depleted rats. *J Am Soc Nephrol* 13: 431-6, 2002.

[7] Reginster F., Jadoul M., van Ypersele de Strihou C. Chinese herb nephropatrhy: presentation, natural history and fate after transplantation. *Nephrol Dial Transplant 12*: 81-86, 1997.

[8] Muniz Martinez M-C., Nortier J., Vereerstraeten P., Vanherweghem J-L. Progression rate of Chinese herb nephropathy: impact of Aristolochia fangchi ingested dose. *Nephrol Dial Transplant 17:* 408-412, 2002.

[9] Vanherweghem JL. Urémie chronique et cancer des voies urinaires secondaires à la prise d'extraits végétaux utilisés en phytothérapie chinoise. *Médecine/Sciences* 18: 1095-1101, 2002.

[10] Vanherweghem JL., Debelle F., Muniz Martinez MC., Nortier J. Aristolochic acid nephropathy after Chinese herbal remedies. *In* De Broe ME., Porter GA., Bennett WM. and Verpooten GA. (eds). *Clinical nephrotoxins*, 2nd edition: 579-586, 2003.

[11] Depierreux M., VAN Damme B., Vanden Houte K., Vanheweghem JL. Pathologic aspects of a newly described nephropathy related to the prolonged use of Chinese herbs. *Am J Kidney Dis* 24: 172-80, 1994.

[12] Nortier J., Deschodt-Lanckman MM., Simon S., et al. Proximal tubular injury in Chinese herbs nephropathy: monitoring by neutral endopeptidase enzymuria. *Kidney Int* 51: 288-293, 1997.

[13] Cosyns JP., Jadoul M., Squifflet JP., DE Plaen JF., Ferluga D., van Ypersele de Strihou C. Chinese herbs nephropathy: A clue to Balkan endemic nephropathy? *Kidney Int* 45: 1680-1688, 1994.

[14] Cosyns JP., Jadoul M., Squifflet JP; van Cangh PJ., van Ypersele de Strihou C. Urothelial malignancy in nephropathy due to Chinese herbs. *Lancet* 344: 188, 1994 (letter).

[15] 15. Vanherweghem JL., Tielemans C., Simon J., Depierreux M. Chinese herbs nephropathy and renal pelvic carcinoma. *Nephrol Dial Transplant* 10: 270-273, 1995.

[16] 16. Lord GM., Cook T., Arlt VM., Schmeiser HH., Williams G., Pusey CD. Urothelial malignant disease and Chinese herbal nephropathy. *Lancet* 358: 1515-1516, 2001.

[17] Cosyns JP., Jadoul M., Squifflet JP., Wese F-X., van Ypersele de Strihou C. Urothelial lesions in Chinese-herb nephropathy. *Am J Kidney Dis* 33: 1011-1017, 1999.

[18] Nortier JL, Schmeiser HH, Muniz Martinez MC, et al. Invasive urothelial carcinoma after exposure to Chinese herbal medicine containing aristolochic acid may occur without severe renal failure. *Nephrol Dial Transplant* 18: 426-428, 2003.

[19] Cabanne F., Pages A., Billerey C., Oppermann A., Carbillet JP (Eds). *Pathologie génitale masculine: uropathologie.* Masson, Paris 1992, pp.354-355.

[20] Sobin LH., Wittekind C., (Eds). *TNM classification of malignant tumors*, fifth ed..

[21] Wiley-Liss, New York 1997. US Food and Drug Administration Center for Food Safety and Applied Nutrition. Office of Nutritional Products, Labeling, and Dietary Supplements. Revised version May 30, 2000.

[22] Bostwick DG., Eble JN. (Eds). *Urologic Surgical Pathology*. Mossby-Year Book, St Louis 1997, pp 246-247.

[23] Murphy WM., Soloway MS. Urothelial dysplasia. *J Urol* 127: 849-854, 1982.

[24] Richards B., Parmar MKB., Anderson CK., et al. Interpretation of biopsies of « normal » urothelium in patients with superficial bladder cancer. *Br J Urol* 67: 369-375, 1991.

[25] Mengs U., Lang W., Poch J-A. The carcinogenic action of aristolochic acid in rats. *Arch Toxicol* 51: 107-119, 1982.

[26] Schmeiser HH., Pool B.L., Wiessler M. Identification and mutagenicity of metabolites of aristolochic acid formed by rat liver. *Carcinogenesis* 7: 59-63, 1986.

[27] Pezzuto JM., Swanson SM., Mar W., et al. Evaluation of the mutagenic and cytostatic potenital of aristolochic acid (3,4-methylene-dioxy-8-methoxy-10-nitrophenanthrene-1-carboxylic acid) and several of its derivatives. *Mut Res* 206: 447-454, 1988.

[28] Stiborova M., Frei E., Wiessler M., Schmeiser HH. Human enzymes involved in the metabolic activation of carcinogenic aristolochic acids: evidence for reductive activation by cytochrome P450 1A1 and 1A2. *Chem Res Toxicol* 14: 1128-1137, 2001.

[29] Stiborova M., Frei E., Breuer A., Wiessler M., Schmeiser HH. Evidence for reductive activation of carcinogenic aristolochic acids by prostaglandin H synthase – (32)P-labeling analysis of DNA adduct formation. *Mut Res* 493: 149-160, 2001.

[30] Schmeiser H.H., Scherf H.R., Wiessler M. Activating mutations at codon 61 of the c-Ha-ras gene in thin-tissue sections of tumors induced by aristolochic acid in rats and mice. *Cancer Lett* 59: 139-143, 1991.

[31] Arlt VM., Stiborova M., Schmeiser HH. Aristolochic acid as a probable human hazard in herbal remedies: a review. *Mutagenesis* 17: 265-277, 2002.

[32] *International Agency for Research on Cancer* (IARC). Some traditional herbal medicines, some mycotoxins, nephtalene and styrene. In *IARC Monographs on the Evaluation of Carcinogenic Risks of Chemical to Humans.* Volume 82. IARC, Lyon, France; 2002.

[33] Stewart JH., Buccianti G., Agodoa L., Gellert R., MC Credie MRE., Lowenfels AB., et al. Cancers of the kidney and urinary tract in patients on dialysis for end-stage renal disease: analysis of data from the United states, Europe, and Australia and New Zealand. *J Am Soc Nephrol* 14: 197-207, 2003.

[34] Djukanovic L. and Rodovanovic Z. Balkan endemic nephropathy. *In* De Broe ME., Porter GA., Bennett WM. and Verpooten GA. (eds). *Clinical nephrotoxins*, 2nd edition: 587-601, 2003.

[35] Chen K-S., Lai M-K., Huang C-C., Chu S-H., Leu M-L. Urologic cancers in uremic patients. *Am J Kidney Dis* 25: 694-700, 1995.

[36] Swindle P., Falk M., Rigby R., et al. Transitional cell carcinoma in renal transplant recipients: the influence of compound analgesics. *Br J Urol* 81: 229-233, 1998.

[37] Thon WF, Kliem V., Truss MC, et al. Denovo urothelial carcinoma of the upper and lower urinary tract in kidney – transplant patients with end-stage analgesic nephropathy. *World J Urol* 13: 254-261, 1995.

[38] Cohen RA, Brown RS. Microscopic hematuria. *N Engl J Med* 348: 2330-2338, 2003.

[39] *Food and Drug Administration.* Dietary supplements: aristolochic acid. (accessed September 25, 2003, at http://www.cfsan.fda.gov/~dms/ds-bot.html).

[40] Gold L.S., Slone T.H. Aristolochic aid, an herbal carcinogen, sold on the Web after FDA alert. *N Engl J Med* 349:1576-1577, 2003.

[41] Vanherweghem J.L. Nephropathy and herbal medicine. *Am J Kidney Dis* 35: 330-332, 2000.

In: Trends in Kidney Cancer Research
Editor: Kelvin R. Nunez, pp. 89-102

ISBN 1-59454-141-8

Chapter VII

Nephrectomy and Resection of the Liver with the Inferior Vena Cava for Recurrences of Adrenal Cortical Carcinoma over Ten Years after the Adrenalectomy: Report of a 14-year-survived Case with Good Quality of Life

Koho Akimaru**, *Takashi Tajiri*,
Kazuo Shimizu and Kiichiroh Uchiyama*
Department of Surgery, Nippn Medical School, Tokyo
Ebina General Hospital*, Kanagawa

Abstract

Background: Aggressive resection of the vena cava infiltrated by malignancy may yield good results.
Case: A 61-year-old Japanese man who underwent right adrenalectomy for non-hormonal cortical adenoma with indeterminate malignant potential at the age of 51, then right nephrectomy for recurrent and invasive growth of the initial tumor diagnosed as adrenal cortical carcinoma at the age of 56, was admitted to our hospital for another recurrence in August, 1998. He tolerated resections of the liver and inferior vena cava for the invasiveness. He had been alive and well for 4 years since the last surgery, but eventually died of metastases to the spine, hepatic hilum and lung in August 2003.

* Corresponding author: Koho Akimaru, M.D., Professor of Surgery, Transplantation Surgery, Nippon Medical School Hospital, 1-1-5 Sendagi, Bunkyo-ku, Tokyo, JAPAN 〒113-8603; Fax: +81-3-5685-0989; E-mail: akimaru@nms.ac.jp

Besides the surgeries, no any other chemotherapy or radiation therapy as an adjuvant or main strategy was given throughout the entire disease course.
Conclusion: Since this patient with adrenal cortical carcinoma survived the curative resections for 14 years, aggressive surgery can yield a good quality of life and long survival for a patient who had resections of slow-growing malignancy and subsequent recurrences.

Key words: adrenal cortical carcinoma, adrenalectomy, local neoplasm recurrence, nephrectomy. hepatectomy, recontructive surgical procedures, inferior vena cava, blood vessel prosthesis implantation.

Introduction

In the selected patient in whom the inferior vena cava (IVC) had been infiltrated by a primary or metastatic liver tumor, renal cell carcinoma, or adrenal carcinoma, an aggressive excision of the vena cava or caval tumor thrombus with the primary lesion yielded good results (1~4). We have treated a man with adrenal cortical carcinoma (ACC), who had right adrenalectomy for adenoma first, then right nephrectomy for its local recurrence, and subsequent hepatectomy with resection of the vena cava for local and metastatic lesions during the 10 years after the first surgery (5). They were all successful, and enabled the patient to survive more than 14 years with a fair quality of life. A Discrepancy between the histology of the primary adrenal tumor and the histological diagnoses of the subsequent surgical specimens for the recurrences, and aggressive surgery for the invaded vena cava in terms of patient's benefit will be discussed.

Case Report

(1). A 61 year-old Japanese male patient, complaining of distress in the upper abdomen and weight loss of 4 kg over several months before presentation, was admitted to the Nippon Medical School Hospital, Tokyo in August 1998 for diagnosis and treatment. His family and past histories were unremarkable except for an appendectomy at the age of 20, and pulmonary tuberculosis treated with medication at the age of 30. His present illness began with a right adrenalectomy for non-hormonal cortical adenoma at the age of 51 in October 1989. That was a huge round mass measuring 15×13×8 cm, with the findings of non-invasivness, mitotic rate 4/50 HPF, and no remarkable cellular or nuclear atypia. The Weiss score (6) was 2. The tumor was retrospectively thought to be one of indeterminate malignant potential (7). At the age of 56, he underwent right nephrectomy for local recurrence of the tumor with invasiveness and atypia with mitotic rate 4/50 HPF. Since then he had been well until several months prior to this admission.

(2). Physical examinations upon admission showed him to be an emaciated but not lethargic medium-sized man, 169 cm tall and 52 kg in weight. He had no fever or jaundice but anemic palpebral conjunctiva and decreased skin turgor. The abdomen was concave with

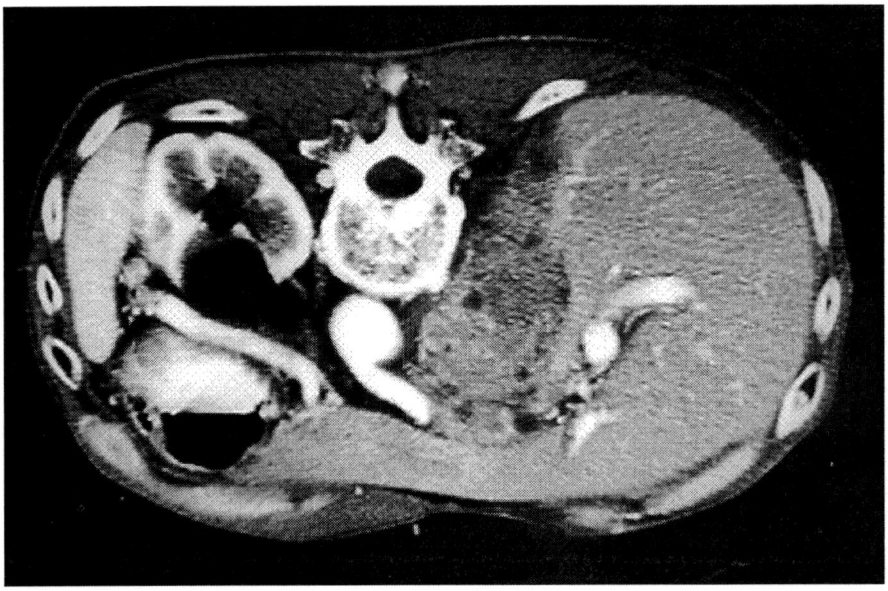

Figure 1. Enhanced computerized tomogram of the abdomen disclosed the main tumor in the hepatic hilum and posterior segment of the liver. It is oppressing the common hepatic artery, left lateral segment, and hepatic hilum forward, and invading the caudate lobe and right posterior segment, mainly subsegment 7. By the tumor encased is the retro-hepatic portion of the inferior vena cava. Enhancement and density varied throughout the tumor with some necrosis. Reprinted from Akimaru K, et al. Resection of the liver, inferior vena cava, and right kidney for recurrences over 10 years after right adrenalectomy for carcinoma. *Eur J Surg 2002; 168*: 130-133 (with permission).

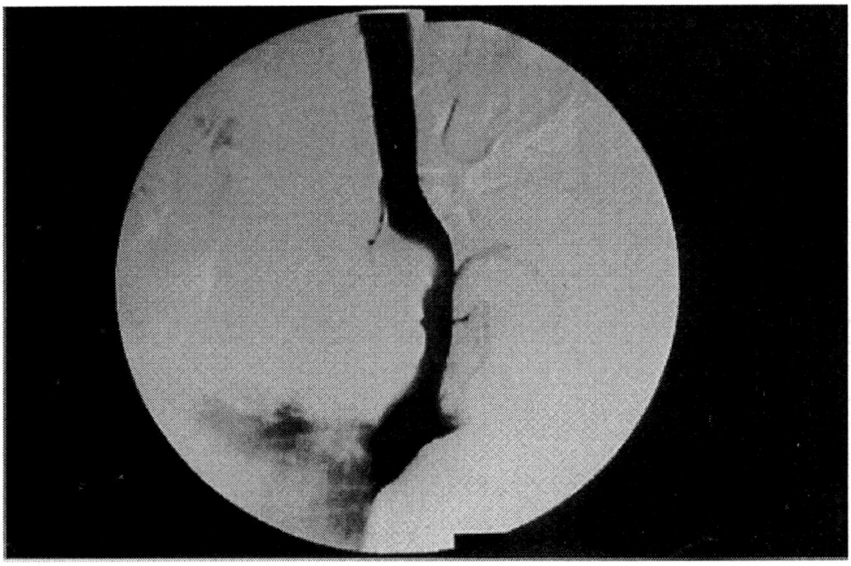

Figure 2. Preoperative venogram of the inferior vena cava showed a deviated and tortuous retro-hepatic portion with invasiveness by the tumor. Confluence of the cava with the right hepatic vein is preserved. As the patient was asymptomatic for the narrow IVC, no fluid collection, disturbed renal function or edema was noted in anywhere. Reprinted from Akimaru K, et al. Resection of the liver, inferior vena cava, and right kidney for recurrences over 10 years after right adrenalectomy for carcinoma. *Eur J Surg 2002; 168*: 130-133 (with permission).

surgical scars, and a fist-sized mass was indirectly palpable almost in the epigastrium. Laboratory data showed mild anemia, malnutrition, and increased lactate dehydrogenase and alkaline phosphatase, but no biochemical evidence of excess steroid production. A computerized tomogram (CT) of the abdomen disclosed a large tumor in the right posterior aspect of the IVC encasing the retrohepatic portion, oppressing the liver anteriorly, and invading the caudate lobe and posterior segment (Figure 1). There were also three metastases within the left lateral segment. In addition, a venogram of the cava (Figure 2) showed that its retrohepatic portion was narrowed by the involvement of the main tumor but it did not seem to extend to the aspect confluencing with the right hepatic vein. The patient was asymptomatic for the narrowed IVC, and had no fluid collection, disturbed function in hemi-renal status, or edema noted anywhere. Magnetic resonance image (MRI) of the upper abdomen (Figure 3) showed that the heterogeneously imaged tumor was oppressing the hilum of the liver forward, but preserving the right hepatic vein influx. These tumors were considered to be recurrences of the relatively slow growing ACC. No metastases were noted elsewhere. He underwent total removal of the tumors on September 16th 1998 (Figure 4).

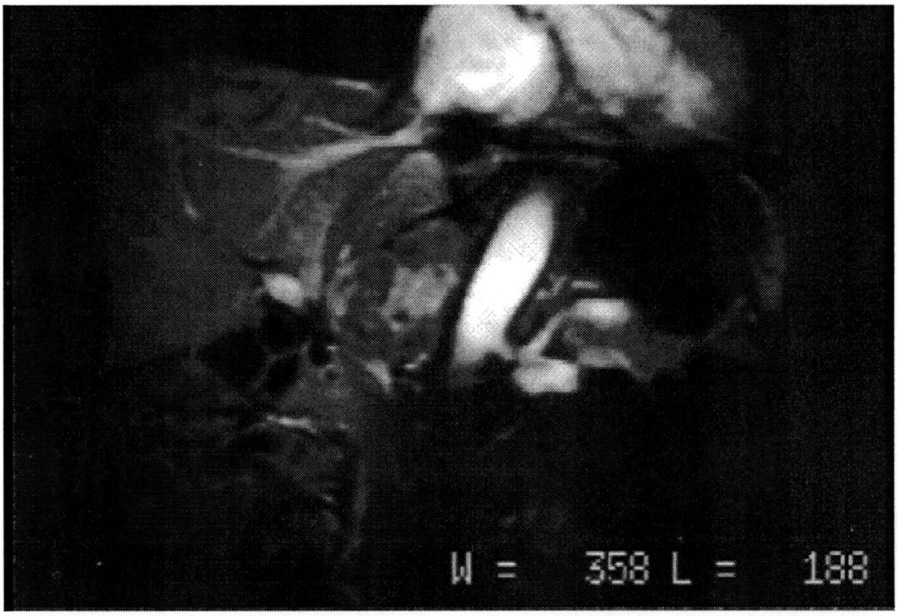

Figure 3. Frontal plane in magnetic resonance image of the upper abdomen revealed the heterogeneously enhanced tumor right to the aorta, which was encasing the cava, and oppressing the hilus hepatis anteriorly. The abdominal aorta, a part of the portal trunk, and the well preserved right hepatic vein were clearly visible. Reprinted from Akimaru K, et al. Resection of the liver, inferior vena cava, and right kidney for recurrences over 10 years after right adrenalectomy for carcinoma. *Eur J Surg 2002; 168*: 130-133 (with permission).

(3). The upper abdomen was opened by a Mercedes (three-armed stellate) incision to expose the intestines adequately, as they were firmly adherent to the liver and retroperitoneum as results of the previous operations. The adhesions between the liver and the transverse colon and duodenum were freed, and the gall bladder was removed. Then the whole liver with the tumors was separated from its surroundings by sharp dissections and excision of contiguously invaded part of the diaphragm. Then the main tumor mass with the invaded caudate lobe and posterior segment was separated from the liver by dissecting the parenchyma using forceps. The vessels in the hepato-duodenal ligament, the supra-hepatic and supra-renal aspects of the IVC, the hepatic veins, and the left renal vein were thoroughly exposed and taped individually. Then, the mass firmly encasing the retro-hepatic portion of the IVC, rather than forming an intracaval tumor thrombus was resected en-bloc, while the IVC was cross-clamped at sites just underneath the junction of the hepatic veins and below the left renal vein inflow and the root of the left renal vein was clamped. The IVC was reconstructed with a polytetrafluoroethylene (PTFE) graft. Veno-venous bypass was not used because the circulation was stable and the renal vein did not distend with clamping. Lastly, after the metastatic nodules in the left lateral segment were excised, the defect of the diaphragm was repaired with a PTFE sheet. Drains were placed in the thorax, right subphrenic space and in the foramen of Winslow.

The resected main tumor (Figure 5) measuring 13×8×4.5 cm was histologically diagnosed as adrenal cortical carcinoma (Figure 6) with a mitotic rate 3/50 HPF, similar to the findings of the previously resected tumors except for invasiveness, and had invaded the diaphragm and wall of the vena cava without intracaval extension. Variously sized tumor cells had bright and partly eosinophilic cytoplasm, and equally round nuclei with seldom seen moderate anisokaryosis and prominent nucleoli, less atypism than in other findings, but with some necrosis in places. Then, the Weiss score was 4.

The patient's postoperative course was uneventful except for early occlusion of the synthetic IVC graft (Figure 7) and mildly risen serum creatinine (1.25~1.5 mg/dl), for which no particular treatment was administered. He was discharged in October 1998. Since then, he had been very well, resuming his usual life style in a tumor free status without renal dysfunction or edematous lower extremities. In July 2001, he started to complain of lumbago, and had a compression fracture of the 12th thoracic vertebra in the next month. He was examined later with an MRI and had a diagnosis of tumor metastases to the 12th thoracic and 1st lumbar vertebrae in June 2002. No chemotherapy or radiation was applied. Gait disturbance with muscle weakness of the lower extremity developed in September 2002, and was followed by intractable pain in the extremity, which needed narcotics and a wheelchair for ambulation. In July 2003, his lower extremity was paralyzed with disturbed urination and defecation, and accompanied by edema and ascites. Eventually in the next month, he expired of pneumonia. Autopsy revealed metastases to the hepatic hilum, vertebrae, and lung with severe bilateral pneumonia. He survived 14 years after the first surgery.

DISCUSSION

Adrenal cortical carcinoma (ACC) is rare, composing only 0.02~0.2% of malignant tumors (8, 9). There does not appear to be a significant racial predilection, although a recent epidemiologic study showed a trend of increased rate among blacks (10). ACC can occur at any age, but there is a bimodal age incidence of ACC with the disease peaking in the first and fourth (11) or fifth (12) decade of life. In adults such as ours, individuals in the fourth and fifth decades of life are most frequently affected. ACC occurring in adults presents a mixed Cushing and virilizing syndrome, with overproduction of corticoids and androgens, and a far

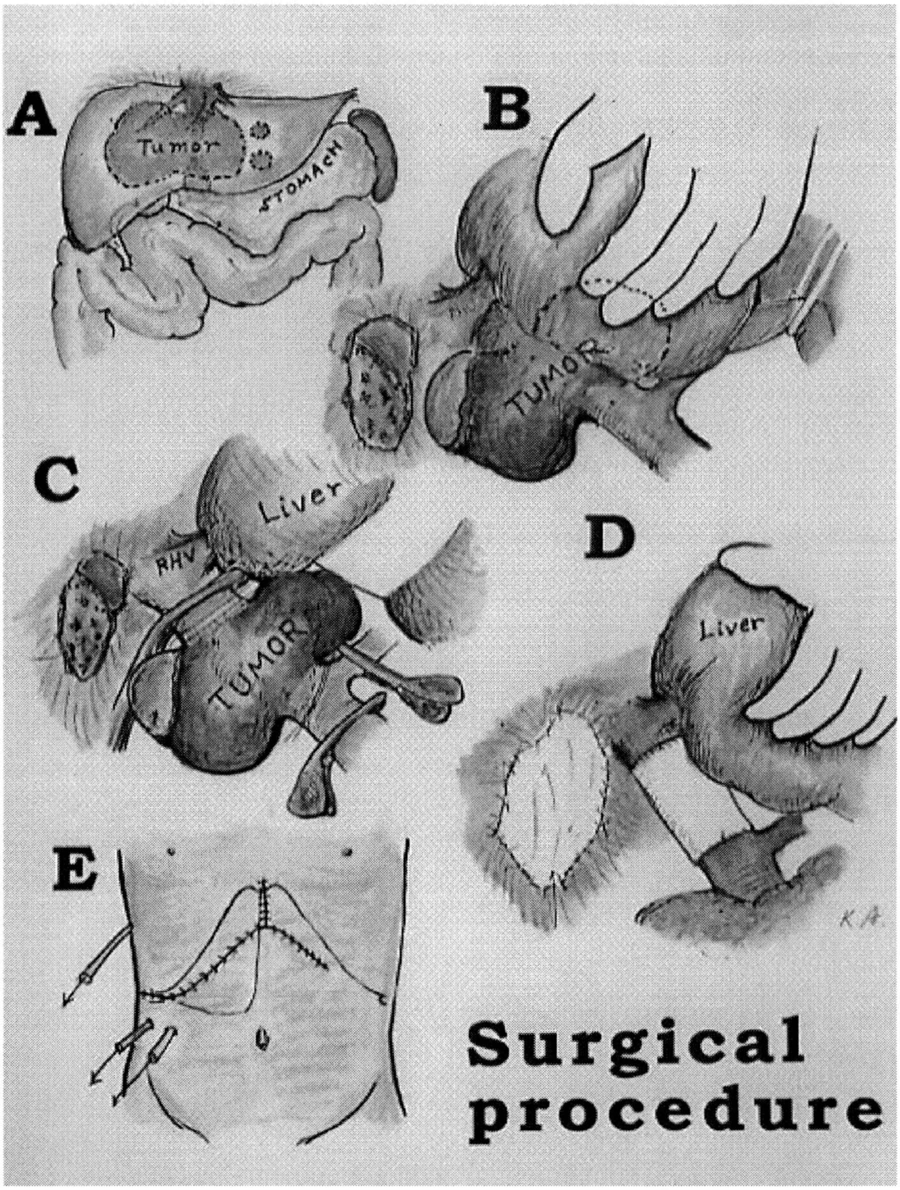

Figure 4. Procedure of the third excision.
The main tumor invading the caudate lobe and posterior segment with metastatic nodules in the left lateral segment, compressed the liver anteriorly, encircled the IVC, and invaded the diaphragm (A). The liver was lifted from the right after resection of the partially invaded diaphragm, and the main tumor was partly exposed. Then, right portion of the main tumor was separated from the posterior segment by dissecting the parenchyma (B). After left portion of the main tumor was completely freed from the liver by dissecting the left lateral segment, three cross-clamps were placed over just under the hepatic vein confluences, at the infra-renal aspect, and on the left renal vein, respectively. The IVC with the main tumor mass was excised with clear margins (C). The IVC was reconstructed with a PTFE tube graft. The diaphragm was repaired with a PTFE sheet, and 3 metastases in the left lateral segment were excised individually (D). The Mercedes skin incision over the previous surgical incisions was closed after a suctioning drain had been placed in the right thorax, soft tube drains in the right subphrenic space, and the foramen of Winslow (E). Modified figure with coloration from Akimaru K, et al. Resection of the liver, inferior vena cava, and right kidney for recurrences over 10 years after right adrenalectomy for carcinoma. *Eur J Surg 2002; 168*: 130-133 (with permission).

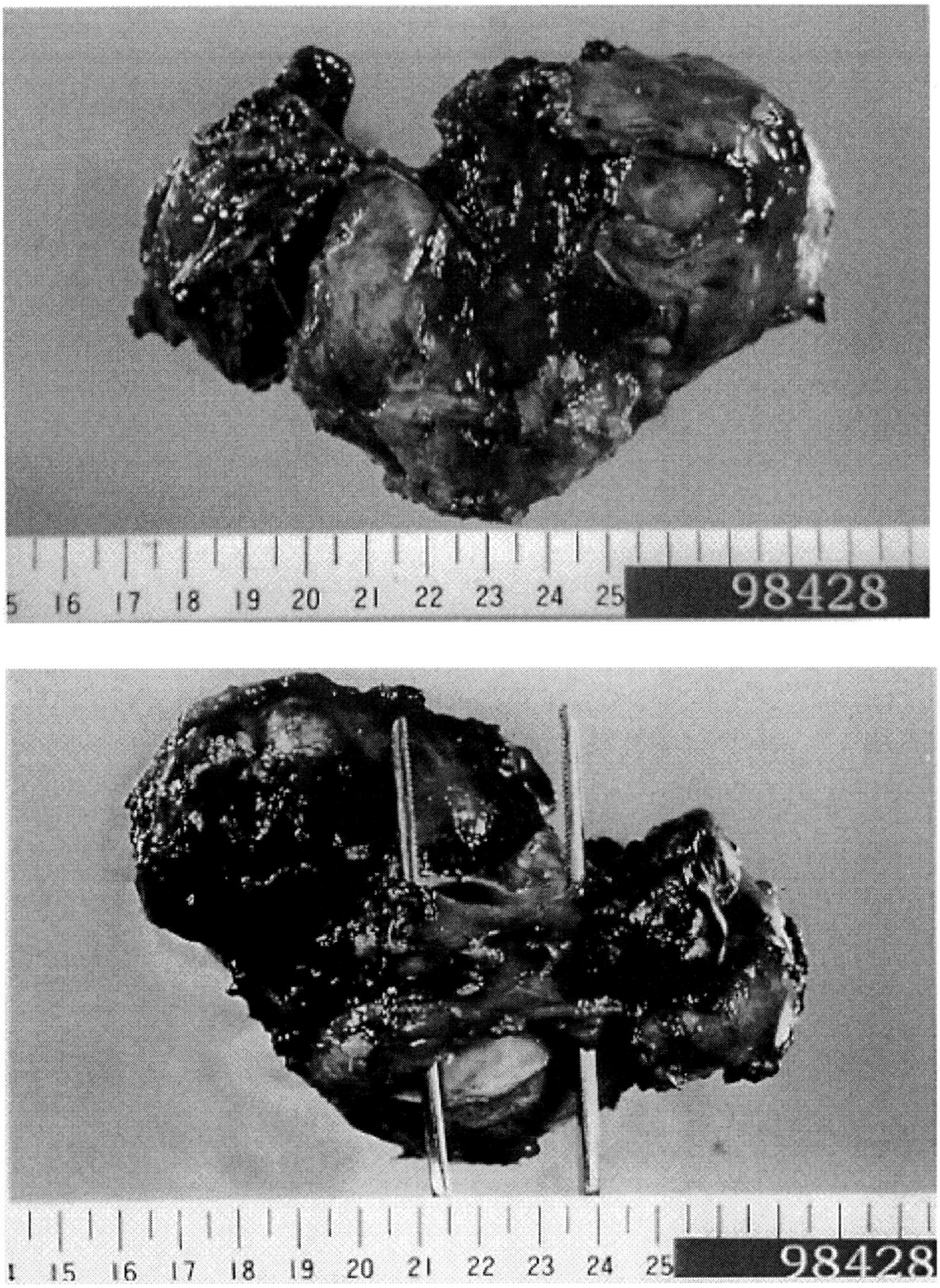

(a)

(b)

Figure 5. Anterior view of the resected tumor specimen, (a) measuring 13×8×4.5 cm, shows the tumor invading a part of the lateral segment and Spiegel lobe (on the right), and the subsegment 7 and paracaval portion of the caudate lobe (on the left). (b) Because of the obvious tumor involvements, the diaphragm (over the top) and retrohepatic portion of the vena (in the center) were simultaneously resected. Anterior aspect of the cava shows partial expansibility as proven by insertion and release of the forceps, while the other parts were firmly invaded with thick tumor tissue.

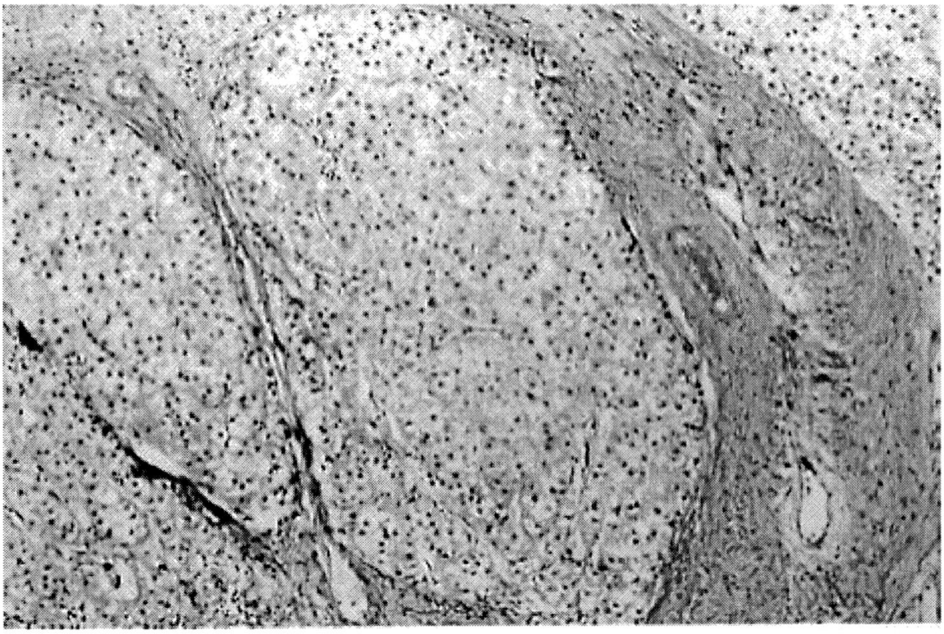

(a)

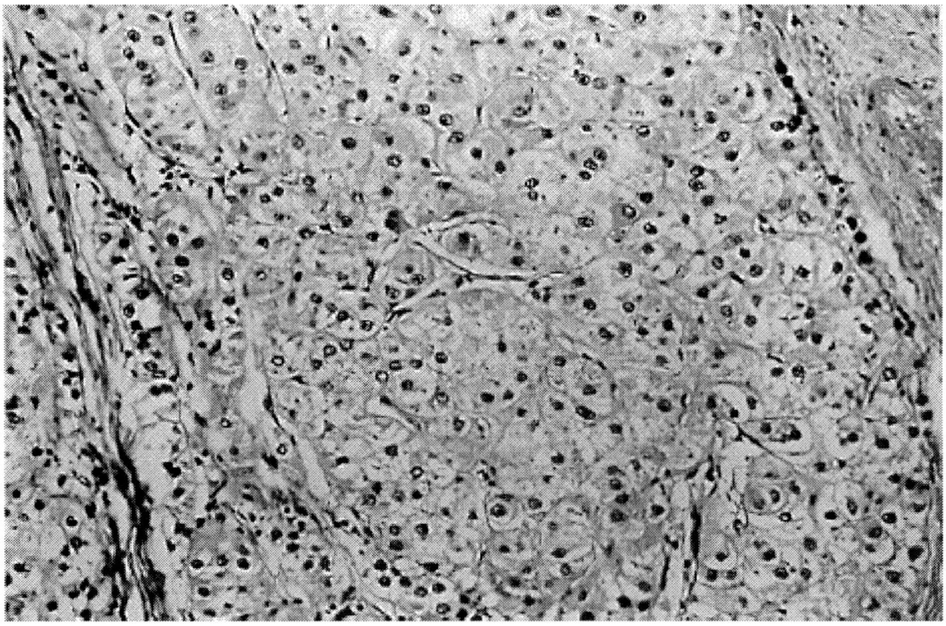

(b)

Figure 6. Histologically diagnosed as adrenal cortical carcinoma, similar to the findings of the previously resected tumor. Trabecular and alveolar clusters of tumor cells were separated by thin fibrous connective tissue (6a). The variously sized tumor cells with bright and partly eosinophilic cytoplasm had equally round nuclei, seldom seen moderate anisokaryosis, prominent nucleoli, and less atypism. Mitotic figure could hardly been seen (6b; high power magnification).

more aggressive clinical course, leading to rapid death within months or years (11). Men develop non-functioning malignant adrenal tumors more commonly than women, while women develop functional ACC more commonly than men (8, 10). As in our case, ACC was reported to be nonfunctional in 26 to 76% of cases from the collected data (10), especially in 85.6% of male patients older than 30 years (12). Most patients show initial signs of abdominal or flank pain, discomfort or fullness, and up to 30% may have a palpable abdominal mass (9, 10). On initial presentation, metastases have been noted in 15% to 38% of patients (10, 13). Another study of 42 patients with ACC showed distant metastases in 52% at diagnosis (14). Pulmonary, skeletal, or mediastinal metastases were noted on an initial chest X ray in 24 % of patients (15). In addition, an extraordinarily higher incidence rate of metastases (67%) at the time of tissue diagnosis has been reported on a series of 21 patients with ACC (16).

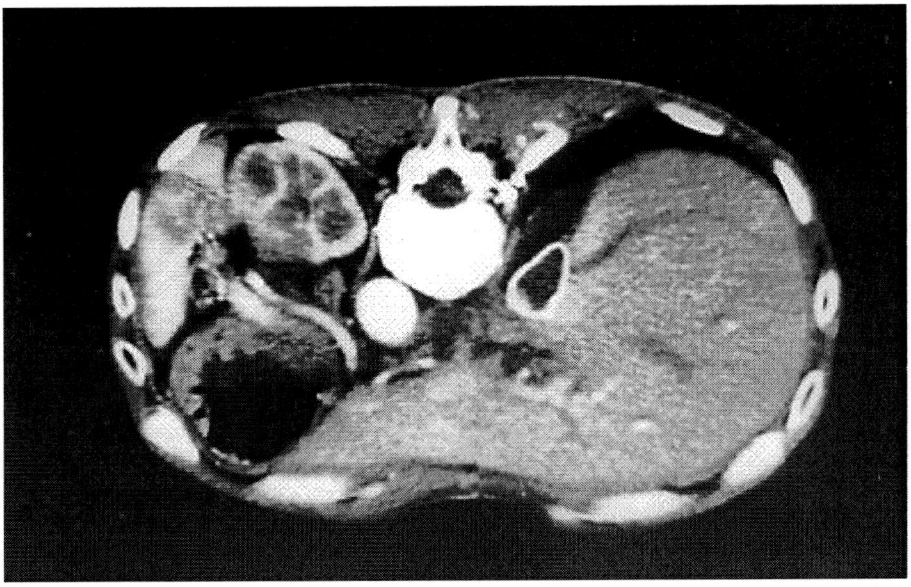

Figure 7. Enhanced computerized tomogram of the abdomen on postoperative day 21 showed positive contrast in the aorta, portal vein, left kidney, and hepatic veins. But, no contrast could be seen within the well expanded PTFE tube graft for the retrohepatic IVC reconstruction. The graft was fully thrombosed not to show the contrast at all, but did not induce renal failure on account of collaterals. Reprinted from Akimaru K, et al. Resection of the liver, inferior vena cava, and right kidney for recurrences over 10 years after right adrenalectomy for carcinoma. *Eur J Surg 2002; 168*: 130-133 (with permission).

ACC is often a bulky neoplasm with an average weight in several series being 510 g to 1210 g (10). Tumor weight has been reported to be an important prognostic factor (9, 10, 17), and all tumors weighing 95 g or more were malignant, while tumors less than 50 g were benign. Clearly, there are exceptions since some tumors weighing less than 50 g metastasize, and some in excess of 1000 g fail to do so on prolonged follow-up. The first adrenal tumor in our case measured 15×13×8 cm, and was estimated to weigh more than 800 g at malignancy. But, its histological diagnosis was cortical adenoma, since the findings were noninvasiveness, low mitotic rate, and no remarkable cellular or nuclear atypia. But, the actual biological behavior and the recurred tumor histology showed malignancy. Then, the original histological diagnosis could appropriately be designated as "adrenal cortical neoplasm of indeterminate malignant potential"(7).

Histological grading of ACC has been based upon extent of cellular pleomorphism (anaplastic versus differentiated) (16), but has not been uniform due to the variability in criteria used. More objective criteria have been proposed such as mitotic rate: ACCs having 20 or less mitoses per 50 HPF are low grade with a median survival of 58 months, and tumors with more than 20 mitoses per 50 HPF are high grade with a median survival of 14 months (7, 18). This is compatible with the few mitoses in our case having the long survival. We saw 3/50 HPF of the first tumor, 4/50 HPF of the second tumor, and 4/50 HPF of the last tumor, respectively. Venous invasion as well as mitotic activity correlated highest with metastasizing or recurring tumors (6, 8, 10), although our primary tumor used to be an adenoma showing no invasiveness at first and 2 points of Weiss criteria (6).

Weiss reported a comparative histological study of 43 adrenocortical tumors, and summarized a number of microscopic criteria found useful in separating metastasizing and recurring tumors from non-metastasizing and non-recurring ones. The useful criteria are: 1. nuclear grade III or IV, 2. mitotic rate greater than 5/50 HPF; 3. atypical mitoses, 4. clear cells comprising 25 % or less of the tumor; 5. a diffuse architecture; 6. microscopic necrosis; 7. invasion of venous structures; 8. invasion of sinusoidal structures; and 9. invasion of tumor capsular structures. It was concluded that none of the 24 tumors with two or less of those criteria metastasized or recurred, while all but one of the 19 tumors with four or greater of those criteria either recurred or metastasized. But, as Weiss mentioned, the median follow-up was 11 years and on occasion adrenocortical tumors can recur or metastasize in a longer period of time. Our case had the first recurrence in the kidney at 5 years, a second recurrence at the vena cava with liver metastases in 4 years after the nephrectomy, and carcinomatosis with bone and lung metastases in another 5 years after the resections of the tumor invading the IVC diaphragm and caudate lobe of the liver, and the multiple metastatic nodules in the lateral segment. A case report of metastatic ACC to the brain in a 9-year-old female patient has been reported with the same histology and biological behavior (19). She had adrenalectomy for Cushing's syndrome at the age of 4 years (the tumor weighed 290 g). She was then totally asymptomatic for 5 years until she presented with blurred vision caused by brain metastasis which was successfully removed. No recurrence or metastasis occured for 2 years while she retained her normal life. The histologic pattern of the brain metastasis was almost identical to the originally classified adrenocortical neoplasm without malignant features, and showed the tumor resuming the normal adrenal cortical architecture with little cellular pleomorphism and neither vascular nor capsular invasions with only few small areas of necrosis. The primary tumor in this case could not be diagnosed as ACC as in our case. Although Weiss criteria (6, 11) and the mitotic rate (18, 20) appear to be the best indicator of prognosis (11), the low scores of Weiss criteria and low mitotic rates in all the resected tumors from our patient and the girl could not predict their prognoses in some aspects. These cases have two common points of similarities, the benign histological findings and the large size of the primary tumors.

Resection of localized ACC can be curative. In Didolkar and a coworkers' report (14), 16 (38%) out of 42 patients could have a curative resection, while 80 (76%) patients of 105 patients with ACC were able to undergo surgery for cure reported by Luton et al. (21), who mentioned 12 months as a median postoperative disease-free interval. It invades adjacent organs or tissues, and may require en bloc removal of invaded structures, which is still the best individual factor for a good prognosis and prolonged survival (13, 14, 22). And even debulking improves prognosis.

ACC metastasized to lung (71%), lymph node (68%), liver (42%), bone (26%), and gastrointestinal tract (26%) in that order at autopsy in 31 patients (14). Another autopsy series of 50 patients (22) showed the distributions of distant metastases of ACC, which were liver (92%), lung (78%), lymph node (58%), retroperitoneum (48%), IVC (28%), bone (18%), peritoneum (16%), kidney (12%), diaphragm (12%), and so forth.

Fortunately our patient tolerated the second and third operations for recurrences in the kidney after 5 years, and for liver metastases with involvement of the IVC at 9 years, respectively, and had lived 14 years after the right adrenalectomy. In the report by van Slooten et al. (23), 93% of the patients developed metastases within 10 years after diagnosis. Death from metastatic ACC often occurs within the first 12 months after diagnosis (8), and overall five-year survival is between 20% and 35% (8, 10, 22, 24). ACC with IVC involvement has been reported in 78 patients identified by MEDLINE (25). Although the prognosis is often poor, aggressive surgery for local recurrence at the IVC as intracaval or wall invasive tumor growth or metastatic cancer has been reported (8) with good functional results (2) and better quality of life, as our case has shown.

The IVC involved with the tumor can be removed with cardiopulmonary bypass (25, 26), veno-venous (4) or without any bypass (2, 3, 27, 28, 29). Because of long-term stenosis or obstruction of the cava, patients tolerate venous congestion with collaterals. We did not use veno-venous bypass or test clamping of the IVC (30) in our case having only the left kidney, and resection of the IVC was accomplished safely because of collaterals. In our case, it was unnecessary to use cardiac bypass technique (26) because of no possibility of intracaval tumor extension which might cause tumor thrombus migration through the cava to the heart and lung. We used a PTFE graft for reconstruction of the IVC. Its patency is said to be satisfactory in terms of postoperative functional results (2), especially when reinforced grafts and anticoagulants are used. Without graft reinforcement or adequate anticoagulant treatments, ours failed to remain patent, but the patient's postoperative course was uneventful because of collaterals as the adrenal, lumbar and gonadal veins up to the hemi-azygos vein, and he had no subsequent renal dysfunction or leg edema. This phenomenon was observed in the first case to survive by Clark (31) after excision of a kidney, segmental resection of the vena cava, and division of the opposite renal vein. Our replacement of the occluded IVC with a tube graft might have been unnecessary as the case reported by Huguet et al (2). Their case involved a 21 year-old male patient who had en bloc resection of adrenal carcinoma with the suprarenal inferior vena cava under hepatic vascular exclusion, and had no venous problems at all after the resection without reconstruction of the cava on account of marked collateral circulation. Fortunately, our patient's IVC was invaded by ACC without formation of intra-caval tumor thrombi, and could be resected with clear margins without danger (10) of inducing tumor emboli by intra-operative manipulation. In a limited series of ACC with IVC tumor thrombus extension (27), three of six patients who had undergone removal of the primary tumor and the venous tumor thrombus were able to survive 5 years. One of them had pulmonary metastasis a year after the surgery, which was resected, and she subsequently died of brain and lung metastases 5 years later. The results of such aggressive surgery (1, 2, 27) can be appreciated for longer survival of patients and excellent performance status. Some patients with ACC invading the vena cava are candidates for aggressive surgery such as resection of the vena cava, which may offer the only possibility for tumor control, as in our case. We have learned from our patient that the primarily diagnosed adenoma might change behavior, recur and invade with malignant potentiality, and metastasize to distant organs during the long courses after the each radical surgery. After resection of adrenal tumors we have to be observant about the postoperative biological behavior for a long time, not only with consideration of the histology but tumor size as well. When it recurred the patient must be able to tolerate aggressive and well designed surgery by positive and careful surgeons, and can live an ordinary life longer.

Chemotherapy of ACC was not evaluated well by Didolkar et al. in 1981 (14); they showed a low response rate of 11% (3 of 28 patients) with relatively short durations of complete and partial responses, and high incidence of toxicity. But, in the report by Luton et al. among 80 patients who underwent surgery, 59 (74%) patients also received the adrenal cytotoxic agent mitotane (21), by which hormonal secretion was controlled in 75% of the patients, and 8 (22%) of 37 patients with measurable disease had partial tumor regression. The regression in all eight patients was transient. In 1993, Wooten and King (12) reviewed the literature concerning the treatment of ACC with mitotane from 1965 to 1992, and found that 35.2% (194 of 551) of patients had at least some response to mitotane. But, the definition of clinical response was too varied and broad to evaluate its efficacy uniformly. And, it is unclear if tumor response or shrinkage correlates with prolonged patient survival. They concluded that treatment of ACC with mitotane was insufficient therapy for most patients with the carcinoma, whether the agent was given alone or in combination with other forms of chemotherapy. In 1998, approximately 20% to 25% of ACC patients were reported to respond to mitotane with prolonged survival (24). Another review by Kopf et al. (22) in 2000 disclosed that the efficacy of mitotane treatment and outcome were heterogenous, and those discrepancies might be due to the time course of treatment and the dosage. In addition, as there is a dose-response relationship between mitotane serum levels and survival, the primary tumor as well as recurrent tumor responded well to serum levels of more than 15 mg/l, while no response was noted in patients with lower serum levels. Although our case with bone metastases in the last year might have responded somewhat to chemotherapy, other chemotherapeutic agents are now used in recurrent or progressive disease despite treatment with mitotane and in patients with primarily unresectable lesions or recurrent tumors after initially radical surgery. They are 5-fluorouracil, doxorubicin, cisplatin, and etoposide, used in combination each other or with mitotane.

In conclusion, we have learned that a histologically diagnosed adenoma which looks too deceivingly benign to be treated by complete resection at first, can then change to be a ACC and recur, invade and metastasize. Aggressive surgery may be indicated for recurrences of slow growing malignancy to yield a good quality of life and longer survival such as the 14 years shown in our case.

REFERENCES

[1] Bower TC, Nagorney DM, Toomey BJ, Groviczki P, Pairolero PC. Hallett JW Jr, Cherry KJ Jr. Vena cava replacement for malignant disease: Is there a role? *Ann Vasc Surg 1993; 7*: 51-62

[2] Huguet C, Ferri M, Gravelli A. Resection of the suprarenal inferior vena cava. - The role of prosthetic replacement. *Arch Surg 1995; 130*: 793-7

[3] Skinner DG, Pfister RF, Colvin R. Extension of renal cell carcinoma into the vena cava: the rationale for aggressive surgical management. *J Urol 1972; 107*: 711-716.

[4] Miyazaki M, Ito H, Nakagawa K, Ambiru S, Shimizu H, Okuno A, Nukui Y, Yoshitomi H, Kusashio K, Furuya S, Nakajima N. Aggressive surgical resection for hepatic metastases involving the inferior vena cava. *Am J Surg 1999; 177*: 294-298.

[5] Akimaru K, Onda M, Tajiri T, Umehara M, Yoshida H, Nomura T, Masuda G, Uchiyama K, Shimizu K, Ochi M. Resection of the liver, inferior vena cava, and right kidney for recurrences over 10 years after right adrenalectomy for carcinoma. *Eur J Surg 2002; 168*: 130-3.

[6] Weiss LM. Comparative histological study of 43 metastasizing and nonmetastasizing adrenocortical tumors. *Am J Surg Pathol 1984; 8*: 163-169

[7] Pathak IC. Survival after right nephrectomy, excision of infrahepatic vena cava and ligation of left renal vein: a case report. *J Urol 1971; 106*: 599-602.

[8] Norton JA, Le HN. Adrenal tumors. In: DeVita VT Jr, Hellman S, Rosenberg SA, ed. *Cancer: principles & practice of oncology.* Sixth edition. Vol. 2. Philadelphia: Lippincott Williams & Wilkins; 1999. P 1777-80

[9] DeLellis RA. The adrenal glands. In: Sernberg SS, ed. *Diagnostic surgical pathology.* Third edition. Vol. 1. Philadelphia: Lippincott Williams & Wilkins; 1999. P 589-623.

[10] Lack EE. Tumors of the adrenal gland and extra-adrenal paraganglia (3rd series, fascicle 19). In: Rosai J, Sobin LH, editors. *Atlas of tumor pathology.* Washington, DC: Armed forces institute of pathology; 1997. P 123-52.

[11] Wajchenberg BL, Pereira MAA, Medonca BB, Latronico AC, Carneiro PC, Alves VAF, Zerbini MCN, Lieberman B Gomes GC, Kirschner MA. Adrenocortical carcinoma: clinical and laboratory observations. *Cancer 2000; 88*: 711-736.

[12] Wooten MD, King DK. Adrenal cortical carcinoma. Epidemiology and treatment with mitotane and a review of the literature. *Cancer 1993; 72*: 3145-55.

[13] Bellantone R, Ferrante A, Boscherini M, Lombardi CP, Crucitti P, Crucitti F, Favia G, Borrelli D, Boffi L, Capussottil L, et al. Role of reoperation in recurrence of adrenal cortical carcinoma: results from 188 cases collected in the Italian National Registration fo Adrenal Cortical Carcinoma. *Surgery 1997; 122*: 1212-8.

[14] Didolkar MD, Bescher RA, Elias EG, Moore RH. Natural history of adrenal cortical carcinoma: a clinicopathologic study of 42 patients. *Cancer 1981; 47*: 2153-61.

[15] King DR, Lack EE. Adrenal cortical carcinoma: a clinical and pathologic study of 49 cases. *Cancer 1979; 44*: 239-44.

[16] Hogan TF, Gilchrist KW, Westring DW, Citrin DL. A clinical and pathological study of adrenocortical carcinoma: therapeutic implications. *Cancer 1980; 45*: 2880-3.

[17] Hough AJ, Hollifield JW, Page DL, Hartmann WH. Prognostic factors in adrenal cortical tumors: a mathematical analysis of clinical and morphologic data.; *Am J Clin Pathol 1979;72*: 390-99.

[18] Weiss LM, Medeiros LJ, Vickery AL Jr. Pathologic features of prognostic significance in adrenaocortical carcinoma. *A J Surg Pathol 1989; 13*: 202-6.

[19] Romaguera RL, Minagar A, Bruce JH, Jagid JR, Falcone S, Curless RG, Ragherb J, Morrison G. Adrenocortical carcinoma with cerebral metastasis in a child: case report and review of the literature. *Clin Neurol Neurosurg 2001; 103*: 46-50.

[20] Medeiros LJ, Weiss LM. New developments in the pathological diagnosis of adrenal cortical neoplasms. A review. *Am J Clin Pathol 1992; 97*: 73-83.

[21] Luton JP, Cerdas S, Billaud L, Thomas G, Guilhaume B, Bertagna X, Laudat MH, Louvel A, et al. Clinical features of adrenocortical carcinoma, prognostic factors, and the effect of mitotane therapy. *N Engl J Med 1990; 322*: 1195-201.

[22] Lack EE, Travis WD, Oertel JE. Adrenal cortical neoplasms. In: Lack EE, ed. Pathology of the adrenal glands. *New York: Churchill Livingstone, 1990*: 115-71.

[23] van Slooten H, Schaberg A, Smeenk D, Moolenaar AJ. Morphologic characteristics of benign and malignant adrenaocortical tumors. *Cancer 1985; 55*: 766-73.

[24] Demeure MJ, Somberg LB. Functioning and nonfunctioning adrenocortical carcinomas: clinical presentation and therapeutic strategies. *Surg Oncol Clin N Am 1998; 7*: 791-805.

[25] Chesson JP, Theodorescu D. Adrenal tumor with caval extension: case report and review of the literature. *Scand J Urol Nephrol 2002; 36*: 71-73.

[26] Hedican SSP, Marshaall FF. Adrenocortical carcinoma with intracaval extension. *J Urol 1997; 158*: 2056-2061.

[27] Figueroa AJ, Stein JP, Lieskovsky G, Skinner DG. Adrenal cortical carcinoma associated with venous tumour thrombus extension. *Brit J Urol 1997; 80*: 397-400.

[28] Clayman RV, Gonzalez R, Fraley EE. Renal cell cancer invading the inferior vena cava: clinical review and anatomical approach. *J Urol 1980; 123*: 157-163.

[29] Lack EE, Travis WD, Oertel JE. Adrenal cortical neoplasm. In: Lack EE, ed. Pathology of the adrenal gland. New Yorl: *Churchil Livingstone, 1990*: 115-71.

[30] Lord RSA The trial clamping before division of the left renal vein. *Surgery 1982; 91*: 409-412.

[31] Clark CD. Survival after excision of a kidney, segmental resection of the vena cava, and division of the opposite renal vein. *Lancet 1961; 2*: 1015-6.

In: Trends in Kidney Cancer Research
Editor: Kelvin R. Nunez, pp. 103-118

ISBN 1-59454-141-8

Chapter VIII

Quality of Life of Metastatic Renal Carcinoma Patients Receiving Subcutaneous Interferon or Intravenous Interleukin-2

Sylvie Négrier [1*], ***Sandrine Touzet*** [2], ***Frédéric Gomez*** [2], ***Jean-Yves Douillard*** [3], ***Alain Ravaud*** [4], ***Christine Chevreau*** [5], ***Alice Dazord*** [6] ***and Bernard Escudier*** [7], ***for the Groupe Français d'Immunothérapie.***

[1] Medical Oncology Department, Centre Léon Bérard, 28 rue Laennec, 69008 LYON, France.

[2] Public Health Department, Centre Léon Bérard, 28 rue Laennec, 69008 LYON, France

[3] Medical Oncology Department, Centre Gauducheau, Boulevard Jacques Monod, 44805 NANTES Saint-Herblain Cedex, France

[4] Institut Bergonié, 180, rue de Saint-Genès, 33076 BORDEAUX Cedex, France.

[5] Medical Oncology Department, Centre Claudius Régaud, 20-24 rue du Pont Saint-Pierre, 31052 TOULOUSE Cedex, France.

[6] SCRIPT-INSERM, Hôpital Saint-Jean-de-Dieu, 290 route de Vienne, 69008 LYON, France.

[7] Immunotherapy Unit, Institut Gustave Roussy, Rue Camille Desmoulins, 94805 VILLEJUIF Cedex, France.

* Correspondent: Sylvie Négrier, M.D., Medical Oncology Department, Centre Léon Bérard, 28 rue Laënnec, 69373 Lyon Cedex 08, France; tel. (33) 478 78 27 51; fax: (33) 478 78 27 16; e-mail: negrier@lyon.fnclcc.fr

ABSTRACT

Purpose: Despite interleukin-2 and interferon treatments, the survival of metastatic renal carcinoma patients remains poor. Unlike treatment toxicity, the quality of life of these patients has seldom been investigated.

Materials and methods: Quality of life was evaluated on patients of the CRECY trial randomized to intravenous interleukin 2 or subcutaneous interferon, or a combination of both drugs. Investigators had initially hypothesized that quality of life was better in patients receiving interferon alone. Quality of life was assessed using a 17-item questionnaire investigating 4 domains of everyday life: health, relationships, inner life, material conditions. The degree of importance or satisfaction attributed by patients to each parameter, and the degree of change experienced were measured. Questionnaires were given 12 weeks after treatment start; 182 patients returned the questionnaire. Results were submitted to different correlation tests, principal component analyses, and survival analyses.

Results: Contrary to expected findings, no difference was revealed between interferon or interleukin-2 patients. Overall, quality of life seems relatively poor. The profiles of satisfaction and change are close: relationships were judged positive and improved, whereas physical activities were labeled negative and worse. No significant correlation was found with patients' features, except age.

Conclusions: We demonstrate that patients with metastatic renal carcinoma receiving cytokines, either subcutaneous interferon at home or intravenous interleukin-2 in the hospital, have equally impaired quality of life.

Keywords: quality of life; renal carcinoma; interleukin-2; interferon; cytokine

INTRODUCTION

The 5-year survival rate of patients suffering metastatic renal carcinoma (MRCC) remains below 10% [1-3]. In the past two decades, high confidence was placed in cytokine treatments, mainly interleukin-2 and interferon alfa-2a, which accounts for the large number of trials that evaluated these agents. Interleukin-2 and interferon alfa-2a finally proved capable of inducing tumor regressions, a few of these being complete and durable [4-6]. However, the benefit obtained in terms of survival is still questionable. The results of large phase III trials were only recently published and represent a very limited part of the literature [3,7,8]. The 5-year survival rates are low (10% or less) and the median survival duration is between 12 and 18 months in the best series. Since the improvement in terms of survival has not yet been fully established, it seems important to consider the psychosocial aspects of MRCC beside evaluating the medical aspects of the disease. Therefore, quality of life represents an important issue for these patients.

Quality of life is more and more frequently investigated in patients suffering from advanced cancers. However, if the side-effects induced by cytokines are well-known and were largely reported in the past, data concerning the quality of life of patients treated with interferon alfa-2a or interleukin-2 are not frequent [8-14].

From 1992 to 1995, the Groupe Français d'Immunothérapie conducted a large multicenter randomized trial, the CRECY trial, which investigated the respective roles of interleukin-2, interferon alfa-2a, or both cytokines, in patients with MRCC. The main therapeutic results have already been reported in details [7]. The assessment of patients' quality of life was a secondary endpoint of the trial. The present paper reports the results of this quality of life investigation.

PATIENTS AND METHODS

Patients and Treatment Protocol

Patients between 18 and 65 years were eligible if they had histologically confirmed, clearly progressive metastatic renal-cell carcinoma. Patients who required nephrectomy were invited to enter the trial only after they had undergone the operation. Eligible patients were randomly assigned to receiving either intravenous recombinant human interleukin-2 alone (group 1), subcutaneous recombinant human interferon alfa-2a alone (group 2), or intravenous interleukin-2 combined with interferon alfa-2a (group 3).

In group 1, recombinant human interleukin-2 (Proleukin®, Chiron Therapeutics, Suresnes, France) was administered as a continuous intravenous infusion from day 1 to day 5 and from day 10 to day 15. In group 2, recombinant human interferon alfa-2a (Roferon®, Roche, Neuilly-sur-Seine, France) was given subcutaneously thrice a week for the first 12 weeks. In group 3, a combination of group 1 regimen with subcutaneous interferon alfa-2a thrice a week from day 1 to day 15 was performed. Treatment cycles with interleukin-2 were repeated once after a 3-week rest. Tumor was assessed 12 weeks after the beginning of treatment in each group. All patients gave informed consent prior to randomization. They were concurrently informed of the quality-of-life questionnaire. Details of the trial were previously reported [7].

Assessment of Quality of Life

The investigators of the CRECY trial hypothesized that patients receiving ambulatory subcutaneous interferon alfa-2a would have a better quality of life than patients treated with one of the intravenous interleukin-2 regimens requiring hospitalization.

Twelve weeks after the beginning of treatment, patients enrolled in the trial received anonymous self-administered questionnaires investigating their quality of life. Completed questionnaires were to be returned by pre-paid mail within the following weeks. We used the only French questionnaire available at the time when the CRECY trial was designed: the Subjective Quality of Life Profile (SQLP) questionnaire initially developed by the SCRIPT-INSERM (National Institute Health and Medical Research, Lyon, France) of which both the

French and English versions were subsequently validated [15-17]. This self-administered questionnaire may be used in healthy volunteers as well as in patients; it was previously tested and validated in both types of populations, including patients with different cancer types [18,19]. The questionnaire makes it possible for investigators to explore the various facets of patient quality of life. It is characterized by its multidimensional pattern and subjective approach. For each item, the SQLP takes into account patients' aptitude to change, degree of satisfaction, importance attributed to various domains of life, as well as their expectations concerning these domains. Quality of life is evaluated in terms of the patients' satisfaction with change compared with their life before treatment.

Internal consistency as well as construct validity have been verified using principal component analysis. Predictive validity had also been checked against other existing quality of life questionnaires [16,18]. The SQLP comprises a 'core-questionnaire' that must be entirely completed by each patient and an 'optional questionnaire' including a variable number of questions chosen by the investigator among a 'bank' of items. The other items included are dependent on the pathology studied. Here, we have used 17 items of the core questionnaire that take into consideration 4 different domains: health, relationships, inner life and material conditions. Table 1 summarizes the items used in the present study. Each item was scored for satisfaction from -2 (very dissatisfied) to +2 (very satisfied); the answer 'indifferent' scored zero. In the questions assessing the importance attributed to each dimension of quality of life, the lowest score was zero (unimportant) and the highest score was 3 (extremely important). In the questions assessing patient's expectations for change, scores varied from -2 ('change for the worse') to +2 ('change for the better'); the answer 'no change' scored zero. The various aspects of quality of life, such as physical and psychological well-being or inter-individual and social relationships were also recorded. The total score was calculated as the mean of all sub scores for satisfaction, attributed importance and expectation. The degrees of change and satisfaction were weighted by importance. The usual statistical tests and comparisons between populations could then be performed. Moreover, the influence of discrete as well as continuous covariates such as sex, age, etc. on the quality of life score could readily be studied [16].

Table 1: The Subjective quality of life profile. List of the 17 items used in the study

1. Your physical abilities (or difficulties) to perform the movements you usually do every day.
2. Your abilities (or difficulties) to go out or move about outside the house.
3. Your overall fitness.
4. How you feel physically (pain for example).
5. Your relationships with other people.
6. Your sleep.

Table 1 – Continued

7. Your ability (or difficulty) to think or focus your attention.
8. Your sexuality.
9. People's attitude toward you.
10. Your meals, what you can eat.
11. Your income or the money that you have available.
12. Your personal or inner life (reflection, reading, meditation, day-dreaming).
13. Your physical appearance.
14. The fact that you have (or do not have) relationships with close family or friends.
15. The fact that you have (or do not have) personal activities or leisure.
16. The fact that you live (or do not live) with someone (as a couple, as a family, as a single person...).
17. What is happening in the world.

Statistical analysis was performed using different correlation tests: chi square test, Kruskal-Wallis test, Spearman test. The descriptive statistics of the variables was analyzed using the chi-square test. The scores obtained from the questionnaires were analyzed using non parametric statistical tests (e.g., Wilcoxon signed rank test) or Spearman Rho test for correlations. The usual threshold for significance ($p < 0.05$) was used. We conducted a univariate analysis of factors that might potentially influence the degrees of change and satisfaction such as age, sex, and treatment groups: treatment assigned by randomization or patients receiving an interleukin-2-containing regimen versus others. A principal component analysis (multivariate analysis) using the varimax rotation method was performed in order to summarize all the responses to the quality-of-life questionnaire under a limited number of items (SPSS Advanced Statistics software, Chicago, MI, USA).

Principal component analysis has marked advantages over other factorial methods used for questionnaires, such as multiple correspondence analysis, for instance. Indeed, principal component analysis takes into account the ordinal nature of the variables whereas multiple correspondence analysis considers the variables as nominal. The ordinal nature of the variables is not a problem for principal component analysis, since this analysis can be performed using a rank correlation matrix. In addition, principal component analysis summarizes correlated variables into a reduced number of non correlated factors, thus making other phenomena, independent from the size effect, detectable on the other factors. There is no absolute hypothesis about the nature or distribution of the variables in the method of principal components.

Survival analysis was performed using the Kaplan-Meier method, and comparisons of survival were performed using the log-rank test.

RESULTS

From March 1992 to July 1995, a total of 425 patients were randomized into the CRECY trial; 138 were randomly assigned to the interleukin-2 group, 147 to the group receiving interferon alfa-2a, and 147 to the group receiving interleukin-2 plus interferon alfa-2a. There were no statistically significant differences in patient characteristics among the three treatment groups. Most patients (77 percent) had a performance-status score of 0, and most (93 percent) had undergone nephrectomy. The therapeutic results were previously reported [7]. Briefly, a significant advantage was found in favor of the combination group (interleukin-2 combined with interferon alfa-2a) in terms of response rate and event-free survival, but no gain in overall survival was detected.

Of the 182 patients who eventually returned the SQLP questionnaire, 54 (29%) had received interleukin-2 alone, 74 (40%) had been treated with subcutaneous interferon alfa-2a, and 54 (29%) with a combination of both cytokines.

The characteristics of patients who returned the questionnaire were not statistically different from those who did not (table 2).

Table 2: Characteristics of patients according to whether they have returned the quality of life questionnaire or not.

Patients characteristics	Questionnaires were not returned	Questionnaires were returned	P value (chi square test)
Age ≤ 56	52.9 %	50.0 %	
Age > 56	47.1 %	50.0 %	NS
Female	68.2 %	70.7 %	
Male	31.8 %	29.3 %	NS
Prior chemotherapy	2.1 %	1.6 %	
No prior chemotherapy	97.9 %	98.4 %	NS
Prior radiotherapy	12.9 %	14.3 %	
No prior radiotherapy	87.1 %	85.7 %	NS
Time tumor-metastases			
> 1 year	31.8 %	34.1 %	
≤ 1 year	68.2 %	65.9 %	NS
Performance status			
ECOG score = 0	55.0 %	57.7 %	
ECOG score < 0	45.0 %	42.3 %	NS
Weight loss < 10 %	86.8 %	90.7 %	
Weight loss ≥ 10 %	13.2 %	9.3 %	NS

Table 2 - Continued

Patients characteristics	**Questionnaires were not returned**	**Questionnaires were returned**	**P value (chi square test)**
One metastatic site ≥ 2 metastatic sites	20.9% 79.1%	34.6% 65.4%	.002
No lung metastasis Lung metastases	28.9% 71.1%	23.6% 76.4%	NS
No hepatic metastasis Hepatic metastases	78.5% 21.5%	81.9% 8.1%	NS
No bone metastasis Bone metastases	64.0% 36.0%	78.0% 22.0%	.002
No mediastinal lymph node Mediastinal lymph nodes	63.6% 36.4%	68.1% 31.9%	NS
No grade 4 toxicity Grade 4 toxicity	24.4% 75.6%	25.3% 74.7%	NS
Objective response or stabilization Progression Not evaluable	33.1% 56.6% 10.3%	49.5% 47.8% 2.7%	NS

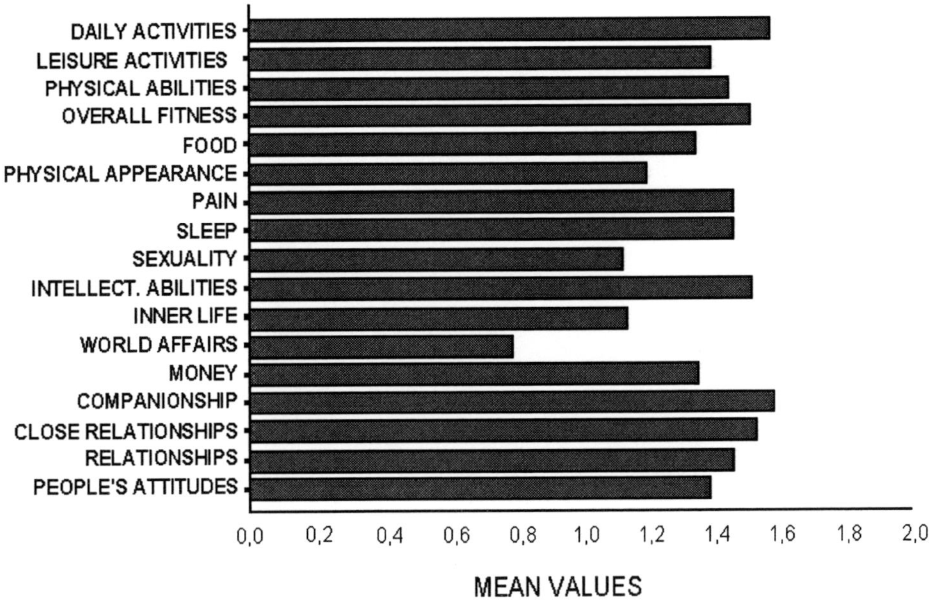

Figure 1: Mean levels of importance attributed to each parameter.

The degree of importance attributed to each item was rather similar for all the patients, with a mean score of 1.34 (Figure 1). The degree of importance given to the world affairs was the only parameter scored under 1, with a mean value of 0.79.

The degree of satisfaction and the degree of change had a mean score of -0.014 and 0.002, respectively. Since the degree of importance attributed to the different items appears rather similar, the degrees of change and satisfaction were weighted by the degree of importance in further analyses.

Mean values of the satisfaction scores are given in Figure 2. Parameters concerning relationships (companionship, close relationship, relationship, people's attitudes) have obtained the highest positive values. Conversely, items investigating different physical activities show overall negative values.

The profile of change is close to the satisfaction profile, indicating that relations with others were improved while physical activities worsened (Figure 2).

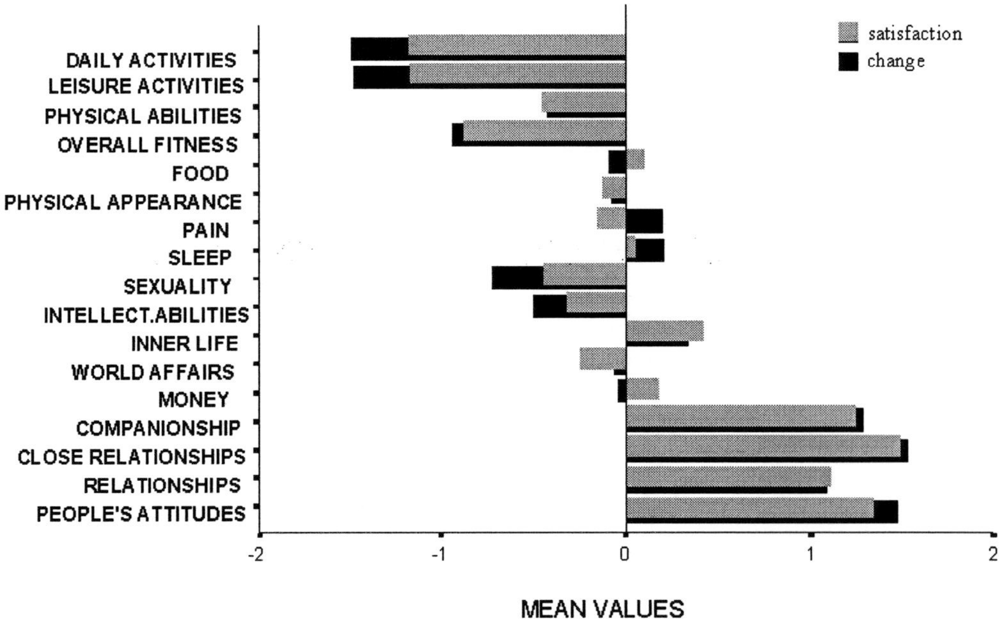

Figure 2: Mean rates of satisfaction (gray scale) and change (black scale) weighted by importance given to each parameter.

A univariate analysis was performed to identify factors that might potentially influence the degrees of change and satisfaction. No significant correlation with the patients' characteristics was found, except for the age of the patients. We analyzed the results according to a threshold value of 56 years of age, which was the median age of the patients enrolled in the CRECY trial. A significant correlation was found in 9/17 parameters, indicating that younger patients felt more unsatisfied than their older counterparts (Table 3). In addition, age may influence the degree of importance given to some parameters. For instance, patients under 56 assigned a priority to sexuality (P=0.001), leisure activities (P=0.023), income and money (P=0.024) and companionship (P=0.043).

Table 3: Parameters showing a significant correlation with age (threshold value: 56) according to the results of the univariate analysis

Variables		P value (Spearman correlation test)
Sexuality	change* satisfaction*	0.015 0.014
Leisure	change* satisfaction*	0.021 0.011
Money	change* satisfaction*	0.026 0.049
Daily activities	change* satisfaction*	0.011 0.030
Fitness	satisfaction*	0.006
Physical aspect	satisfaction*	0.018
Pain	satisfaction*	0.014
Intellectual abilities	change* satisfaction*	0.004 0.015
Inner life	change* satisfaction*	0.034 0.014

Younger patients felt more unsatisfied.

- degrees of change and of satisfaction were weighted by importance.

Table 4: Results of the univariate analysis according to treatment group, when all patients receiving interleukin-2 were pooled.

	Interferon alfa-2a mean values	Interleukin-2 ± interferon alfa-2a mean values	P. Value (Kruskal-Wallis test)
Food change* satisfaction*	 -0.66 -0.46	 0.17 0.45	 0.009 0.017
Pain satisfaction*	 -0.71	 0.25	 0.017
Physical aspect change* satisfaction*	 0.29 0.18	 -0.51 -0.49	 0.003 0.021
Sleep	0.48	-0.32	0.040

* degrees of change and of satisfaction were weighted by importance.

Finally, the impingement of the treatment group was analyzed. No difference was noted in the degree of importance attributed to items, but a few significant correlations were observed in the satisfaction or change profiles: only 4 parameters correlated with one of the two treatments, when both groups of patients receiving interleukin-2 were pooled together (Table 4). Patients treated with interferon alfa-2a considered 2 aspects unfavorably: food and pain, while interleukin-2 -treated patients gave negative values to their physical aspect and sleep. No significant difference was detected in the other 13 parameters.

Principal component analyses performed according to the degrees of change and of satisfaction weighted by importance gave virtually similar results.

The 4 main components according to the degree of change weighted by importance are indicated in Table 5. They are responsible for 56.7% of the total variance. Aspects of everyday life are gathered in the first component, personal life, social life and external world are mostly included in components 2, 3 and 4, respectively.

The results of the principal component analysis confirm the discrepancy in the physical status of the patients and the concurrent improvement in the relationship aspects (data not shown).

Table 5: Results of the principal component analysis of the degree of change weighed by importance

Component 1 **Everyday life**	*Component 2* **Personal life**	*Component 3* **Social life**	*Component 4* **External world**
Physical abilities Fitness Pain Sleep Food intake Daily activities Leisure activities	Intellectual abilities Sexuality Inner life Physical aspect	Close relationships Relationships Companionship People's attitudes	Money World's affairs

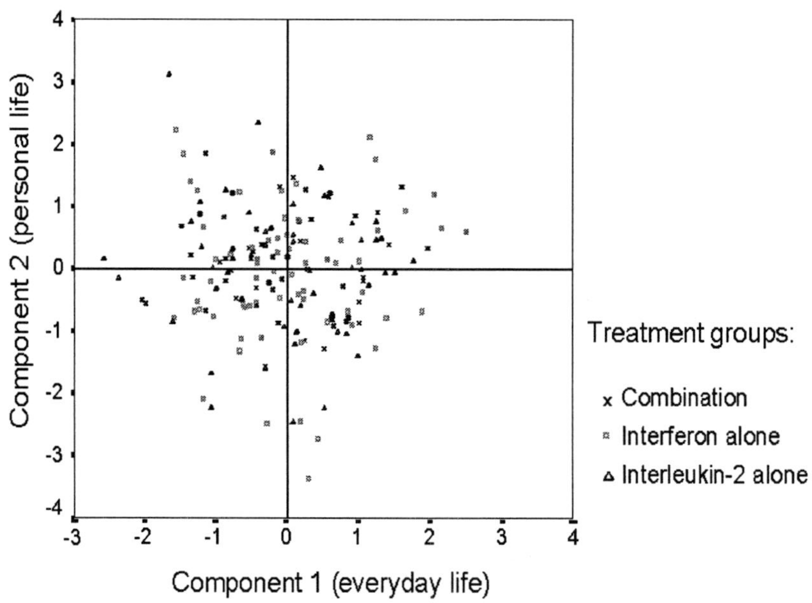

Figure 3: Graphic representation of the patients according to the major 2 components identified by the analysis in terms of change weighted by importance and for each treatment group.

The graphic representation (Figure 3) of the patients plotted according to treatment group within the major two domains identified by the analysis in terms of change, illustrates that no significant difference was observed between treatment groups, since all spots appear to be scattered over the four graph areas.

DISCUSSION

Numerous trials using cytokines were conducted in the past 10 years. They have generated a complete view of cytokine-induced toxicities. Conversely, only few and recent data dealing with the quality of life of patients treated with cytokines are available. Most studies were performed on limited numbers of patients [9-13]. Only one was performed during a large randomized trial [8], but it has only been reported as part of the overall results.

One of the largest phase III trial testing cytokines in patients with MRCC, the CRECY trial, has included the evaluation of quality of life by the way of a self-administered questionnaire as a secondary objective. The major goal of the study was to gain knowledge on the quality of life of patients with limited survival who underwent impairing treatments. Moreover, the group of investigators had initially raised the hypothesis of a better quality of life in patients receiving interferon alfa-2a treatment than in patients treated with intravenous interleukin-2. The toxicity profile of these drugs is clearly different; in addition, interferon alfa-2a is administered at home, while iv. interleukin-2 requires hospitalization and a rigorous management.

When the CRECY trial was designed, no validated quality-of-life questionnaire written in French was available in the literature. We had an opportunity to use the Subjective Quality of Life Profile questionnaire which had previously been used and formalized in French patients [16].

Quality of life was also investigated in another randomized trial performed by investigators from the Medical Research Cancer Group [8]. In this trial, patients with MRCC were randomized to receive subcutaneous interferon alfa-2a for 12 weeks or oral medroxyprogesterone acetate, which was supposed to act somewhat like a placebo treatment, for the same period of time. Approximately half of the 111 patients enrolled returned a quality-of-life questionnaire; a minority of parameters (7/24) were judged significantly different by the patients according to the treatment group they belonged to.

These results could support the hypothesis that advanced disease, as well as cytokine treatment, is responsible for impaired quality of life. This was also the conclusion from another study [13], although on a more limited number of patients with MRCC. This, to our opinion, must be taken into account by the physicians at the time of deciding to use a cytokine treatment.

The second important result of our study is that, conversely to what was expected by the investigators, patients treated with interferon alfa-2a alone did not feel much better than their interleukin-2 -treated counterparts. The results of the univariate analysis, as well as the patients' distribution in the principal component analysis, concordantly show an absence of differences between treatment groups. At least two other reports [12,14] demonstrated the deleterious effect of interferon alfa-2a treatment in these patients. The investigators who had made the hypothesis of a better quality of life in patients receiving ambulatory interferon alfa-2a than in those receiving interleukin-2, had probably based their initial judgement on the significant difference of toxicities induced by each cytokine [7]. As demonstrated by other authors [18-21], if physicians correctly estimate the adverse effects of treatments as well as the performance status of patients, their appraisal of the quality of life of these patients is not so accurate.

Despite these overall negative results some particular points are worth being noted. First, as mentioned by other authors in the past [21,22], younger patients appear to be more affected by their condition than older patients. Second, patients indicated that some aspects of their lives had improved and were judged satisfying: namely, relations with spouse, relatives or others. This can be considered as a positive effect of the disease which induces support from friends or relatives. As previously shown by other authors [23], family concerns are frequently rated as very important by the patients.

The concept of quality of life is complex. Most misunderstandings and difficulties with quality of life studies in medicine arise from uncertainty about which aspects of the concept are being considered: either objective aspects of everyday life (including patient's health status, functional capabilities, or material considerations), or subjective aspects (dealing with the person's own inner experience), or both.

Health-related quality of life is a multidimensional construct encompassing perceptions of both positive and negative aspects of dimensions such as physical, emotional, social, and cognitive functions, as well as the negative symptoms produced by a disease or its treatment. However, the literature provides many examples of studies indexed under the term quality of life, but in which only unidimensional or bidimensional instruments were used [22]. Authors frequently refer to the quality of life of patients in clinical studies in which either physical performance status or psychological well-being was the only dimension measured.

In therapeutic trials, quality of life studies are usually based on a health model, which results in a restrictive view. Therefore, it is important to clearly define the concept of quality of life, since ambiguous concepts may alter the results. The key to this problem is to make a clear distinction between the two components of the quality of life, i.e. subjective and objective. This latter component is the only one considered in the current medical approach. The reference to subjective quality of life would introduce a number of methodological problems that do not exist when only objective quality of life is assessed, and would thus require a specific model that can be derived from the model of life goals used by sociologists[15].

A limitation for European researchers is that most QOL questionnaires are only available in English and tend to focus primarily on health – as their names suggest, i.e., Sickness Impact Profile, Nottingham Health Profile, ... Consequently, researchers recognized the need to develop a mental health QOL instrument that would reflect their specific language and culture. In France, the subjective quality of life profile (SQLP) – a patient administered questionnaire assessing subjective quality of live – was developed. Intuitively, it seems reasonable to assume that since quality of life is a subjective concept, it is the patients' opinions that should be sought. Self-rating by patients is preferable to observer ratings. Generally, physicians or other observers assign lower score to the patients' quality of life than the patients themselves. There is considerable variability in scores among observers [22].

The SQLP was endorsed and tested on more than 13,000 subjects recruited outside of any medical context, and not suffering from any somatic or psychological pathology. It is an evaluation tool that uses a psychometric approach. The patients evaluate their position in relation to their goals in life. It is not the actual distance between their position and goal that is important in this approach, but rather how the patients feel about this distance. At inclusion, the patients are asked to describe the degree of discomfort or satisfaction they experience in different areas of life, and the importance they attach to it. During the follow-up period, the patients are asked their feelings about the changes that occur in these areas and their satisfaction with these changes (or lack of change). The degree of satisfaction is a better expression of subjective quality of life than the change itself.

The results are of interest in several domains. They make it possible 1) to specify the demands and complaints of subjects afflicted, 2) to demonstrate the impact of various factors on quality of life, 3) to observe patients' evolution following long-term or difficult therapy.

The Functional Living Index Cancer (FLIC) instrument [24] comprises 22 items covering psychological, social, vocational and somatic areas. This instrument has been widely used although it has been criticized as being unable to detect differences in clinical trials. The European Organization for Research and Treatment of Cancer (EORTC) developed a core questionnaire for use in cancer which incorporates physical, emotional and social factors [25].

The results of quality of life assessments in oncology can give unexpected results. In some situations, e.g., where treatment is likely to be curative, temporary declines in quality of life related to the treatment are likely to be acceptable to patients in the knowledge that the ultimate result will be an improvement in both quantity and quality of life. If this is true, then such treatment may be considered not to be overly aggressive. However, it is important to ascertain what patients feel about the trade-offs between improvement in quality of life and toxicity where there is a significant potential for long-term side effects that may result in less than an optimum quality of life [22].

Most so-called "quality of life" questionnaires tend to cover mainly the health domain, and questionnaires such as Karnofsky's, which investigates health more than quality of life, tend to be able to show differences between treatment groups in clinical trials.

In conclusion, patients with metastatic renal cancer treated with a less toxic ambulatory treatment do not seem to judge their quality of life much better than patients receiving interleukin-2 on an in-patient basis. We think these results must be taken into account when deciding to treat MRCC patients with cytokines.

Acknowledgments

In addition to previously mentioned authors, the following investigators and centers from the Groupe Français d'Immunothérapie also participated in this study:

Christine Lasset, Frank Chauvin and Thierry Philip (Centre Léon Bérard, Lyon); Thomas Tursz (Institut Gustave Roussy, Villejuif); Jean Peny (Centre François Baclesse, Caen); Mireille Mousseau (Hôpital Michalon, Grenoble); Bernard Coronel (Hôpital E. Herriot, Lyon); Jean-François Rossi (Centre Hospitalier Universitaire, Montpellier); Michel Fabbro

(Centre P. Lamarque Montpellier); Jean-Pierre Bergerat (Centre Hospitalier Universitaire, Strasbourg); Armelle Caty (Centre O. Lambret, Lille); Daniel Baume (Institut P. Calmettes, Marseille); Joël Fleury (Centre J. Perrin, Clermont-Ferrand); Jean-Marc Ferrero, Antoine Thyss (Centre A. Lacassagne, Nice); Rémi Delva (Centre P. Papin, Angers); Nicole Tubiana-Mathieu (Hôpital de la Timone, Marseille); Bruno Coudert and Pierre Fargeot (Centre G.F. Leclerc, Dijon); Thierry Lesimple (Centre E. Marquis, Rennes); Thierry Dorval (Institut Curie, Paris); Marie-Brigitte Orgerie (Hôpital Minjoz, Besançon); Thierry Conroy (Centre A. Vautrin, Nancy); Alain Goupil (Centre R. Huguenin, Saint-Cloud); Elhani Khenifar (Hôpital Saint-Jacques, Besançon); Bruno Audhuy (Centre Hospitalier, Colmar); Jean-Christophe Eymard (Institut J. Godinot, Reims).

We thank Jacqueline Savary and Karine Pignard for their excellent trial monitoring and data management. We acknowledge Ian Tannock, M.D., Ph.D., for helpful advice, and Marie-Dominique Reynaud for editorial assistance.

Financial support: This work was supported by a grant from the Association pour la Recherche contre le Cancer.

REFERENCES

[1] Motzer RJ, Bander NH, Nanus DM. Renal cell carcinoma. *N Engl J Med* 335: 865, 1996.

[2] Elson PJ, Witte RS, Trump DL. Prognostic factors for survival in patients with recurrent or metastatic renal cell carcinoma. *Cancer Res* 48: 7310, 1988.

[3] Pyrhönnen S, Salminen E, Ruutu M, Lehtonen T, Nurmi M, Tammela T, et al. Prospective randomized trial of interferon alfa-2a plus vinblastine versus vinblastine alone in patients with advanced renal cell cancer. *J Clin Oncol* 17: 859, 1999.

[4] Rosenberg SA, Yang JC, White DE, Steinberg SM. Durability of complete responses in patients with metastatic cancer treated with high-dose interleukin-2: identification of the antigens mediating response. *Ann Surg* 228: 307, 1998.

[5] Fyfe GA, Fisher RI, Rosenberg SA Sznol M, Parkinson DR, Louie AC. Long-term response data for 255 patients with metastatic renal cell carcinoma treated with high-dose recombinant interleukin-2. *J Clin Oncol* 14: 2410, 1996.

[6] Négrier S, Maral J, Drevon M, Vinke J, Escudier B, Philip T. Long-term follow-up of patients with metastatic renal cell carcinoma treated with intravenous recombinant interleukin-2 in Europe. *Cancer J Sci Am* 6: S93, 2000.

[7] Négrier S, Escudier B, Lasset C, Douillard JY, Savary J, Chevreau C, et al. Recombinant human interleukin-2, recombinant human interferon alfa-2a, or both in metastatic renal-cell carcinoma. *N Engl J Med* 338: 1272, 1998.

[8] Medical Research Council Renal Cancer Collaborators. Interferon-α and survival in metastatic renal carcinoma: early results of a randomised controlled trial. *Lancet* 353: 14, 1999.

[9] Heinzer H, Mir TS, Huland E, Huland H. Subjective and objective prospective, long-term analysis of quality of life during inhaled interleukin-2 immunotherapy. *J Clin Oncol* 17: 3612, 1999.

[10] Kroger MJ, Menzel T, Gschwend JE, Bergmann L. Life quality of patients with metastatic renal cell carcinoma chemo-immunotherapy, a pilot study. *Anticancer Res* 19: 1553, 1999.

[11] Litwin MS, Fine JT, Dorey F Figlin RA, Belldegrun AS. Health related quality of life outcomes in patients treated for metastatic kidney cancer: a pilot study. *J Urol* 157: 1608, 1997.

[12] Wong M, Goldstein D, Woo H, Testa G, Gurney H. Alpha-interferon 2a and 13-cis-retinoic acid for the treatment of metastatic renal cell carcinoma. *Intern Med* 32:158, 2002.

[13] Cohen L, de Moor C, Parker PA, Amato RJ. Quality of life in patients with metastatic renal cell carcinoma participating in a phase I trial of an autologous tumor-derived vaccine. *Urol Oncol* 7:119, 2002.

[14] Motzer RJ, Murphy JA, Bacik J, Schwartz LH, Nanus DM, Mariani T, et al. Phase III trial of interferon alfa-2a with or without 13-cis-retinoic acid for patients with advanced renal cell carcinoma. *J Clin Oncol* 18:2972, 2000.

[15] Gerin P, Dazord A, Boissel J, Chifflet R. Quality of life assessment in therapeutic trials: rationale for and presentation of a more appropriate instrument. *Fundam Clin Pharmacol.* 1992;6(6):263-76.

[16] Dazord A. Quality of life assessment in medicine. Presentation of a new instrument (SQLP: subjective quality of life profile) and first results. *Eur Respirat Rev* 5: 66, 1995.

[17] Bonomi AE, Patrick DL, Bushnell DM, Martin M. Validation of the United States' version of the World Health Organization Quality of Life (WHOQOL) instrument. *J Clin Epidemiol.* 2000 Jan; 53(1): 1-12.

[18] Slevin ML, Stubbs L, Plant HJ, Wilson P, Gregory WM, Armes PJ, Downer SM. Attitudes to chemotherapy: comparing views of patients with cancer with those of doctors, nurses, and general public. *Br Med J* 300: 1458, 1990.

[19] Olver IN, Matthews JP, Bishop JF, Smith RA. The roles of patient and observer assessments in anti-emetic trials. *Eur J Cancer* 30A: 1223, 1994.

[20] Bjordal K, Freng A, Thorvik J, Kaasa S. Patient self-reported and clinician rated quality of life in head and neck cancer patients; a cross sectional study. *Eur J Cancer* 31B: 340, 1995.

[21] Kahn SB, Houts PS, Harding SP. Quality of life and patients with cancer: A comparative study of patients versus physicians perceptions and its implications for cancer education. *J Cancer Educ* 7: 241, 1992.

[22] Osoba D. Lessons learned from measuring health-related quality of life in Oncology. *J Clin Oncol* 12: 608, 1994.

[23] Waldron D, O'Boyle C, Kearney M, Moriarty M, Carney D. Quality of life measurement in advanced cancer: assessing the individual. *J Clin Oncol* 17: 3603, 1999.

[24] Schipper H, Clinch J, Powell V. *Definition and conceptual issues*. Quality of life assessments in clinical trials. B. Spilker Ed. Raven Press Ltd. New York, 1990.

[25] Aaronson NK, Ahmedzai S, Bergman B, Bullinger M, Cull A, Duez NJ, Filiberti A, Flechtner H, Fleishman SB, de Haes JC, et al. The European Organization for Research and Treatment of Cancer QLQ-C30: a quality-of-life instrument for use in international clinical trials in oncology. *J Natl Cancer Inst.* 1993 Mar 3;85(5):365-76.

In: Trends in Kidney Cancer Research
Editor: Kelvin R. Nunez, pp. 119-132
ISBN 1-59454-141-8

Chapter IX

Implementation of a Web-Based Clinical Pathway for Radical Nephrectomy to Improve Health Outcomes

Phei Lang Chang,* Ke Hung Tsui, Sheng Hui Lee, Chien Lun Chen, Biing Yir Shen and Mei Yin Lin

Department of Surgery, Division of Geriatric Urology,
Chang Gung Bioinformatics Center, Chang Gung Memorial Hospital,
Chang Gung University, Taipei, Taiwan

Abstract

Radical nephrectomy is a conventional method of treating patients with renal cell carcinoma. The implementation of clinical pathways has been used to monitor health outcomes. Recently, many advantages of web-based technologies have been reported. Therefore, this study develops a web-based clinical pathway for radical nephrectomy and applies it to improve patient care quality.

The web-based clinical pathway for radical nephrectomy was a daily special form that scheduled consultation, discharge plan, elimination, medication, nutrition, psychosocial support, teaching, laboratory test, treatment, and variance times. Daily patient activities were tracked via the web-based clinical pathway. The clinical pathway variations were identified and recorded using the Internet. Following patient discharge, the web-based clinical pathway was completed and the results were stored on the web server. The analyzed data, including variations, then were e-mailed to the clinical physicians and nurses for reference.

* Corresponding author: Phei Lang Chang, M.D., Chair, Department of Surgery, Professor, Department of Urology, Director, Chang Gung Bioinformatics Center, Chang Gung Memorial Hospital, No. 5, Fu-Shing Street, Kweishan, Taoyuan 333, Taiwan. TEL: 886-3-3281200-2137; FAX: 886-3-3274541; E-mail: henryc@cgmh.org.tw

From July 2000 to August 2001, 63 consecutive patients with renal cell carcinoma were treated using the web-based clinical pathway for radical nephrectomy. After implementing the web-based clinical pathway, the mean hospital stay reduced significantly from 11.4 to 9.9 ($p = 0.0063$) days compared to before clinical pathway implementation. Average admission charges also reduced significantly ($p = 0.0075$). The percentage of patients with variances reduced from 38.3% to 23.8% ($p = 0.232$) compared to the first-year paper-based pathway. Notably, no significant differences were noted in variances between the web-based and paper-based pathways. However, the variance detection time in the web-based implementation was significantly ($p = 0.0162$) less than that in the paper-based pathway.

A previous report confirmed the improvement in care quality when using a paper-based clinical pathway. The web-based clinical pathway improved care quality by a quantity equal to that reported for the paper-based pathway in 2002. In this study, one of the four quality indicators was continuously improved ($p = 0.0006$) in the implementing web-based pathway. Additionally, the web-based clinical pathway captured the data directly in an electronic format, facilitating and accelerating analysis.

Implementation of a web-based clinical pathway for radical nephrectomy can improve health outcomes by reducing mean hospital stay and average admission charges, and by improving care quality. Such a web-based pathway is as efficient as the paper-based pathway. However, the web-based clinical pathway is superior to the paper-based pathway in variance detection.

INTRODUCTION

History

The New England Medical Center in Boston and the Hillcrest Medical Center in Tulsa have pioneered efforts to implement clinical pathways [1, 2]. They described their managed care strategy as a project management tool based on particularly standards of care. At Hillcrest, the clinical pathway was designed to guide patient care. Recently, the main goal of clinical pathways implementation has been used to reduce system failures, enhance collaboration among health care team members and minimize unnecessary variations in patient care practices [3-5].

Clinical pathways were created based on a multidisciplinary model, and patient care under pathways was performed in a standard way. Many variations were noted when the process defined in the clinical pathway was compared with actual practice. These variations cause differences in practical decisions that exert varying influences on health outcomes. Clinical pathways have been implemented in various fields [6-9]. This methodology aims to identify and reduce variations in clinical results. Clinical pathway implementation has been shown to reduce average length of hospital stay (LOS) and admission charges for many procedures and diseases [10-12]. Most organizations are interested in implementing clinical pathways to manage their clinical care processes. Moreover, various clinical pathways have been implemented in home health care, perioperative services, and ambulatory care [13, 14].

In January 1995, a Clinical Pathway Development Team (CPDT) was established to design the Clinical Pathways at Chang Gung Memorial Hospital (CGMH). CGMH, located in Lin-Kou, is a medical center close to Taipei city, equipped with around 3,600 beds. The Department of Urology of CGMH has been running a Clinical Pathway for Transurethral Resection of Prostate (TURP) since February 1995. Favorable results were reported for implementing a clinical pathway for TURP [15]. Since April 1997, the CPDT has progressively designed 18 clinical pathways for urological surgeries. Improving urological practice performances and facilitating medical care following the implementation of the 18 clinical pathways has been reported in 2002 [16]. From our previous study, we believe that continued implementation of the clinical pathway can continuously improve the practices of physicians [17].

Web-Based Technologies

Recently, web-based technologies have been used in the field of medical information. Accordingly, the quantity of retrievable medical information available on the web has grown. Numerous web-based education systems have been developed for physicians, nurses, and patients [18-20]. These web-based technologies provide a tool for communication among physicians, nurses, and patients [21, 22]. Numerous advantages have been reported for web-based medical information [23-25]. In implementing clinical pathways, nurses must review the daily activities of patients and make records on the sheet of the clinical pathway. Computerization of the records for clinical pathway implementation can increase the accuracy of such records and reduce the error rate. Therefore, in July 2000, a web-based clinical pathway for radical nephrectomy was developed and implemented to enhance health outcomes.

Radical nephrectomy is the primary treatment for localized renal cell carcinoma. 26]. This investigation selected radical nephrectomy for clinical pathway study because it is one of the relatively high volume diagnostic-related groups used in our department. A paper-based clinical pathway for radical nephrectomy was developed in 1997. Moreover, differences in health outcomes between web-based and paper-based implementations of a clinical pathway for radical nephrectomy were reported in 2002 [21]. The present study evaluate health outcomes before and after the implementation of web-based clinical pathways for radical nephrectomy.

Materials and Methods

From April 1997 to June 2000, patients with renal cell carcinoma were treated using a paper-based clinical pathway for radical nephrectomy. Furthermore, a web-based clinical pathway for radical nephrectomy was developed and implemented from July 2000 to August 2001. This study compares the LOS, admission charges, variances, and quality indicators in the obtained results both before and after the implementation of the web-based clinical pathway for radical nephrectomy.

Patients

Patients were classified into five groups: (1) those treated with radical nephrectomy in the year preceding implementation of the clinical pathway (April 1996-March 1997); (2) those treated with the first-year paper-based pathway from April 1997 to March 1998; (3) those treated with the second-year paper-based pathway from April 1998 to March 1999; (4) those treated with the third-year paper-based pathway from May 1999 to June 2000; (5) those treated with the web-based pathway from July 2000 to August 2001.

Web-Based Clinical Pathway

The web-based clinical pathway was developed using Active Server Pages (ASP), Structured Query Language (SQL) Server 7.0, and the hypertext markup language used on the Web (HTML). Figure 1 displays the special form of web-based clinical pathway for radical nephrectomy. This pathway included daily special forms of time schedule for patient activities, consultation, discharge plan, elimination, medications, nutrition, psychosocial support, teaching, laboratory tests, treatments, and variance. Special education was provided for regular nurses in urological wards to help them familiarize themselves with the web-based clinical pathway for radical nephrectomy.

Clinical Pathway Implementation

Generally, all preoperative laboratory tests were performed immediately following patient admission to hospital. In the urological ward, an assigned nurse educated the patient and his/her family members, including education regarding likely treatment outcomes. The nurse reviewed the daily patient activities and made records on the web-based clinical pathway for radical nephrectomy. When variation existed between the web-based clinical pathway and actual management, the assigned nurse was expected to either resolve the variance immediately or alternatively to record it on the pathway. The ward nurses were separated into three groups according to working time: group 1 (from 8 am to 4 pm), group 2 (from 4 pm to 12 am), and group 3 (from 12 am to 8 am). Patients' activities were recorded on the web-based clinical pathway mainly by the nurses in group 2 and the records were checked by nurses in group 3.

Radical nephrectomy was generally performed on the second admission day. The intravenous fluid was generally started during the early morning of the day of surgery and discontinued postoperatively one day after the patients started on a diet. In the implementation of web-based clinical pathway, the daily record was completed and sent to the web server everyday, and could not be changed. Following patient discharge, the nurse completed the clinical pathway, including the variance. Subsequently, the variances were discussed in regular meetings. The CPDT then analyzed the treatment data. The data was stored on the web server, and analytical results were e-mailed to the clinical physicians and nurses for reference.

Radical nephrectomy	**Day 1**	**Day 2**	**Day 3**	**Day 4**	**Day 5**	**Day 6**	**Day 7**	**Day 8**	**Day 9**
Activity		Bed rest	Ambulate with assistance	Ambulate independently	Cont.	Cont.	Cont.	Cont.	D/C
Consults	Anesthesia permit Nursing preparation Op. permit	Consult R/T			Dietary				Discharge
Discharge planning	Admit assessment							Review discharge instructions	
Elimination	Fleet enema			Supp. prn	Cont.	Cont.	Cont.	Cont.	D/C
Medications	Send antibiotics to OR with patient CM	Analgesics IM IV Antibiotics Foley care	Cont. Cont. Cont.	Cont. Cont. D/C	Cont.(oral) Cont.(oral) Laxative	Cont. Cont. Cont.	Cont. Cont. Cont.	Cont. Cont. Cont.	D/C D/C D/C D/C
Nutrition	NPO since midnight	NPO	NPO	NPO	Diet as tolerated after flatus passage	Cont.	Cont.	Cont.	D/C
Psychosocial support	Pat./family support	Cont.	Cont.	Cont.	Cont.	Cont.	Cont.	Cont.	D/C
Teaching	Orientation Pre/post-op education	Cont. D/C	Cont.	Cont.	Cont.	Cont.	Cont.	Cont.	Review discharge medications Review discharge instruction F/U appoi.
Tests	CBC/DC U/A BUN Cr GOT Sugar PT APTT Chest PA EKG	Ht Hb K prn Sugar prn Cr prn	Ht prn Hb prn Sugar prn Cr prn						
Treatments	Weight Vital sign IV fluid Prepare blood	D/C q1hx2, q2hx2, q4h IV fluid On NG tube prn Record I/O q8h On Foley	q8h Cont. Cont. Cont. Cont.	Ordinary Cont. Cont. Cont. Remove Foley Remove Penrose	Cont. Cont. Remove NG prn D/C	D/C D/C			Remove stitches
Variance									

Figure 1. Special form of web-based clinical pathway for radical nephrectomy

Variances

Variances were defined as deviations from the clinical pathway, which will alter the outcomes. For comparison, this study classified variances as in previous studies. Patient-related variances included psychosocial delays, changing clinical regimen, and clinical complications. Moreover, physician-related variances included nurse delay, physician ordered delay, and support service delay. Additionally, hospital-related variances included equipment workload and breakdown. Finally, discharge variances included service non-availability, inadequate home support, and unresolved health concerns.

Our previous investigation compared the undetected, correctable, and uncorrectable variances between implementing the third-year paper-based and web-based clinical pathways [25]. Undetected variances were defined as those discovered following patient discharge. Meanwhile, correctable variances were defined as those that can be corrected by an assigned nurse immediately without influencing health outcomes. Uncorrectable variances were defined as those that cannot be corrected or are obsolete. Finally, variance detection time was defined as the period from the scheduling time until identification of variance.

Care Quality

Continued implementation of the paper-based clinical pathway for radical nephrectomy was reported to continuously enhance care quality [17]. The eight quality indicators used in this investigation included: (1) the percentage of patients with incomplete preoperative tests on admission day; (2) the percentage of patients to whom fluid was intravenously administered for over one day following their starting on a diet postoperatively; (3) the percentage of patients requiring acute pain management for over 24 hours postoperatively; (4) the percentage of patients requiring intravenous antibiotic administration for over four days; (5) the percentage of patients undergoing postoperative blood transfusion; (6) the percentage of patients with complications; (7) the percentage of patients suffering in-hospital mortality; and (8) the percentage of patients readmitted within two weeks of discharge. Implementation of a web-based clinical pathway for radical nephrectomy was also reported to improve care quality as much as a paper-based clinical pathway [25]. The six quality indicators used included: (1) the percentage of patients to whom fluid was intravenously administered for over one day following their starting on a diet postoperatively; (2) the percentage of patients with Foley catheterization for over three days postoperatively; (3) the percentage of patients with drainage tube insertion exceeding five days; (4) the percentage of patients experiencing complications; (5) the percentage of patients suffering in-hospital mortality; and (6) the percentage of patients readmitted within two weeks of discharge. This study used four quality indicators to compare care quality before and after using the web-based clinical pathways. These four quality indicators included: (1) the percentage of patients to whom fluid was intravenously administered for over one day following their starting on a diet postoperatively; (2) the percentage of patients with complications; (3) the percentage of in-hospital mortality; and (4) the percentage of patients readmitted within two weeks of discharge. Table 1 lists the quality indicators in detail.

Table 1. The Quality Indicators Used for Evaluation of Clinical Pathway for Radical Nephrectomy

	Quality Indicators
1.	The percentage of patients with incomplete preoperative tests on admission day
2.	The percentage of patients to whom fluid was intravenously administered for over one day following their starting on a diet postoperatively
3.	The percentage of patients requiring acute pain management for over 24 hours postoperatively
4.	The percentage of patients requiring intravenous antibiotic administration for over four days
5.	The percentage of patients undergoing postoperative blood transfusion
6.	The percentage of patients with Foley catheterization for over three days postoperatively
7.	The percentage of patients with drainage tube insertion exceeding five days
8.	The percentage of patients with complications
9.	The percentage of patients suffering in-hospital mortality
10.	The percentage of patients readmitted within two weeks of discharge.

Statistical Analysis

Differences in mean LOS, average admission charges, variances, and quality indicators were determined in the five patient groups. Moreover, a Chi-squared test was used to assess the differences in variances. Analysis of variance (ANOVA) for correlated proportions was also used to measure the statistical significance of differences among the groups. Finally, statistical analysis was performed using commercial software.

RESULTS

The total number of patients in the various groups was 37, 47, 55, 61, and 63 for groups 1 to 5, respectively. The five groups did not differ significantly ($p = 0.608$) in the number of patients undergoing radical nephrectomy. The proportions of men and women ($p = 0.289$) and the mean patient age ($p = 0.574$) also exhibited no statistically significant differences among the groups. The mean LOS was 11.4 days before clinical pathway implementation. The LOS decreased significantly by 14.0% ($p = 0.0048$) following the first year of implementation of paper-based clinical pathway for radical nephrectomy, and by 15.8% ($p = 0.0014$) following the second year of implementation. Moreover, the mean LOS was 10.1 days following the third year implementation of paper-based pathway, and did not differ significantly ($p = 0.3145$) compared to the LOS of the second-year pathway. The mean LOS of patients treated using the web-based clinical pathway was 9.9 days. Notably, the LOS did not differ significantly ($p = 0.6914$) between the web-based and third-year paper-based pathways. However, following implementation of the web-based clinical pathway, the mean hospital stay decreased significantly from 11.4 to 9.9 days ($p = 0.0063$) compared to before clinical pathway implementation. Total admission charges following the first-year of implementation of paper-based clinical pathway decreased significantly (p = 0.001), by 19%, compared to before clinical pathway implementation. Moreover, total admission charges following the second-year of implementation decreased still more significantly (p < 0.0001), by 27.9%, compared to before clinical pathway implementation. After implementing the web-based pathway, the admission charges decreased significantly (p = 0.0075), compared to the results before paper-based pathway implementation. However, the admission charges did not differ significantly (p = 0.7330) between the implementation of the web-based clinical pathway and the third-year of the paper-based pathway. Table 2 lists the details.

Table 2. Demographic Characteristics of Patients, Length of Hospital stay (LOS), and Admission Charges for the Five Study Groups

	Before pathway implementation	1st-year pathway	2nd-year pathway	3rd-year pathway	Web-based pathway	P
No. Patients	37	47	55	61	63	0.608
No. Men	20	21	34	39	38	
No. Women	17	26	21	22	25	
Mean age (range)	58(33-74)	60(32-89)	62(32-91)	58(25-82)	56(19-80)	0.574
LOS (days)	11.4*	9.8	9.6	10.1	9.9	
Admission charges (NT$)	91501†	74151	65981	77512	75178	

* There was significantly different when compared to the 1st-year (p = 0.0048), 2nd-year (p = 0.0014), and web-based (p = 0.0063) pathways.

† There was also different significantly when compared to the 1st-year (p = 0.001), 2nd-year (p < 0.0001), and web-based (p = 0.0075) pathways.

When implementing the web-based pathway, the proportion of patients with variances decreased from 38.3% to 23.8% compared to the first-year paper-based pathway. However, no significant (p = 0.392) difference in variances existed among groups. The most common variances in the implementation of paper-based clinical pathway were patient-related, followed by physician-related, discharge-related and finally hospital-related. However, the discharge variances in the implementation of web-based clinical pathway were less than the hospital-related variances. The number of variances did not differ significantly (p = 0.299) between the paper-based and web-based pathway implementation.

The number of undetected variances in the web-based pathway implementation was significantly (p = 0.0193) less than for the first-year paper-based pathway. The correctable variances were 48.2% in the third-year paper-based pathway implementation and 59.5% in the web-based pathway. Meanwhile, the uncorrectable variances were 29.6% in the third-year paper-based pathway and 33.3% in the web-based pathway. The correctable and uncorrectable variances did not differ significantly (p = 0.7698, p = 0.6059) between the two groups. The average variance detection time in the web-based implementation was 0.48 days, significantly (p = 0.0162) less than in the third-year paper-based pathway. Table 3 details the patients with variances originating from the paper-based and web-based clinical pathways.

The quality indicator, percentage of patients remaining on intravenous fluid administration for over one day after starting on a diet postoperatively, significantly (p = 0.007) improved following the first-year implementation of a paper-based clinical pathway.

Table 3. Patients with Variances from the Clinical Pathways

	1st-year pathway	2nd-year pathway	3rd-year pathway	Web-based pathway	P
Total number of patients with variances	18	11	20	15*	0.392
Patient-related variances	8	6	9	8	0.876
Physician-related variances	2	1	6	3	0.320
Hospital-related variances	3	1	4	3	0.665
Discharge variances	5	3	1	1	0.112
Correctable variances			26(48.2%)	25(59.5%)	0.7698
Uncorrectable variances			16(29.6%)	14(33.3%)	0.6059
Undetected variances			12(22.2%)	3(7.2%)	0.0193
Average variance detection time (days)			0.79	0.48	0.0162

*P = 0.407 compared to the data of the 3rd-year pathway.

The quality indicator improved continuously following the second-year implementation. After implementation of the web-based clinical pathway, the quality indicator improved significantly (p = 0.0006) compared to before paper-based pathway implementation. However, the quality indicator did not differ significantly between the web-based and third-year implementation of the paper-based pathway. Ten patients in each group were intravenously administered fluid for over one day after starting on a diet postoperatively. Meanwhile, the mean period of intravenously administering fluid after starting on a diet postoperatively was 1.18 days in the third-year implementation of the paper-based pathway compared to 1.16 days in the web-based pathway implementation.

Table 4. Quality Indicators for the Five Study Groups

Quality Indicator	Before pathway implementation	1st-year pathway	2nd-year pathway	3rd-year pathway	Web-based pathway
Percentage of patients who had intravenously administered fluid for over one day after starting on a diet postoperatively	31*	14	12	10	10
Percentage of patients with complications	1	1	1	3	2
Percentage of in-hospital mortality	0	0	0	0	0
Percentage of patients readmitted within 2 weeks	1	0	0	0	0

*There was significantly different when compared to the 1st-year (p = 0.007), 2nd-year (p = 0.001), and web-based (p = 0.0006) pathways.

Few surgical complications occurred after radical nephrectomy. The complication rates were too low for statistical comparison, and no in-hospital mortality occurred in these groups. The numbers of patients requiring rehospitalization within two weeks of hospital discharge did not increase after implementing the clinical pathways. Table 4 details the comparisons of quality indicators among these groups.

DISCUSSION

Clinical pathway has been assessed as a tool for monitoring health outcomes, and has emerged as a strategy for enhancing medical care quality [27, 28]. The hospital, patients and family can all benefit from using clinical pathways [29-33]. In our department, the first clinical pathway for TURP has been used for eight years, and the other 17 clinical pathways for urological operations have been implemented for six years. Our previous studies demonstrated that implementing clinical pathways could improve practical results by reducing LOS and average admission charges, and improving the care quality [34].

Many health care providers are now making their medical information available on the World Wide Web (WWW) because this can reduce turnaround times and costs. Moreover, the use of Web-based medical education materials has achieved good results [35-37]. In 2002, it was reported that the implementation of a web-based clinical pathway for radical nephrectomy could improve health outcomes as much as a paper-based clinical pathway. However, the web-based clinical pathway is more accurate and faster than the paper-based pathway in detecting variances [21].

Nurses must review daily patient activities on the Web when implementing web-based clinical pathways for radical nephrectomy. Although most nurses are familiar with personal computers, designing an usable web-based clinical pathway remains challenging. The development of a web-based clinical pathway should focus on increasing functional accessibility [21]. Nurses thus are intensively trained before implementing the web-based clinical pathway for radical nephrectomy. Physicians and health care staffs were educated to familiarize them with the web-based pathway. A personal computer at the urological nurse station was used only for implementing the web-based clinical pathway. Meanwhile, a nurse assigned to a patient can record patient activity on the web-based pathway form at any time. Implementing a web-based clinical pathway is more convenient for nurses than implementing a paper-based pathway.

Patient numbers, proportions of men and women and the mean age of patients who underwent radical nephrectomy did not differ significantly among the five study groups. The demographic characteristics of patients in the web-based clinical pathway for radical nephrectomy group are the same as those of the patients in the paper-based pathway group. The previous report by the authors demonstrated that continued implementation of the paper-based clinical pathway for radical nephrectomy could improve practical results achieved by physicians by reducing the LOS and average admission charges [25]. In this study, the LOS and the admission charges following web-based clinical pathway implementation reduced significantly compared to before paper-based pathway implementation. However, significant differences did not exist between implementing the web-based and the third-year paper-based clinical pathway. Therefore, implementing a web-based clinical pathway for radical nephrectomy can improve health outcomes as much as implementing the paper-based pathway.

Implementing clinical pathways is a complex task. Pathway variances must be analyzed to evaluate their effectiveness. Variances were defined as any deviation from the pathway with the potential to influence health outcomes. Minor deviations were corrected immediately by nurses or surgical residents. Meanwhile, major deviations were recorded and discussed at a subsequent meeting. In the study, less patients in the second-year paper-based pathway had variances than in the first-year pathway. However, the differences were not significant. The total number of patients with variances, and the causes of variances did not differ significantly between the paper-based and web-based clinical pathways. In correctable and uncorrectable variances, the number of patients also did not differ significantly between the third-year paper-based and web-based pathways. However, there were significantly fewer undetected variances with the web-based clinical pathway than with the third-year paper-based pathway. Variance detection time was measured to compare the efficiency of the detection of variances between the implementation of the paper-based and web-based pathways. The average variance detection time in the web-based clinical pathway was significantly less than in the third-year paper-based pathway. In variance detection, the web-based clinical pathway is faster and more accurate than the paper-based pathway. The web-based clinical pathway thus has obvious advantages.

Implementation of clinical pathways is designed mainly to enhance care quality. The continued improvement in the care quality owing to continued implementation of a paper-based clinical pathway was demonstrated in previous investigations [23-25, 34]. This study found that one important indicator of patient care quality displayed improved continuously when web-based clinical pathways were employed. Moreover, previous investigations showed that implementing the web-based clinical pathway for radical nephrectomy improved care quality as much as the paper-based pathway [17].

The goal of care quality improvement is to reduce variations from the clinical pathway by removing the causes of the variations. In improving suitability of clinical pathway implementation, three pathway improvement steps were followed including understanding the pathway, designing improvements and monitoring the results. We discovered ways to improve the clinical process and integrated these improvements into the development of clinical pathway. The CPDT monitored the pathway implementing results using pathway variance data and other sources of outcomes information. The CPDT modified clinical pathway for radical nephrectomy every year.

After implementing the web-based clinical pathway for radical nephrectomy, health care staff, nurses and physicians became familiar with the web-based technologies. The results of implementing the web-based clinical pathway can be disseminated to enhance health care outcomes. Notably, implementing web-based clinical pathways for radical nephrectomy can also offer numerous advantages. For example, nurses can record daily patient activities at any time. Web-based implementation positively influences health outcomes, as does the paper-based clinical pathway. Moreover, any variances in the web-based pathway are easily and quickly identified. Nurses can easily complete the web-based pathway and forward it to the clinical pathway development team. In implementing the web-based clinical pathway for radical nephrectomy, the data are obtained directly in electronic format, facilitating and accelerating analysis.

The analytical results of this study reveal that a web-based clinical pathway for radical nephrectomy can improve health outcomes as much as the paper-based clinical pathway. Furthermore, the web-based clinical pathway is superior to the paper-based pathway in terms of detection of variance.

REFERENCES

[1] Zander, K.: Managed care and nursing case management. In: Patient Care Delivery Models. Edited by G.G. Mayer, M.J. Maddin and E. Lawrenz, M.D. Rockville: *Aspen Publications*, p.38, 1990.

[2] Mckenzie, C.B., Torkelson, N.G. and Holt, M.A. Care and cost: nursing case management improves both. *Nursing Management* 1989; 20:30-4.

[3] Heacock, D. and Brobst, R. A. A multidisciplinary approach to critical path development: a valuable CQI tool. *J Nurs Care Qual* 1994; 8:38-41.

[4] Barnes, R. V., Lawton, L. and Briggs, D. Clinical benchmarking improves clinical paths: experience with coronary artery bypass grafting. *Jt Comm Qual Improv* 1994; 20: 267-76.

[5] Shikiar, M. S. and Marner, P. Selecting financial indices to measure critical path outcomes. *Nursing Management* 1994; 25:58-60.

[6] Richards, J.S., Sonda, L.P., Gaucher, E., Kocan, M.J. and Ross, D.A. Applying critical pathways to neurosurgery patients at the University of Michigan Medical Center. *Qual Lett Healths Lead* 1993; 5:8-10.

[7] Nelson, M.S. Critical pathways in the emergency department. *J Emerg Nurs* 1993; 19:110-4.

[8] Latini, E.E. and Foote, W. Obtaining consistent quality patient care for the trauma patient by using a critical pathway. *Crit Care Nurs Q* 1992; 15:51-5.

[9] Metcalf, E.M. *The orthopedic critical path. Orthop Nurs* 1991 Nov-Dec; 10(6):25-31.

[10] Neidig, J.R., Megel, M.E. and Koehler, K.M. The critical path: an evaluation of the application of nursing case management in the NICU. *Neonatal Netw* 1992; 11:45-52.

[11] Strong, A.G. and Sneed, N.V. Clinical evaluation of a critical path for coronary artery bypass surgery patients. *Prog Cardiovasc Nurs* 1991; 6:29-37.

[12] Fisher AA, Poole RL, Machie R, Tsang C, Baugh N, Utley K, Kerner JA Jr. Clinical pathway for pediatric parenteral nutrition. *Nutr Clin Pract* 1997; 12:76-80.

[13] Gooldy J and Duncan B. Home care's role in clinical pathways. *J Home Health Care Practice* 1994; 6:63-9.

[14] Spath PL. Critical paths: maximizing patient care coordination. *Today's OR Nurse* 1995; 17:13-20.

[15] Chang, P.L., Huang, S.T., Hsieh, M.L., Wang, T.M., Chen, J.I., Kuo, H.H., Chuang, Y.C. and Chang, C.H. Use of the transurethral prostatectomy clinical path to monitor health outcomes. *J Urol* 1997; 157:177-83.

[16] Chang PL, Lee SHH, Hsieh ML, Huang ST, Tsui KH, Lai RH. Improvement of practice performance in urological surgery via clinical pathway implementation. World *J Urol* 2002; 20:213-8.

[17] Chang PL, Wang TM, Huang ST, Hsieh ML, Chuang YC, Chang CH. Improvement of health outcomes after continued implementation of a clinical pathway for radical nephrectomy. *World J Urol* 2000; 18:417-21.

[18] Dgawa H, Yonezawa Y, Maki H, Hahn AW, Caldwell WH. A web-based home helper support system. *Biomed Sci Instrum* 2001; 37:95-9.

[19] Relan A, Uijdehaage S. Web-based assessment for students' testing and self-monitoring. *Acad Med* 2001 May; 76(5):551.

[20] Demiris G, Finkelstein SM, Speedie SM. Considerations for the design of a Web-based clinical monitoring and educational system for elderly patients. *J Am Med inform Assoc* 2001; 8:468-72.

[21] Baldwin CD, Gephart D, Maulitz R. Collaborative planning of a web-based learning resource for primary care education. *Acad Med* 2001 May; 76(5):549-50.

[22] Schleyer TKL, Forrest JL. Methods for the design and administration of Web-based surveys. *J Am Med Inform Assoc* 2000; 7:416-25.

[23] Embi PJ, Bowen JL, Singer E. A web-based curriculum to improve residents' education in outpatient medicine. *Acad Med* 2001 May; 76(5):545.

[24] Dornan T, Lee C, Stopford A. Skills base: a web-based electronic learning portfolio for clinical skills. *Acad Med* 2001 May; 76(5):542-2.

[25] Chang PL, Li YC, Lee SH. The differences in health outcomes between Web-based and paper-based implementation of a clinical pathway for redical nephrectomy. *BJU Int* 2002; 90:522-8.

[26] Robson CJ. Radical nephrectomy for renal cell carcinoma. *J Urol* 1963; 89:37-42.

[27] Strassner L. Critical pathways: the next generation of outcomes tracking. *Orthoped Nurs suppl.* 1997; 16:56-61.

[28] Archer SB, Burnett RJ, Flesch LV, Hobler SC, Bower RH, Nussbaum MS, Fischer JE. Implementation of a clinical pathway decreases length of stay and hospital charges for patients undergoing total colectomy and ileal pouch/anal anastomosis. *Surgery.* 1997; 122:699-705.

[29] Cohen J, Stock M, Andersen P, Everts E. Critical pathways for head and neck surgery. Development and implementation. *Arch Otolaryngol Head Neck Surg* 1997; 123:11-4.

[30] Colucciello ML, Mangles LM. Clinical pathways in subcuate care settings. *Nurs Manage* 1997; 28:52-4.

[31] Lykins TC. Nutrition support clinical pathways. *Nutr Clin Pract* 1996; 11:16-20.

[32] Coffey RJ, Richards JS, Remmert CS, LeRoy SS, Schoville RR, Baldwin PJ. An introduction to critical paths. *Qual Manage Health Care* 1992; 1:45-54.

[33] Mateo MA, Newton C. Managing variances in case management. *Nurs Case Management* 1996; 1:45-51.

[34] Chang PL, Wang TM, Huang ST, Hsieh ML, Tsui KH, Lai RH. Effects of implementation of 18 clinical pathways on costs and quality of care among patients undergoing urological surgery. *J Urol* 1999; 161:1858-62.

[35] Branger PJ, Duisterhout JS. Communication in health care. *Meth Inform Med* 1995; 34:244-52.

[36] Berry E, Parker-Jones C, Jones RG, Harkin PJR, Horsfall HO, Nicholls JA, Cook NJA. Systematic assessment of World Wide Web materials for medical education: online, cooperative peer review. *J Am Med inform Assoc* 1998; 5:382-9.

[37] Hersh WR, Junium K, Mailhot M, Tidmarsh P. Implementation and evaluation of a medical informatics distance education program. *J Am Med inform Assoc* 2001; 8:570-84.

In: Trends in Kidney Cancer Research
Editor: Kelvin R. Nunez, pp. 133-158

ISBN 1-59454-141-8

Chapter X

SURGICAL MANAGEMENT OF RENAL CELL CARCINOMA WITH INFERIOR VENA CAVA TUMOR THROMBUS AND REVIEW OF THE LITERATURE

Sadi Kaplan*
Department of Thoracic and Cardiovascular Surgery, Faculty of Medicine, Hacettepe University, Ankara, Turkey
Department of Cardiovascular Surgery, Yuksek Ihtisas Hospital of Turkey, Ankara, Turkey
Sinan Ekici
Department of Urology, Faculty of Medicine, Hacettepe University, Ankara, Turkey

ABSTRACT

Background: The successful excision of a renal cell carcinoma (RCC) invading the inferior vena cava (IVC) remains a technical intraoperative challenge and requires careful preoperative surgical management planning. Although a radical operation remains the mainstay of the therapy for RCC, optimal management of patients with RCC causing IVC tumor thrombus remains unresolved. In this chapter, we review our experience over the past 12 years with 18 patients who had RCC causing IVC tumor thrombus.

Methods: Between July 1990 and October 2001, 18 patients with RCC with IVC tumor thrombus underwent surgical treatment. The mean patient age was 54.2 years and the male to female ratio was 1. The cephalad extension of the tumor was infrahepatic in 9 patients, intrahepatic in 6, and suprahepatic with right atrial extension in 3 patients. All

* Corresponding author: Sadi Kaplan, M.D, Dedeefendi Altay sok, 4/11, Kurtulus, 06600, Ankara, Turkey. Tel: +90-312-433-8801; Fax: +90-312-229-0148; E-mail address: skaplan@bir.net.tr

tumors were resected via the inferior vena cava isolation and, when necessary, extended hepatic mobilization and Pringle maneuver, with primary or patch closure of the vena cavotomy. Cardiopulmonary bypass (CPB) and deep hypothermic circulatory arrest (DHCA) were used in 3 patients.

Results: The mortality rate was 5.5 % (1 patient was lost on the 11th postoperative day). Complications occurred in 5 patients. The remaining 17 patients (94.4 %) were successfully discharged from the hospital. Two of them died of tumor progression at the 43rd and 54th postoperative months. The 10-year Kaplan-Meier survival estimate was 75.6, with a mean follow-up of 64.1 months. The presence of lymph node metastases and perinephric spread seemed to possess an adverse effect on the survival in our patients. Although the groups in this series included small numbers of patients, there was no significant difference in survival with regard to the different levels of tumor thrombus extension into the vena cava.

Conclusions: Surgical treatment is the preferred approach to patients with RCC and IVC tumor thrombi as it provides markedly better results when compared with the other therapeutical modalities. Our experience confirms that RCC with extension into the IVC is a potentially curable condition provided complete removal is achieved. The level of extension of the tumor thrombus dictates the surgical techniques used for successful removal of the tumor thrombus. The treatment of patients with caval involvement and metastatic disease at presentation needs to be carefully individualized. We believe that complete surgical excision of the tumor and the resulting thrombus and metastases, if present, with appropriate preoperative staging and a well-planned surgical approach, using CPB and DHCA when necessary, provide an acceptable long-term survival with a good quality of life expectation.

Keywords: Renal cell carcinoma; tumor thrombus; vena cava invasion; renal tumor metastases; surgery; experience; prognosis.

INTRODUCTION

Renal cell carcinoma (RCC) is the most common malignancy arising in the adult kidney, representing 2% of all malignancies and 2% of cancer-related deaths [1, 2]. It is a clinicopathologically heterogeneous disease, subdivided into clear, papillary, granular, spindle, and mixed cell variants based on cytoplasmic features [3]. Although there can be some variations, the prognosis of RCC is mainly based on tumor staging and histological grading [4], and patients with metastatic RCC (30% of all RCC cases) have a life expectancy averaging around 12 months [5,6]. Lung and bones are the most common sites of metastases. Lung lesions are seen in up to 60% of patients with metastases and bone lesions are seen in up to 40% [7], as 20% with concomitant improvements in cancer specific survival [8]. However, currently it is not clear whether the basic biology underlying either the pattern of metastatic spread or the specific site of metastatic disease leads to differences in the response to therapy or predicts eventual differences. Unfortunately, to date there is little understanding of the underlying molecular mechanisms that cause this variety in prognoses [9].

Renal cell carcinoma is an unusual cancer with the propensity to invade not only the renal vein but to propagate into the inferior vena cava (IVC) as a tumor thrombus. The tumor thrombus occasionally extends to the infrarenal IVC. Vena cava involvement by intraluminal extension of tumor mass has been reported to occur in 4% to 10% of patients with renal neoplasms [10-14]. This intracaval extension of tumor thrombus is rather unique, because in the majority of cases, it just extends along the cava without involvement of the wall and has no bearing on distant spread or survival. Although such intravascular growth implies a heightened biologic behavior of the tumor, the presence of a tumor thrombus associated with RCC has not been shown to be a determinant of survival when treated surgically [10, 13, 15-17]. But when present and if not treated, these patients have unfortunately poor survival rates [18]. Previous reports have shown that total resection of this tumor affords the best chance of cure and long-term survival when no distant metastases are present [10, 13, 19]. However, recent reports recommend surgical treatment even in the presence of distant metastases [9, 17, 20-22]. Hence, in the absence of effective alternative treatment, complete surgical removal of the primary tumor with its extension along the vena cava is the only hope for a potential cure. For this reason, an aggressive approach for resection has been advocated for several decades and has remained the mainstay of treatment.

The diagnosis of vena caval invasion and the level of tumoral extension in RCC are important determinants when planning the surgical approach. If present, certain clinical manifestations may indicate complete occlusion of the vena cava by tumor thrombus [23]. However most often the tumor thrombus is nonobstructive or sufficient collaterals have developed so that these signs are seldom detected [13, 19, 23, 24]. Because of that, the diagnosis of vena caval invasion and the level of tumoral extension in RCC are mainly based on radiological examinations [17, 20, 23, 25-28]. The superior margin of the tumor in the IVC is the basis for classification, and several different operations have been advocated depending on the proximal extends of tumor thrombus [10, 13, 15, 16, 18, 29-36]. Although there is a great deal of emphasis on the importance of an aggressive surgical approach in the literature, a uniform operative strategy based on the level of the tumor thrombus has not been established. However, during that time, improvement in surgical experience and surgical techniques derived from liver transplant surgery and cardiac arrest with cardiopulmonary bypass (CPB) have drastically decreased morbidity and mortality, and operative complications associated with extensive involvement of the inferior vena cava with tumor thrombus. Traditional surgical approaches have included resection with or without the use of CPB. When the thrombus is located within the IVC (level I), tumor extraction is usually accomplished after proximal and distal control of the IVC. When the thrombus extends into the intrahepatic IVC (level II) or higher to the right atrium (level III), exposure and isolation of the IVC are more extensive, and sometimes requiring mobilization of the liver with or without the use of CPB. In some circumstances, this must be accompanied by deep hypothermic circulatory arrest (DHCA) [15, 20, 31, 35]. CPB is usually required when the tumor thrombus extends into the heart and required atriotomy for removal because it improves control of immediate blood loss and with circulatory arrest allows for tumor removal in a bloodless field [15, 31, 35, 37]. Herein, we reviewed the literature on this issue and present the results of our experience over the past 12 years with 18 patients who had renal cancer extending to the IVC.

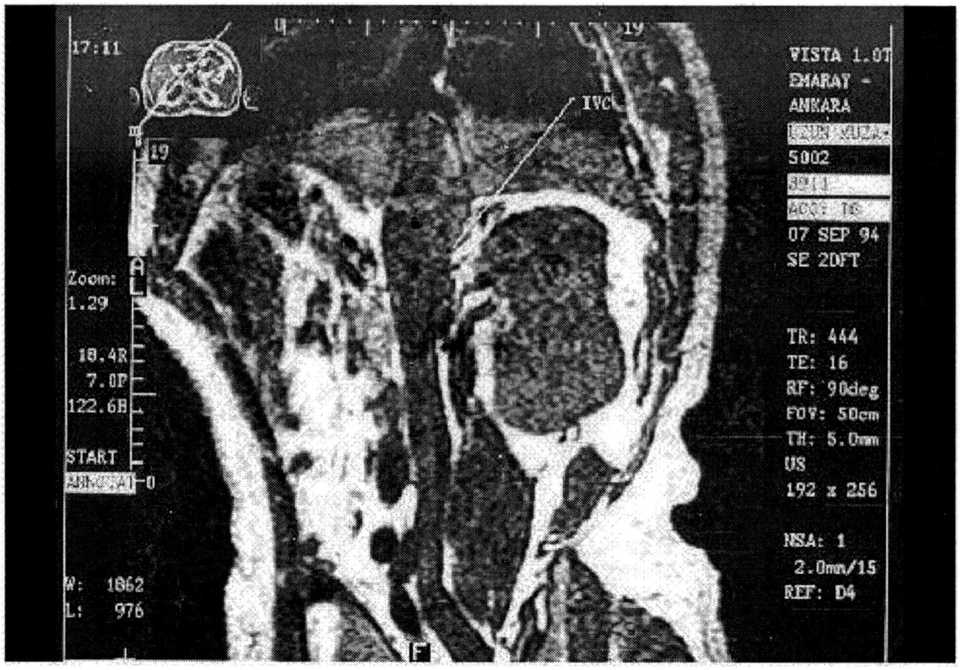

Figure 1. Magnetic resonance image of a suprahepatic inferior vena cava tumor thrombus.

Patients and Methods

From June 1990 to October 2001, a total of 289 patients underwent nephrectomy for cancer at the Hacettepe University Hospital (1990-2001) and the Yuksek Ihtisas Hospital of Ankara (2000-2001). Within this group, 18 patients (6.2 %) had RCC and IVC tumor thrombus. There were 9 males and 9 females, with a mean age of 54.2 years (range 40 to 66 years). The tumor was right sided in 15 patients (83.3 %) and left sided in 3 patients (16.7). All patients presented with symptoms; on initial presentation, 11 patients (61.1 %) had gross or microscopic hematuria, 10 patients (55.5 %) had flank pain, and 9 patients (50 %) had a palpable abdominal mass. The classic triad of hematuria, pain, and lump was present in only 2 patients. None of them had clinical evidence of IVC obstruction. Apart from a detailed history and clinical examination, all patients underwent urine examination for albuminuria, complete biochemistry assessment, and radiological imaging tests to demonstrate the tumor and tumor thrombus. All patients were examined preoperatively with chest radiography, ultrasonography (USG) of the liver and abdomen, chest and abdominal computerized tomography (CT), and isotope bone scan to verify the absence of gross lymph node or metastatic disease. The renal tumor, with its extension to the venous system, was assessed primarily by USG and CT, and in case the tumor thrombus extended above the level of hepatic veins, magnetic resonance imaging (MRI) and echocardiography (ECO) were performed to examine any possible intracardiac extension, and to define the upper limit of the thrombus (Figure 1). Only 2 patients had lung metastases at the time of initial presentation. The levels of tumor thrombus were grouped into three categories according to the extentions of the dissection required to remove the thrombus. The cephalad extension of tumor was infrahepatic (level I) in 9 (50 %) patients, intrahepatic (level II) in 6 (33.3 %) patients, and suprahepatic (level III) in 3 (16.7 %) patients (Figure 2).

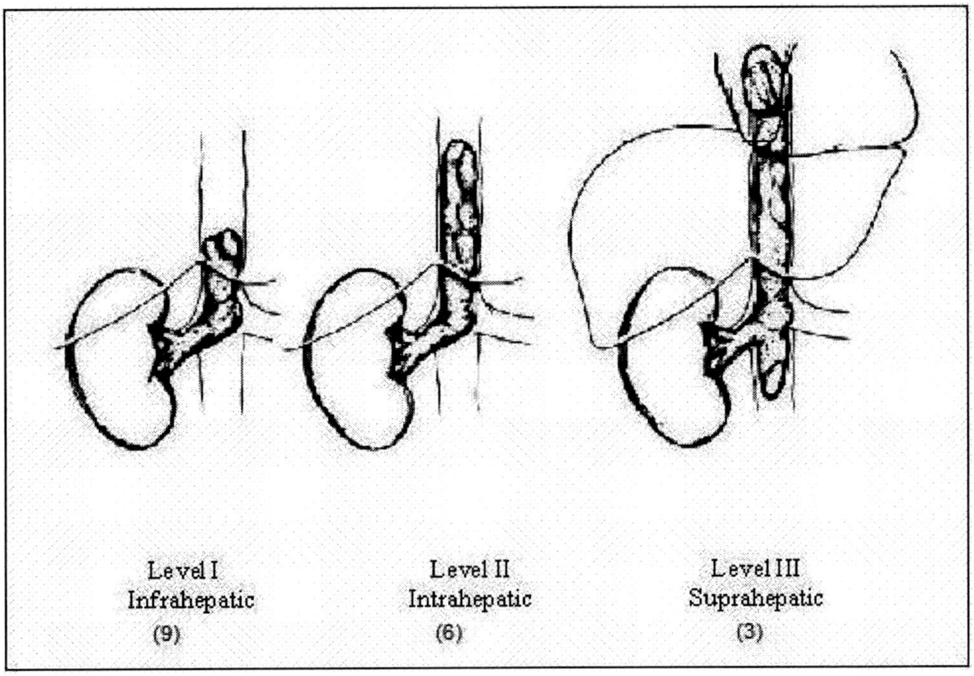

Figure 2. Grouping of 18 patients according to the level of inferior vena cava tumor thrombi.

Surgical Management

In all cases, the renal tumor and IVC tumor thrombus were completely removed. The choice of our surgical approach was dependent upon the categories based on the cephalad extent of the tumor thrombus. The operation was performed through a midline, anterior, abdominal, or chevron incision, and through extended sternotomy in 3 patients for level III tumors. CPB and DHCA were used in 3 patients with level III tumors. Pulmonary metastastectomy was performed in 2 patients, through present sternotomy in 1 and left thoracotomy in the other.

Surgery

The level of extension of the tumor thrombus dictated the surgical techniques used for successful removal of the tumor thrombus. In our experience, a combined team of urology and cardiothoracic - vascular surgeons performed all procedures. For level I tumor, after establishing vascular control of vena cava distal and proximal to the thrombus and the opposite renal vein, vena cavotomy and extraction of tumor thrombus was performed. Partial vena caval resection was performed in 5 patients due to the presence of residual tumor adherent to the IVC wall and high possibility of IVC wall invasion. Patch closure was necessary in 4 of these patients. Regional lymph node resection was performed in 1 patient for the palpable, enlarged, and suspicious-looking lymph nodes and pulmonary metastasectomy was performed in one via left thoracotomy. For level II tumors, control of the IVC above the thrombus at the suprahepatic infradiaphragmatic level was always achieved before any maneuver was performed on the renal vessels. After complete hepatic mobilization, a Pringle's maneuver was performed; the suprahepatic IVC, the infrarenal IVC, the contralateral renal vein, and hepatic vein were occluded in sequence. IVC was opened along its anterolateral aspect to the level of the hepatic veins. The tumor thrombus was removed en bloc as completely as possible, the inferior vena cava was irrigated and adherent tissue was peeled from the endothelial surface. Suture closure began proximally. When the inferior venacavotomy below the hepatic veins was closed, a vascular cross-clamp was applied immediately below the veins across the IVC and across the suture line, the Pringle's maneuver was released, the hepatic vein tourniquet and suprahepatic cross-clamp was removed to minimize hepatic ischemia time. When IVC was closed to the level of the infrarenal segment, cross-clamps were repositioned to allow drainage of the contra lateral renal vein. In 1 patient, partial cavectomy was performed due to the presence of a residual tumor adherent to the IVC wall. Patch closure was needed in this case. The mean liver and renal ischemia time was 17 minutes (range 8 to 26 minutes). It is clear that Level III thrombus in the inferior vena cava still poses a challenge to the surgeon due to its relative inaccessibility. In the literature, it is seen that a thoracoabdominal approach, median sternotomy, cardiopulmonary bypass with profound hypothermia, and circulatory arrest have been used in patients with intracardiac tumor extension and electively in patients with intrahepatic or IVC extension. In our experience, for level III tumor, CPB and DHCA were used in all patients. The surgical technique followed previously described methods [15, 31, 35, 37]. Briefly, during operation, an index finger was inserted through a purse-string–controlled atriotomy to examine the intra atrial extent and the adherence of the tumor thrombus. After confirmation of the right atrial extension of the tumor thrombus, a decision for CPB and DHCA was made. The aorta, the IVC portion below the thrombus, and the right atrium were cannulated, and CPB was instituted with core cooling. An attempt to push the tumor with a finger backward to the abdominal part of the cava is never made, to avoid inadvertent pulmonary embolism. Besides, the dumbbell situation does not allow for such an attempt for tumor removal. In all cases, the renal tumor and the vena caval tumor thrombus could be completely removed. In addition to this, solitary lung metastases were resected in 1 patient. The circulatory arrest time ranged from 14 to 38 minutes, with a mean of 24 minutes. All patients were staged by pathological examination and all tumors were pathologically staged according to the Robson classification system [38]: stage I, tumor confined by renal capsule; stage II, tumor extension to perirenal fat or ipsilateral adrenal but confined to Gerato's fascia; stage IIIa, renal vein or IVC involvement; stage IIIb, lymphatic involvement; stage IIIc, combination of IIIa and IIIb; stage IVa, spread to contiguous organs except ipsilateral adrenal; stage IVb, distant metastases. By virtue of their tumors extending into the renal vein and IVC, all patients in this review had tumors categorized as stage III. Two patients had stage IV disease. A complete blood count, serum biochemistry panel, chest radiograph, bone scan, and abdominal USG and CT were repeated at 6- to 12-month intervals postoperatively. The follow-up interval ranged from 27 to 160 months, with a mean of 64.1

months (5.34 years) and complete follow-up data were obtained for all patients. Cancer-free status was determined by negative findings on these follow-up examinations. Survival times were calculated from date of operation to date of death or last contact and were analyzed by the KaplanMeier method.

RESULTS

In all cases, renal tumor and the vena caval tumor thrombus could be completely removed. As a result of tumor extension into the renal vein or IVC, all patients in this study had stage IIIa, IIIb, or IVb tumors according to the Robson classification. More specifically, sixteen patients had stage III and 2 patients had stage IV renal cell carcinoma. Preoperative evaluation with USG and CT raised suspicion for renal vein and vena caval invasion by tumor thrombi in all cases. In three cases, the upper level could not be visualized; therefore MRI and ECO were used for confirmation of the upper extent of intracaval tumor thrombus. Mean renal tumor size measured by CT was 77.8 mm (range from 30 to 120 mm) and there was no correlation between the renal tumor size, stage, location, and the level of the tumor thrombus. Pathological study of the surgical specimens confirmed RCC along with the inferior vena caval tumor thrombus. Further histopathological study revealed capsular penetration of the tumor in 2 patients and perinephric fat involvement in 2 patients. The enlarged retroperitoneal lymph nodes resected at the time of operation, was positive for renal cell carcinoma in one patient. The excised metastatic lung nodules, which were detected preoperatively, contained RCC in two patients. Local caval resection was performed in 6 patients, necessitating patch closure in 5 of them. Histopathological study confirmed that two of these 6 patients had tumor invasion of the inferior vena cava wall. Unfortunately, in our study, IVC wall invasion, perinephric spread and retroperitoneal lymph node metastases could not be recognized by preoperative radiological examinations. Complications occurred in 5 patients; one patient developed profound hypotension with the induction of anesthesia, resulting in hypoxic encephalopathy, and died at the 11th postoperative day. Liver laceration in one patient, wound infection in one patient, ileus in one patient and mediastinal bleeding requiring immediate reoperation in another with the resultant prolonged ventilatory support were the other major important complications. Transient renal insufficiency was observed in several patients but none of them required dialysis.

Surgicopathological Findings and Survival According to the Levels

Of 9 level I patients, 7 patients had tumors confined to the kidney, but 1 patient had tumoral invasion of the IVC wall, as confirmed by pathological study of the specimens. He is alive and free of disease at 160 months postoperatively. One patient had perinephric spread and solitary lung metastases, and the tumor relapsed in the lungs and bones 20 months after surgery. He received immunotherapy with interferon and died at 43 months after surgery. The remaining patient had retroperitoneal lymph node metastases and perinephric spread. The tumor relapsed in the lungs and liver at 32 months after surgery she received radiotherapy and immunotherapy after a second metastatectomy, but died at 54 months postoperatively. Currently, 7 of 9 patients (77.8 %) are alive and disease free between 27 to 160 months (mean 55.6 months). There were 6 level II patients, who had tumors confined to the kidney. However, one patient had tumoral invasion of the IVC wall, as confirmed by pathological study of the specimens. He is alive and free of disease at 28 months postoperatively. Currently, all of the patients from this group are still alive and disease free between 27 and 160 months (mean 70.5 months). There were 3 level III patients who had tumors confined to the kidney; and there were solitary lung metastases in 1, diagnosed preoperatively by CT, resected, and confirmed by pathological study of the specimens. He died at the 11th postoperative day of hypoxic encephalopathy and after complications. The other 2 patients (66.7 %) are alive and disease free between 110 and 136 months (mean 123 months). The mean operation time for the 18 patients was 3 hours 12 minutes (range 1.5 to 5.5 hours), and the mean circulatory arrest time was 24 minutes (range 14 to 38). The average blood unit number transfused perioperatively was 4.1 units (range 1 to 9 units). When one exceptional case was excluded, the mean intensive care unit stay was 2.7 days (range 1 to 38), and the mean hospital stay was 11 days (range 6 to 48). The blood loss and subsequent transfusion requirement increased with the higher levels of vena caval involvement and for left-sided tumors than the right-sided ones. The level of involvement did not affect the discharge time from the intensive care unit and hospital. There was 1 perioperative death (mortality, 5.5%). Among the discharged 17 patients, 2 died of tumor progression 43 and 54 months after surgery. Currently, 15 patients—more specifically 7 patients of level I, 6 patients of level II, and 2 patients of level III—are alive and enjoying a good quality of life without evidence of disease with a mean follow-up of 64.1 months (range 27 to 160). The 10-year Kaplan-Meier survival estimate was 75.6% with a mean follow-up 64.1 months. Although the groups in this study include a small number of patients, there was no significant difference in survival time based on the different levels of tumor thrombus extension into the vena cava.

COMMENTS

Renal cell carcinoma is a relatively rare tumor, accounting for approximately 2 to 3% of malignancies in adults, but is the most common tumor of the kidney and the third most common tumor seen by urologists [1, 2, 28]. It is a clinicopathologically heterogeneous disease [3], and unfortunately, it is refractory to most traditional oncologic treatments, including chemotherapy, radiation therapy, and hormonal therapy. Although there can be some variations, the prognosis of RCC is mainly based on tumor staging and histological grading [4]. It is prone to metastasize, and local metastases via direct invasion and distant metastases via hematogenous and lymphatic spread can be seen [9]. Metastatic renal cell carcinoma (RCC) accounted for more than 30,000 new cases of cancer and led to 12,000 deaths in the United States in 2001 [3]. Metastatic disease to the lung and bone represent the two most common sites of advanced disease and patients with metastatic RCC (30% of all RCC cases) have a life expectancy averaging around 12 months [5, 6]. Currently, it is not clear whether the basic biology underlying either the pattern of metastatic spread or the specific site of metastatic disease leads to differences in the response to therapy or predicts eventual differences. To date, there is little understanding of the underlying molecular mechanisms that may cause this variety in prognoses of the disease.

Vena caval tumor thrombus extension in a renal cell carcinoma is a relatively uncommon event occurring in 4% to 10% of all patients with renal cell carcinoma [10-13, 17, 39]. Within this group, 2% to 16% will have tumors extending into the right atrium [10, 11, 17, 39]. In our series, the incidence of venous extension with macroscopic IVC tumor thrombus and right atrial thrombus involvement were 6.2 % and 16.7 %, respectively. The prognosis for patients with RCC with IVC tumor thrombus extension has been difficult to predict due to a wide variety in clinical behavior. Although involvement of the IVC in renal cancer is generally not a vascular invasion by the malignant tumor but usually intraluminal extension of the tumor mass, such intravascular growth implies an increased biologic behavior of the tumor. It is suggested that patients with inferior vena caval tumor thrombus should be regarded as being at high risk with a higher potential for metastatic spread [40, 41]. It is reported that patients with tumor thrombus had a higher rate of metastasis at diagnosis than those without tumor thrombus (63% versus 25%) [41]. Therefore, when vena caval tumor thrombus is present and if patients are left untreated, poor survival rates are expected [18, 19]. However, the majority of the reports in the literature suggest that tumor thrombus into the inferior vena cava is not necessarily associated with a worse prognosis and patients with tumor thrombus but no metastasis can achieve long-term survival after complete surgical extirpation [10, 13, 18, 42-46]

In 1688, Blancardus described inferior vena caval involvement by tumor [47]. In 1913, Berg first described nephrectomy and vena cavotomy for RCC that extended into the IVC [48]. He performed the first phlebotomy of the vena cava and thrombus removal in a patient with renal cell carcinoma [48]. In 1922 Rehn resected the vena cava to remove a tumor thrombus adhering to the inferior vena cava and reimplanted the left renal vein into the stump [49]. In the early period of surgical experience, except for the few sporadic reports of successful excision of tumor thrombus in the inferior vena cava of Berg [48], Rehn [49] and Walters and Priestley [50], this operation was considered futile since operative mortality was excessive. At that time, one important factor was the lack of accurate preoperative knowledge of the presence and extent of inferior vena caval thrombus. The other important limiting factor was the lack of a system of staging. Because of that, many clinicians at that time concluded that extension into the inferior vena cava was synonymous with an incurable stage. In 1949, Robson defined renal cell carcinoma staging [38]. As time passed, various investigators reported either an optimistic or fatalistic outlook, depending on their own results [44, 51-53]. However, most of these reports on the surgical therapy of this entity were generally pessimistic except for sporadic accounts of long-term survivors [19, 54, 55]. Sosa et al. reported that there were no survivors at the end of 1 year when patients underwent nephrectomy alone, without removing the tumor mass in the IVC [19]. In 1972, after the report of Skinner et al., it was recognized that venous extension by tumor thrombus was a potentially curable lesion with a 55% 5-year survival rate, provided that complete removal could be achieved [44]. After this report, several investigators have reported favorable outcomes and suggested that vascular extension per se did not indicate a more aggressive form of tumor and total resection of the renal tumor and IVC tumor thrombus affords the best chance of cure and long-term survival when no distant metastases are present

[10,11,13,19,52,53]. Fortunately, recent reports suggest that even distant metastases do not have significant adverse effects on survival rates, when the tumor is excised completely from the IVC [9, 17, 20-22, 40, 41]. The results of these reports support the philosophy of an aggressive approach in patients with IVC involvement from renal cancer with or without distant metastases. Satisfactory long-term survival rates of previous surgical studies have generated a lot of interest in the subject and poor results of nonoperative treatments have encouraged many to handle such thrombi surgically. Since Berg's first report, radical nephrectomy with vena cavotomy has become a safe and effective treatment of RCC with IVC thrombus, with operative mortality rates ranging from 2.7% to 13% [10, 18-20, 39].

The diagnosis of vena caval tumoral invasion and the level of it in IVC are important when planning the surgical approach; hence, accurate preoperative determination of the level of tumor extension is essential [10, 20, 29, 37]. If present, certain clinical manifestations; recurrent pulmonary emboli, deep vein thrombosis, lower extremity edema, renal or hepatic dysfunction, malabsorption, weight loss, anorexia, varicocele, engorgement of abdominal wall veins may indicate complete occlusion of the vena cava by tumor thrombus [23]. However, most often the tumor thrombus is nonobstructive or sufficient collaterals have developed; therefore these signs are seldom detected [13, 19, 23, 24]. It is clinically important that in patients with complete IVC obstruction, collateral circulation usually provides sufficient venous drainage so that obstructive symptoms are uncommon. For this reason, the diagnosis of vena caval invasion and level of tumoral extension is mainly based on radiological examinations [17, 20, 23, 25-28]. Ultrasonography and CT are extremely useful and quite precise in demonstrating the extent of the thrombus in the majority of the patients [17, 20, 23, 25, 26, 39]. Additionally, CT can be helpful in preoperative detection of otherwise occult metastatic disease [26, 28, 56]. However, CT is not always accurate in delineating the superior margin of the tumor in the IVC. MRI can reliably demonstrate a tumor thrombus and its extension, and it can rule out IVC wall invasion so the exact surgical procedure can be planned [27]. Fortunately, the availability of MRI has made accurate noninvasive evaluation of tumor extension in the IVC possible. The ability to scan patients in coronal, sagittal, and axial planes provides visualization of tumor and caval patency without the use of contrast agents [27, 57]. Avoidance of contrast agents is particularly important in this group of patients who are about to lose one kidney; therefore, MRI is the test of choice for evaluation of tumor extension into the IVC [27, 57]. Current technology of Gradient Recall Acquisition in Steady State (GRASS) imaging can differentiate a tumor from a blood clot, as well as identify invasion of the vena cava wall by the tumor [27]. Recently, color-coded Doppler sonography has also been shown to differentiate tumor mass from bland thrombus. Demonstration of a patchy vascularization pattern on color-coded Doppler is considered pathognomonic for tumor thrombus [25]. Transesophageal echocardiography was described by Treiger et al. as an accurate diagnostic technique to determine the superior extent of the intracaval thrombus [58]. A transesophageal 4 chamber cardiac view delineates atrial extension of the thrombus during surgery. Hence, after the recent advances in sophisticated noninvasive radiological studies, the surgeon can now make an accurate preoperative assessment of the nature and extent of kidney tumors and the level of IVC tumor thrombus. It is noteworthy that avoidance of contrast agent is particularly important in this group of patients who are about to lose one kidney.

In our study, all patients presented with symptoms: 11 patients (61.1%) had gross or microscopic hematuria, 10 patients (55.5%) had flank pain, and 9 patients (50%) had palpable abdominal mass. The classic triad of hematuria, pain, and lump existed only in 2 patients (11.1%). None of our patients had clinical evidence of IVC obstruction. In our study, 100% of the vena caval thrombi were diagnosed by the combined use of USG and CT, which is a percentage in line with reports by others [17, 20, 59]. In 3 patients, based on CT findings of IVC involvement, MRI and ECO were needed for better definition of the upper extent of intracaval tumor thrombus. However, in our study, none of the radiological examinations were able to demonstrate IVC wall invasion by the tumoral process and retroperitoneal lymph node involvement. Contrast studies, like vena cavography, have been used in some other series, but we have not found them to be additive to USG, CT, and MRI, and it increases the risk of contrast associated renal injury in a patient with one functioning kidney [10, 13, 17, 20]. We also performed cardiac evaluation of patients with level III tumor thrombus preoperatively.

The key point in the surgical management of RCC with IVC tumor thrombus is the correct assessment of the extension of the endocaval thrombus. Once the diagnosis is made, the level of tumor thrombus involvement determines planning of the operation. Surgical treatment of the patients with a thrombus that extends above the diaphragm is a greater technical challenge. The surgical strategy depends on the level of inferior vena caval involvement and also surgical experience of the surgeon. Main objectives of operative management include: (1) maintenance of complete resection of tumor and tumor thrombus (2) prevention of tumoral embolism, (3) minimizing blood loss, (4) maintenance of hemodynamic stability, and (5) prevention of vital organ ischemia. In performing surgical removal of the IVC thrombus, it is essential to obtain control of the cava above the thrombus before manipulating the intracaval tumor mass to prevent intraoperative embolization of tumor fragments. Although level I tumors do not require any complex maneuvers, except for control of the IVC above and below the tumor, level II and III tumors require a complex maneuver and multi-team approach. Whereas temporary occlusion of the infrahepatic IVC can safely be done for level I tumors, the occlusion of the suprahepatic IVC often causes a profound decrease in venous return resulting in hypotension. Additional disadvantages of the latter maneuver when removing a caval thrombus include back bleeding from hepatic and lumbar veins and occasional swelling of the liver from venous congestion, which interferes with the exposure. Because of that, numerous different method 5 of management have been reported for level II and III tumors [10, 15, 16, 18, 20, 29-35, 37]. The surgical strategy and type of incision (the incision usually depends on surgeon preference) depending on the level of inferior vena caval involvement is given in details elsewhere [30]. However, currently in contrast to variations in surgical approach a few common principles, stated previously, can be important in the surgical treatment of RCC with IVC tumor thrombus. Briefly, in 1994, Swierzewski et al. stated certain principles that apply to vena caval surgery for renal cell carcinoma thrombus regardless of the level of the thrombus [16]. They reported that this surgery was primarily a vena cava operation, and therefore, the surgical approach should be based on this idea, and surgery should be done with minimal manipulation of the inferior vena cava and renal vein and tumor thrombus [16].

In our experience, a midline, anterior, abdominal, or chevron incision was used; and they provided an adequate surgical field for the safe dissection in the abdomen, distal control of the vena cava, and mobilization of the kidney with the tumor in the majority of our cases. Therefore, these were our standard surgical approaches. In the literature, many reports favored a midline incision since it precludes blood loss from the lateral, engorged, superficial abdominal collaterals and intercostal veins. Additionally, the midline incision also allowed abdominal exploration for metastatic disease and it could be extended cephalad to create a sternotomy if cardiopulmonary bypass were required. In addition, during the midline approach, the patient is in the supine rather than the flank position, so the possibility of cardiac arrest from acute thrombus obstruction of the tricuspid valve is less (likely). Hence, because of its advantages, in our experience there is a trend toward the midline incision. In this study, control of the IVC above the thrombus was always achieved before any maneuver was performed on the renal vessels in level I and level II. Tumor extraction was accomplished after proximal and distal control of the IVC in level I tumor thrombus. In the level II tumor thrombus, the suprahepatic IVC just below the diaphragm (with transabdominal, suprahepatic, and infradiaphragmatic dissection), the infrarenal IVC, the contralateral renal vein, and hepatic vein were occluded, and the extraction of the tumor thrombus was performed. Lumbar venous bleeding, seen after the removal of the tumor, was controlled with a curved vascular clamp. In our experience, resection of level II tumors required interruption of the hepatic and contralateral renal circulation. In our series, liver and renal ischemia time varied from 8 to 28 minutes (mean 18), which is acceptable when compared with reported tolerable normothermic continuous hepatic ischemia time of 15 to 30 minutes [24, 37, 60, 61]. Hence, none of our patients had significant postoperative hepatic and renal dysfunction. Although dissection in all cases required significant manipulation of the vena cava and, thus a greater risk of embolization, we have not encountered tumor embolization in any case.

Surgery for renal cell carcinoma with level III inferior vena caval thrombus is challenging. The management of patients with cardiac extension of the tumor thrombus (level III), that is clearly beyond simple minimal extension into the atrium, must be individualized. It requires accurate preoperative preparation and an experienced surgical team. When properly performed, perioperative morbidity and mortality are relatively low. So it needs a special attention. The surgical approach may differ from surgeon to surgeon, however, currently two alternatives are available. One is to control the hepatic circulation by the Pringle maneuver [62]. The liver can withstand about 30 minutes of warm ischemia without functional impairment [24, 37, 60, 61]. The other alternative is to use a cardiopulmonary bypass with or without deep hypothermic circulatory arrest. Introduction of CPB for the surgical treatment of RCC with IVC tumor thrombus is historically important. Marshall et al. first reported cardiopulmonary bypass but the initial results were poor [63]. In his first experience, significant bleeding from the lumbar or hepatic veins was a problem [63]. However, in his report in 1987, Libertino et al. lent their support to cardiopulmonary bypass for tumor thrombus extending into the right atrium [18]. Vaislic et al. first used circulatory arrest and hypothermia facilitates excision of a tumor thrombus extending into the right atrium by allowing the surgeon to operate in a bloodless field [35]. This experience, usage of hypothermic circulatory arrest in addition to cardiopulmonary bypass, was an evolutionary step. This technique had the advantage of permitting careful, controlled dissection in a virtually bloodless field. It decreased the risk of tumor dissemination and pulmonary embolus. In his report, Marshall et al. described cardiopulmonary bypass with circulatory arrest as a reasonable adjunct for cavo-atrial tumors [31]. In 1988, Marshall et al. summarized a strong argument in favor of cardiopulmonary bypass, hypothermia, cardiac arrest and exsanguinations in patients with tumor thrombus above the hepatic veins [64]. In an editorial comment, Novick wrote that "application of CPB and hypothermia to patients with suprahepatic IVC tumor thrombus is an important advance that has improved the safety and technical efficacy of a difficult surgical undertaking." [65]. The pioneering report of Skinner et al. demonstrated a survival advantage for aggressive surgical resection of inferior vena caval tumor thrombus from renal cell carcinoma and led to a dramatic change in the management of these cases [44]. As time passed, due to an increase in experience, cardiopulmonary bypasses with deep hypothermic circulatory arrest were more frequently used which significantly decreased the morbidity and mortality associated with resection of RCC extending into the right atrium or the IVC at or above the hepatic veins [66,67]. Depending on our experience, we believe CPB is necessary with or without DHCA to safely and completely extract the level III tumor thrombus as well as to visualize and remove all sites of adherent tissue within the right atrium The advantages and potential complications of CPB and DHCA were well defined previously [10,15,18,29,37]. It should be kept in mind that digital manipulation of the tumor in an attempt to push it down into the IVC without the protection by CPB may be hazardous and may result in tumor embolism. In our study, we used CPB and DHCA in 3 patients with level III tumor thrombus and did not encounter any problem inherent to these tools [10, 15, 29, 37]. Based on our data, we believe that this approach is safe and effective, and allows extensive IVC thrombi to be completely removed with an excellent exposure in a controlled operative setting.

Various centers have reported mortality rates of 6% to 9% for IVC extension of RCC [10, 11, 15, 17, 39]. The major cause of death was reported to be due to pulmonary embolism and myocardial infarction or due to complications related to the bypass procedures. However, with better perioperative management and standardization of the surgical techniques and improvement in surgical experience, the mortality rates can be decreased considerably [17, 20, 29]. We had only one death, operative mortality 5.5%, due to hypoxic encephalopathy. Of 18 patients, 3 with intraatrial thrombi required sternotomy for CPB and DHCA and the survival was not different from those presenting with invasion of the lower levels of IVC alone.

Although there is a controversy concerning the prognostic significance of certain factors—namely, the presence of lymph node involvement, perinephric fat invasion, metastatic disease, renal vein or IVC wall invasion, or the level of the vena caval tumor extension and possibility of complete tumoral tissue excision—all these factors may show an impact on prognosis and survival. The presence of tumoral invasion in the regional lymph node and the perinephric fat is reported to be a definitive poor prognostic factor [13, 17, 19, 20, 52, 53]. It has been shown that the patients with RCC extending only into the IVC have significantly better survival rates than those with local spread of the tumor to the lymph nodes or perinephric tissue [17, 20, 41, 52, 53]. Zelman et al. reported that local tumor extension has greater prognostic importance than the level of inferior vena cavil tumor thrombus [40, 41]. Metastatic spread to lymph nodes results in rapid relapse and a short overall survival [53, 52]. Reissigl et al. reported a 15.5- month mean survival rate for patients who had lymph node metastases, with an overall 5-year survival of 62.5% [68]. Libertino et al. found an overall 5-year survival of 59% with an overall 10-year survival of 47% [18]. Patients with no evidence of metastatic disease had a 60% survival rate with follow-up to 16 years but no patient with metastatic diseases or nodal involvement survived beyond 5 years. Hatcher et al. found a 5-year survival of 62% for their patients with completely resected stage IIIa disease [13]. For patients with lymph node metastases, the 5-year survival rate dropped to 17%. However, whether the perinephric spread is the only factor to affect the prognosis adversely in patients with RCC with IVC extension or not is controversial [18, 44, 46, 52, 53]. Libertino et al. reported that perinephric spread, per se, does not affect the survival in patients with IVC thrombus [18]. In contrast, others have reported that the presence of perinephric spread in RCC is a strong poor prognostic parameter [44, 52, 53, 46]. In the report of Skinner et al [44] 4 of the 5 nonsurvivors had perinephric spread. Recently, Glazer and Novick found that mean postoperative survival was significantly improved in patients with no renal capsular penetration by tumors compared with those with perinephric fat involvement (58.1 versus 19.7 months) [46]. The prognostic significance of lymph node metastases and perinephric spread in our study confirms the results of the above-mentioned reports [40, 41, 44, 46, 52, 53]. In our series, both patients who had lymph node metastases and perinephric spread died of tumor progression 43 and 54 months after surgery. In contrast, none of the patients without nodal disease and perinephric spread were dead at follow-up.

Patients with RCC extending into the IVC and metastatic disease at presentation continue to be challenging and the treatment of patients needs to be carefully individualized. Theoretically, the presence of distant metastatic disease at diagnosis in RCC with tumor thrombus represents more aggressive disease and implies poor survival. In addition to these, radical nephrectomy in patients with locally advanced and metastatic RCC is associated with relatively high rates (2% to 16%) of intraoperative and postoperative complications [17, 69, 70]. Patients with metastatic RCC have a poor prognosis, with a median survival expectation of less than 1 year and an associated 5-year mortality rate ranging from 80% to 100%. Most researchers note worse survival for such patients [10, 16, 71-73]. Bissada et al. reported that in their series, all of the 20 nonsurgical patients with metastases at presentation died within 2 years [22]. Using the Cox proportional hazards regression model, Montie et al., found that a patient with metastatic disease was 2.76 times more likely to die than patients without metastases [72]. Some reports suggest that finding a metastatic disease at presentation is an ominous sign, as most patients die within a year of diagnosis, and survival is not increased by doing an adjunctive nephrectomy. Therefore, an aggressive operation is not recommended for this group [11, 19, 51, 52, 73]. Furthermore, several other reports stress that the presence of metastases is a contraindication to vena caval thrombectomy [10, 11, 13, 17, 59, 69, 72, 73]. However, controversial reports from large cancer centers indicating distant metastases did not have a significant adverse effect on survival rates have been published recently [17,20,21,41]. On the other hand, a number of authors espouse the benefit of surgical resection of the primary tumor in patients with or without caval thrombus when performed before or after immunotherapy or in conjunction with resection of solitary metastases [70, 75-79]. Zisman et al. reported that the overall survival of patients with inferior vena caval thrombus was similar regardless of metastatic status in their series [40, 41]. Slaton et al. reported their experience in 15 patients having RCC and IVC tumor thrombus with different organ metastasis, and reported that nephrectomy and vena caval thrombectomy in selected patients with metastatic disease were performed safely and enabled a better quality of life and prolonged survival [21]. It is reported that although the potential for perioperative morbidity may be slightly higher in patients with concomitant metastatic disease and a thrombus, long term survival is comparable to that of patients without a caval thrombus [69, 70, 75, 76].

The most common sites of metastasis renal cell carcinoma are the lung and bones [7, 8, 9]. Zisman et al. reported that patients with tumor thrombus had a higher rate of metastasis at diagnosis than those without tumor thrombus (63% versus 25%) [41]. Most metastases in patents with RCC and tumor thrombus probably develop early and hematogenously rather than through the lymphatic [9, 41, 59, 74]. In the series reported by Zisman et al, of the 207 patients with tumor thrombus 74 (36%) presented with non-lymph node metastasis (N0M1), whereas only 16 (8%) presented with lymph node metastasis (N1M0) [41]. Reports about the prognostic significance of the site of metastases are controversial. Several investigators have reported that the presence of bone metastases was an independent prognostic factor of poor outcome on multivariate analysis [80, 81]. In a review of his patients, Mani et al. reported that patients with bony metastases had a median survival of 6.7 months and 62 patients without bony involvement had a median survival of 15.1 months [80]. Tsuda et al. have found no significant differences in the survival rates of patients with bone metastases compared with patients with lung metastases in their patients [82]. In the report of Han et al, the median survival for patients with lung only and bone only metastatic RCC was 27 months; patients with multiple organ involvement had a median survival of 11 months [9]. They found that survival in patients with disease limited to the lung was similar to that of patients whose disease was limited to bone [9]. However, in their study multivariate analysis confirmed that metastatic disease to more than one organ site was associated with poor prognosis (2.05 risk ratio, P <0.001) [9]. Han et al. eventually reported that number of metastatic sites rather than location dictates overall survival of patients with lymph node-negative metastatic renal cell carcinoma, and patients with metastatic RCC to only one organ site fared significantly better than patients who had evidence of disease in multiple organs [9].

In some reports, as is the case in our study, some patients with metastatic disease have prolonged survival for unexplained reasons [10, 11, 17, 20]. Our series included 2 patients with metastatic disease; 1 of them died just after the operation whereas the other lived for more than 3 years. He was given immunotherapy with interferon in the postoperative period for tumor relapse. However, it is difficult to determine whether this approach influenced his outcome or not. We cannot find a reasonable explanation for the improved survival observed in this isolated case. Whatever the reason, irrespective of the implication of the distant disease and in consideration of the potential for a survival benefit, we believe that metastatic disease should not preclude operative intervention. We recommend the removal of the primary neoplasm along with the extraction of the IVC tumor thrombus to palliate symptoms, especially the obstructive symptoms due to thrombus and pain due to local extension of the primary tumor, to remove an immediately life-threatening focus of disease, reduce tumor burden which may optimize the effect of biologic therapy, and to reduce associated problems such as pulmonary emboli, coagulopathies and hepatic dysfunctions. Following the report of spontaneous regression of metastatic disease after tumor nephrectomy, much attention has been focused on immunotherapeutical modalities for the treatment of metastatic RCC recently. Interleukin-2 (IL-2) and interferon-alpha (IFN-α) were found to be effective as immunoediting agents [83, 84]. However, none of them alone was as effective as combination therapy [85]. Additionally it was determined that although 5-fluorouracil itself is a chemotherapeutic agent, it has synergistic effect with IL-2 and IFN-α [86, 87]. Despite several studies reporting better response rates with IL-2, IFN-α and 5-FU triple therapy, its actual effectiveness is still under investigation [88]. A few reports evaluating the effect of nephrectomy before immunotherapy in patients with renal-cell carcinoma have been published recently [21, 40, 69, 70, 75-77, 89]. The theoretical advantages of nephrectomy prior to immunotherapy include reduction in the number of cancerous cells, removal of a trap for trafficing lymphocytes, prevention of complications during systemic treatment, opportunity to harvest tumor-infiltrating lymphocytes and tumor cells for use in experimental treatments, and reduction of a large and potentially immunosuppressive tumor burden [89]. Other potential advantages include improvement in performance status score of patients, better tolerance and higher probability of response to immunotherapy, elimination of the primary tumor as a possible source of hemorrhage, discomfort, or propagation of metastases, and the fact that responses to immunotherapy in the primary disease site have been rare [89]. Potential disadvantages include growth of metastatic disease in the recovery period that could preclude treatment, and morbidity associated with any major operation [90, 91]. Recently it has been reported that nephrectomy prior to immunotherapy reveals a time to progression and a survival benefit for patients with RCC and IVC tumor thrombus [89, 92]. Recent studies on this issue suggest that the combination of aggressive cytoreductive nephrectomy and immunotherapy may improve survival in patients with M1 disease who have inferior vena caval tumor thrombus [21, 41, 93). Recently, Zisman et al. reported that cytoreductive surgery in patients with tumor thrombus and metastasis was not associated with an increase in the extent of surgery, morbidity or mortality compared with their counterparts with nonmetastatic disease [41). However, randomized prospective studies are needed to evaluate the role of cytoreductive nephrectomy and immunotherapy and the precise timing of cytoreductive therapy in combination with immunotherapy in cases of metastasis and inferior vena caval thrombus extension.

Renal tumors often invade the wall of the vena cava and this invasion itself, regardless of the level of invasion and thrombus development, reflects the biological properties of them [59]. The influence of vein invasion in RCC on metastatic spread and survival is theoretically interesting and has been the subject of much debate. It is well known that vein invasion is an adverse prognostic factor in many tumors [94, 95]. However, the prognostic impact of renal vein and IVC wall invasion in RCC has been unclear, and reports concerning the significance of it and the role of partial vena cavectomy to achieve a surgical cure, have been contradictory [13, 38, 52, 59, 72, 96, 97]. Golimbu et al. reported that renal vein invasion alone did not alter the 5-year survival, and noted that there is no survival difference if the vein was grossly or microscopically invaded by a tumor [96]. In contrast, others have reported that the renal vein and IVC wall invasion in RCC is a strong poor prognostic parameter and when present, the risk of distant metastases and relapse is increased in such patients after surgery [13, 38, 52, 59, 72, 97, 98].

Additionally, these reports suggested that complete resection of the tumor thrombus, regardless of the level of the thrombus, including complete resection of the invaded wall of the IVC, provides a survival benefit [13, 38, 52, 59, 72, 97]. Hatcher et al reviewed 44 patients with RCC and IVC tumor thrombi, and found that the presence of inferior vena caval wall invasion was prognostically significant but that the level of inferior vena caval tumor thrombus involvement was not [13]. Hatcher et al. reported that the incidence of vena cava wall invasion, incidence of distant metastasis, and patient's survival is not related with the level of the tumor thrombus [13]. They also reported that among the patients with localized RCC, survival is improved in those with a mobile intraluminal thrombus compared to those with vena caval wall invasion, and survival in the latter group is improved when the involved portion of the vena cava is completely resected [13]. Novick et al. and Hatcher et al. emphase the significance of invasion of the vena caval wall in their reports [13, 65]. Novick believes that in patients who undergo excision of localized RCC with vena caval involvement, evidence of vena caval invasion should be deligently sought at time of operation [37, 65]. If such invasion is present, every attempt should be made to achieve complete excision of the involved vena caval wall with histological verification by intraoperative frozen sections [13, 37, 65]. Commonly, the presence of direct caval involvement or dense adherence of the tumor thrombus to part of the caval wall necessitate caval wall resection and extent of this resection is determined by the extent of adherence or invasion in the IVC wall. Guidelines for resection of IVC were gradually established through a cumulative effort of many surgeons for over a century. If a major part of the circumference of the IVC is a segment of the IVC it can be removed. More recently, reconstruction of the IVC has been performed. When partial resection of the IVC is needed, the defect can be repaired primarily, if suitable, and by a pericardial or synthetic graft [22, 56, 60]. Sarti et al. first reported total prosthetic replacement of the IVC in 1970 using a tubular polytetrafluoroethylene graft in a patient with advanced Wilm's tumor [99]. This was also used as an alternative method for IVC reconstruction after trauma [100]. Katz et al. used this procedure for suprarenal inferior vena caval replacement in RCC with good prosthetic patency 9 months postoperatively [101]. Okada et al. reported on long-term patency after IVC replacement with an expanded polytetrafluoroethylene tubular graft in 4 patients with tumor thrombi from RCC [102]. In our study, partial vena caval resection was performed in 6 patients due to presence of residual tumor adherent to the IVC wall. The defect was closed with a synthetic patch in 5 of these patients. Histopathological examination of the resected segments confirmed that IVC wall invasion was present in only 2 patients with level I and level II tumor thrombus. These patients are still alive and free of disease at 27 and 160 months postoperatively. However, since the number of our patients is too small to analyze, we cannot comment on the prognostic significance of the wall invasion in patients with RCC and IVC tumor thrombus.

To the best of our knowledge, Ardekani et al. were the first to remove a tumor thrombus from the right atrium. However, part of the primary tumor extending into the inferior vena cava was left inside and the patient died of disease [103]. Fortunately, with current surgical technology, thrombus resection can be performed even when it extends into the right atrium. However, the prognostic implication 5 of the level of the IVC tumor thrombus is still unclear and reports have been contradictory [13, 38, 52, 94,104]. Several investigators have noted a worse prognosis for patients with a tumor thrombus that extends into the atrium than for those with disease that remains within the IVC, and some studies suggested that the risk of metastases and early death is increased with a more cephalad extent of IVC thrombi [10, 13, 19, 37, 45, 46, 60, 64, 72, 105]. Sosa et al. reported a 2-year survival rate of 80% in patients with intrahepatic IVC tumor thrombi compared with only 21% in those with suprahepatic thrombi. However, patients in the latter category were also more likely to have perinephric fat and regional lymph node involvement [19]. Skinner et al. indicated a 5-year survival rate of 35%, after surgical treatment for patients with RCC and subhepatic IVC thrombus, and 5-year survival rates for patients with intrahepatic or atrial tumor thrombi were 18% and 0%, respectively [10]. In the series by Montie et al. patients with intrahepatic extension were 0.49 times less likely to die than those with renal or infrahepatic extension as determined by the Cox proportional hazards regression model [72] According to Glazer, there are 2 important issue to address when evaluating the possible prognostic significance of the cephalad extent of inferior vena caval involvement in patients with renal cell carcinoma: 1) is there a greater incidence of lymph node or distant metastasis at the initial presentation in such cases, and 2) is the risk of early metastasis and death increased following surgical treatment in patients who present with nonmetastatic renal cell carcinoma and an inferior vena cava caval thrombus extending into the right atrium [46]. Glazer and Novick reported that in a review of 18 patients with RCC and inferior vena caval thrombi, they found no difference in the incidence of lymph node or distant metastasis at the initial presentation between patients with an atrial thrombus compared to those with lower levels of inferior vena caval involvement [46].

In the series reported by Marshall et al. the survival ratio was worse in the group of patients with a higher-level tumor thrombus, but the difference was not statistically different [64]. In contrast, most reports in the literature have not shown a significant difference in survival when the tumor thrombus remains below the atrium and therefore have concluded that extension to the vena cava alone has a limited or no impact on survival [10, 13, 17, 24, 37, 41, 51, 52]. Cherrie et al [52], Novick et al [37], and Hatcher et al [13] have also reviewed their experience in similar groups of patients with RCC and IVC thrombi and have not found the level of the tumor thrombus to impact survival. Glazer et al. reviewed the long-term outcome in patients who underwent complete surgical excision for localized RCC and an intra-atrial tumor thrombus [46]. Their results indicated overall and cancer-specific 5-year survival rates of 56.6% and 60.2%, respectively [46]. Their findings indicated that the presence or absence of perinephric fat involvement is an important prognostic factor in such cases. In contrast, the cephalad extent of inferior vena caval involvement did not appear to be prognostically important. They also noted significantly improved extended survival among patients with no renal capsular penetration by tumor compared to those with perinephric fat involvement ($p=0.035$) [46]. Hatcher et al. reported that in the absence of other adverse prognostic factors, the cephalad extension of IVC involvement did not appear to be prognostically important [13]. Recently, Zisman et al. reported that local tumor extension has greater prognostic importance than the level of inferior vena caval tumor thrombus [41]. In the present study, there was no significant difference in survival based on the level of the tumor thrombus. This finding in our study confirms the results of many others [10, 13, 17, 24, 27, 37, 41, 51, 52, 97], while actually contradicting the report of Sosa et al [19].

Patients with incomplete resections (excluding patients with metastatic disease) have a significantly worse prognosis. Similar findings have been shown in many reports, stressing the importance of surgical eradication of disease [10, 11, 13, 17, 20]. Hatcher et al. noted that the prognosis was determined by the ability to perform a complete resection of the tumor, not by the level of tumor thrombus [13]. They also showed the prognostic importance of complete resection in patients with nonmetastatic disease, as the 5-year survival rate drops from 57% to 0% [13]. Skinner et al. identified the importance of complete resection by reporting a 34% 5-year survival for those patients undergoing a complete resection and a 1-year survival of only 8% for those who had incomplete resections [10]. Furthermore, Neves and Zincke noted a difference in 5-year survival between patients with complete thrombus removal (68%) and those with incomplete thrombus removal (17.5%) [11]. Because of that, it has been suggested that every attempt should be made for complete resection and surgical eradication of disease [10, 11, 13, 17, 20, 23, 37]. The 52% 5-year survival rate of patients with localized renal cancer [53] and 25% to 75% overall 5-year survival rates of patients with RCC with tumor thrombus extension to the IVC were reported previously [13, 17, 20, 46,104]. In our study, the 10-year Kaplan-Meier survival estimate was 75.6%, with a mean follow-up of 64.1 months for patients with RCC and IVC tumor thrombus and this result was comparable with the above-mentioned results. Although each group in our study included a few number of patients, lymph node involvement and perinephric spread seem to influence the prognosis adversely, whereas the level of tumor thrombus, stage of disease, distant metastatic disease, and the presence of IVC wall invasion do not.

In conclusion, tumor thrombus associated with renal cell carcinoma is no longer considered to have a detrimental impact on survival. During the last 3 decades there have been steady improvements in surgical techniques and perioperative care, which have dramatically improved the ability to safely remove these tumors. Fortunately, with current surgical technology thrombus resection can be performed even when it extends into the right atrium. Because of that, all patients with RCC and IVC tumor thrombi should be considered for operation regardless of the level of the tumor thrombi in the IVC. No other therapeutical modality has achieved comparable results. These tumors can be totally resected by an aggressive approach, using CPB and DHCA when necessary, with an acceptable morbidity and mortality, and satisfactory long-term survival rates can be achieved. We believe that complete surgical excision of the tumor and its thrombus with accurate preoperative staging and a well-planned surgical approach provides a high survival chance and offers a good quality of life.

REFERENCES

[1] Takahashi M, Rhodes DR, Furge KA, et al. Gene expression profiling of clear cell renal cell carcinoma: gene identification and prognostic classification. *Proc Natl Acad Sci USA 2001*; 98 (17): 9754-9.

[2] Jemal A, Thomas A, Murray T, Thun M. Cancer statistics, 2002. *CA Cancer J Clin* 2002; 52(1): 23-47. Erratum in: *CA Cancer J Clin* 2002; 52(2):119. *CA Cancer J Clin* 2002; 52(3):181-2.

[3] Mostfi FK, Davis CJ. *WHO International Histological Classification of Tumours 1998*, (Springer, Berlin).

[4] Tsui KH, Shvarts O, Smith RB, Figlin RA, deKernion JB, Belldegrun A. Prognostic indicators for renal cell carcinoma: a multivariate analysis of 643 patients using the revised 1997 TNM staging criteria. *J Urol* 2000; 163(4): 1090-5.

[5] Minasian LM, Motzer RJ, Gluck L, Mazumdar M, Vlamis V, Krown SE. *J Clin Oncol* 1993; 11:1368–1375.

[6] Hermanek P, Schrott KM. Evaluation of the new tumor, nodes and metastases classification of renal cell carcinoma. *J Urol* 1990; 144(2 Pt 1): 238-41; discussion 241-2.

[7] Motzer RJ, Bander NH, Nanus DM. Renal-cell carcinoma. *N Engl J Med* 1996; 335:865–75.

[8] Figlin RA. Renal cell carcinoma: management of advanced disease. *J Urol* 1999; 161: 381–87.

[9] Han KR, Pantuck AJ, Bui MH, et al. Number of metastatic sites rather than location dictates overall survival of patients with node-negative metastatic renal cell carcinoma. *Urology* 2003; 61(2): 314-9.

[10] Skinner DG, Pritchett TR, Lieskovsky G, Boyd SD, Stiles QR. Vena caval involvement by renal cell carcinoma. Surgical resection provides meaningful long-term survival. *Ann Surg* 1989; 210(3): 387-92; discussion 392-4.

[11] Neves RJ, Zincke H. Surgical treatment of renal cancer with vena cava extension. *Br J Urol* 1987; 59: 390–5.

[12] O'Donohoe MK, Flanagan F, Fitzpatrick JM, Smith JM. Surgical approach to inferior vena caval extension of renal cell carcinoma. *Br J Urol* 1987; 60: 492–6.

[13] Hatcher PA, Anderson EE, Paulson DF, Carson CC, Robertson JE. Surgical management and prognosis of renal cell carcinoma invading the vena cava. *J Urol* 1991; 145:20–4.

[14] Mootha RK, Butler R, Laucirica R, Scardino PT, Lerner SP. Renal cell carcinoma with infrarenal vena caval tumor thrombus. *Urology* 1999; 54(3): 561.

[15] Klein EA, Kaye MC, Novick AC. Management of renal cell carcinoma with vena caval tumor thrombi via cardiopulmonary bypass and deep hypothermic circulatory arrest. *Urol Oncol* 1991; 18: 445–7.

[16] Swierzewski DJ, Swierzewski MJ, Libertino JA. Radical nephrectomy in patients with renal cell carcinoma with venous, vena caval, and atrial extension. *Am J Surg* 1994; 168: 205–9.

[17] Nesbitt JC, Soltero ER, Dinney CP, et al. Surgical management of renal cell carcinoma with inferior vena cava tumor thrombus. *Ann Thorac Surg* 1997; 63(6): 1592–600.

[18] Libertino JA, Zinman L, Watkins E. Long term results of renal cell cancer with extension into inferior vena cava. *J Urol* 1987; 137: 21–4.

[19] Sosa RE, Muecke EC, Vaughan ED, McCorron JP. Renal cell carcinoma extending into the inferior vena cava: the prognostic significance of the level of the vena cava involvement. *J Urol* 1984; 132: 1097–100.

[20] Tongaonkar HB, Dandekar NP, Dalal AV, Kulkarni JN, Kamat MR. Renal cell carcinoma extending to the renal vena cava: results of surgical treatment and prognostic factors. *J Surg Oncol* 1995; 59: 94–100.

[21] Slaton JW, Balbay MD, Levy DA, et al. Nephrectomy and vena caval thrombectomy in patients with metastatic renal cell carcinoma. *Urology* 1997; 50(5): 673-7.

[22] Bissada NK, Yakout HH, Babanouri A, et al. Long-term experience with management of renal cell carcinoma involving the inferior vena cava. *Urology* 2003; 61(1): 89-92.

[23] Libertino JA. Renal cell cancer with extension into vena cava. In: Dudley H, Carter D, editors. Rob and Smith's operative surgery (urology). 4th ed. London: *Butterworths*, 1986, p 122–7.

[24] Clayman RV, Gonzalez R, Fraley EE. Renal cell carcinoma invading the inferior vena cava: clinical review and anatomical approach. *J Urol* 1980; 123: 157–63.

[25] Hubsch P, Schurawitzki H, Susani M, et al. Color Doppler imaging of inferior vena cava: identification of tumor thrombus. *J Ultrasound Med* 1992; 11(12): 639-45.

[26] Marks WM, Korobkin M, Callan PW, Kaysar JA. Computed tomographic diagnosis of tumour thrombus of renal vein and the inferior vena cava. *AJR Am J Roentgenol* 1978; 131: 843–6.

[27] Myneni L, Hricak H, Carroll PR. Magnetic resonance imaging of renal carcinoma with extension into the vena cava: staging, occuracy and recent advances. *Br J Urol* 1991; 68: 571–8.

[28] El-Galley R. Surgical Management of Renal Tumors. *Radiol Clin North Am* 2003; 41(5): 1053-65.

[29] Babu SC, Mianoni T, Shah PM, Goyal A, Choudhury M, Eshghi M, Moggio RA, Sarabu MR, Lafaro RJ. Malignant renal tumor with extension to the inferior vena cava. *Am J Surg* 1998; 176 (2):137–9.

[30] Vaidya A, Ciancio G, Soloway M. Surgical techniques for treating a renal neoplasm invading the inferior vena cava. *J Urol* 2003; 169(2):435-44.

[31] Marshall FF, Reitz BA, Diamond DA. A new technique for management of renal cell carcinoma involving the right atrium: hypothermia and cardiac arrest. *J Urol* 1984; 131 (1): 103-7.

[32] Fitzgerald JM, Tripathy U, Svensson LG, Libertino JA. Radical nephrectomy with vena caval thrombectomy using a minimal access approach for cardiopulmonary bypass. *J Urol* 1998; 159(4): 1292-3.

[33] Belis JA, Levinson ME, Pae WE Jr. Complete radical nephrectomy and vena caval thrombectomy during circulatory arrest. *J Urol* 2000 Feb; 163(2): 434-6.

[34] Ciancio G, Hawke C, Soloway M. The use of liver transplant techniques to aid in the surgical management of urological tumors. *J Urol.* 2000 Sep; 164(3 Pt 1): 665-72.

[35] Vaislic CD, Puel P, Grondin P, Vargas A, Thevenet A, Fontan F, Deville C, Leguerrier A, Touchot B, Piwnica A, et al. Cancer of the kidney invading the vena cava and heart. Results after 11 years of treatment. *J Thorac Cardiovasc Surg.* 1986 Apr; 91(4): 604-9.

[36] Pritchett TR, Lieskovsky G, Skinner DG. Extension of renal cell carcinoma into the vena cava: clinical review and surgical approach. *J Urol.* 1986 Mar; 135(3): 460-4.

[37] Novick AC, Kaye MC, Cosgrove DM, et al. Experience with cardiopulmonary bypass and deep hypothermic circulatory arrest in the management of retroperitoneal tumors with large vena caval thrombi. *Ann Surg* 1990; 212(4): 472-6; discussion 476-7

[38] Robson CJ, Churchill BM, Anderson W. The results of radical nephrectomy for renal cell carcinoma. *J Urol* 1969;101: 297–301.

[39] Kaplan S, Ekici S, Dogan R, Demircin M, Ozen H, Pasaoglu I. Surgical management of renal cell carcinoma with inferior vena cava tumor thrombus. *Am J Surg* 2002; 183(3): 292-9.

[40] Zisman A, Pantuck AJ, Chao DH, et al. Renal cell carcinoma with tumor thrombus: is cytoreductive nephrectomy for advanced disease associated with an increased complication rate? *J Urol* 2002; 168(3): 962-7.

[41] Zisman A, Wieder JA, Pantuck AJ, et al. Renal cell carcinoma with tumor thrombus extension: biology, role of nephrectomy and response to immunotherapy. *J Urol* 2003; 169(3): 909-16.

[42] Mattos RM, Libertino JA. Survival of patients with renal cell carcinoma invading the inferior vena cava. *Semin Urol Oncol* 1996; 14(4): 223-6.

[43] Skinner DG, Colvin RB, Vermillion CD, Pfister RC, Leadbetter WF. Diagnosis and management of renal cell carcinoma. A clinical and pathologic study of 309 cases. *Cancer* 1971; 28(5): 1165-77.

[44] Skinner DG, Pfister RF, Colvin R. Extension of renal cell carcinoma into the vena cava: the rationale for aggressive surgical management. *J Urol* 1972; 107(5): 711-6.

[45] Quek ML, Stein JP, Skinner DG. Surgical approaches to venous tumor thrombus. *Semin Urol Oncol* 2001; 19(2): 88-97.

[46] Glazer AA, Novick AC. Long-term followup after surgical treatment for renal cell carcinoma extending into the right atrium. *J Urol* 1996; 155(2): 448-50.

[47] Blancardus. Cited by Schecter DC. Cardiovascular surgery in the management of exogenous tumors involving the vena cava. In: Surgery of the Veins. Edited by JJ Bergan and JST Yao. Orlando: Grune & Stratton, chapt. 28, pp. 393–412, 1985 cell carcinoma. *J Urol* 1981; 125: 769.

[48] Berg AA. Malignant hypernephroma of the kidney. Its clinical course and diagnosis, with a description of the author's method of radical operative cure. *Surg Gynecol Obstet* 1913; 17:463.

[49] Rehn E. Gefasskomplikatnen und ihre Beherrschung bei dem hypernephrom. *Z Urol Chir* 1922; 10: 326.

[50] Walters W, Priestley JT. Survey of the inferior vena cava. Clinical and experimental studies. *Ann Surg* 1934; 99:167.

[51] Kearney GP, Waters WB, Klein LA, Richie JP, Gittes RF. Results of inferior vena cava resection for renal cell carcinoma. *J Urol.* 1981; 125(6): 769-73.

[52] Cherrie RJ, Goldman RG, Linder A, deKernion JB. Prognostic implications of vena caval extension of renal cell carcinoma. *J Urol* 1982; 128: 910–12.

[53] Heney NM, Nocks BN. Influence of perinephric fat involvement on survival in patients with renal cell carcinoma extending into the inferior vena cava. *J Urol* 1982; 128: 18–20.

[54] McDonals JR, Priestley JT. Malignant tumor of the kidney: surgical and prognostic significance of the tumor thrombosis of renal vein. *Surg Gynecol Obstet* 1943; 77: 295–9.

[55] Myers GH, Fehrenbaker LG, Kelalis PP. Prognostic significance of renal vein invasion by hypernephroma. *J Urol* 1968; 100(4): 420–3.

[56] Gohji K, Yamashita C, Ueno K, Shimogaki H, Kamidono S. Preoperative computerized tomography detection of extensive invasion of the inferior vena cava by renal cell carcinoma: possible indication for resection with partial cardiopulmonary bypass and patch grafting. *J Urol* 1994; 152(6 Pt 1): 1993-6.

[57] Pritchett TR, Raval JK, Benson RC, et al. Preoperative magnetic resonance imaging of vena caval tumor thrombi: experience with 5 cases. *J Urol* 1987; 138(5): 1220-2.

[58] Treiger BF, Humphrey LS, Peterson CV Jr, et al. Transesophageal echocardiography in renal cell carcinoma: an accurate diagnostic technique for intracaval neoplastic extension. *J Urol* 1991; 145(6): 1138-40.

[59] Ljungberg B, Stenling R, Osterdahl B, Farrelly E, Aberg T, Roos G. Vein invasion in renal cell carcinoma: impact on metastatic behavior and survival. *J Urol* 1995; 154(5): 1681-4.

[60] Marshall FF, Reitz BA. Supradiaphragmatic renal cell carcinoma tumor thrombus: indications for vena caval reconstruction with pericardium. *J Urol* 1985; 133(2): 266-8.

[61] Yellin AE, Chaffee CB, Donovan AJ. Vascular isolation in treatment of juxtahepatic venous injuries. *Arch Surg* 1971; 102(6): 566-73.

[62] Pringle JH. Notes on the arrest of hepatic hemorrhage due to trauma. *Ann Surg* 1908; 48: 541.

[63] Marshall VF, Middleton RG, Holswade GR, Goldsmith EI. Surgery for renal cell carcinoma in the vena cava. *J Urol* 1970; 103(4): 414-20.

[64] Marshall FF, Dietrick DD, Baumgartner WA, Reitz BA. Surgical management of renal cell carcinoma with intracaval neoplastic extension above the hepatic veins. *J Urol* 1988; 139(6): 1166-72.

[65] Novick AC. Editorial comment. *J Urol* 1988; 139: 1172.

[66] Stief CG, Schafers HJ, Kuczyk M, et al. Renal-cell carcinoma with intracaval neoplastic extension: stratification and surgical technique. *World J Urol* 1995; 13(3): 166-70.

[67] Belis JA, Pae WE Jr, Rohner TJ Jr, et al. Cardiovascular evaluation before circulatory arrest for removal of vena caval extension of renal carcinoma. *J Urol* 1989; 141(6): 1302-7.

[68] Reissigl A, Janetschek G, Eberle J, et al. Renal cell carcinoma extending into the vena cava: surgical approach, technique and results. *Br J Urol* 1995; 75(2): 138-42.

[69] Franklin JR, Figlin R, Rauch J, Gitlitz B, Belldegrun A. Cytoreductive surgery in the management of metastatic renal cell carcinoma: the UCLA experience. *Semin Urol Oncol* 1996; 14(4): 230-6.

[70] Rackley R, Novick A, Klein E, Bukowski R, McLain D, Goldfarb D. The impact of adjuvant nephrectomy on multimodality treatment of metastatic renal cell carcinoma. *J Urol* 1994; 152(5 Pt 1): 1399-403.

[71] Linehan WM, Shipley WU, Longo DL, et al. Cancer of the kidney and ureter. In: DeVita VT, Hellman S, Rosenberg SA, editors. Principles and practice of oncology. *Philadelphia: Lippincott*, 1993, p 1023–51.

[72] Montie JE, el Ammar R, Pontes JE, et al. Renal cell carcinoma with inferior vena cava tumor thrombi. *Surg Gynecol Obstet* 1991; 173(2): 107-15.

[73] Suggs WD, Smith RB 3rd, Dodson TF, Salam AA, Graham SD Jr. Renal cell carcinoma with inferior vena caval involvement. *J Vasc Surg* 1991; 14(3): 413-8.

[74] Franklin JR, Figlin R, Belldegrun A. Renal cell carcinoma: basic biology and clinical behavior. *Semin Urol Oncol* 1996; 14(4): 208-15.

[75] Walther MM, Alexander RB, Weiss GH, et al. Cytoreductive surgery prior to interleukin-2-based therapy in patients with metastatic renal cell carcinoma. *Urology* 1993; 42(3): 250-7; discussion 257-8.

[76] Wolf JS Jr, Aronson FR, Small EJ, Carroll PR. Nephrectomy for metastatic renal cell carcinoma: a component of systemic treatment regimens. *J Surg Oncol* 1994; 55(1): 7-13.

[77] Levy DA, Slaton JW, Ellerhorst J, Swanson DA, Dinney CPN. Feasibility of cytoreductive surgery before systemic biologic therapy in carefully selected patients with metastatic renal cell carcinoma. *J Urol* 1997; 157(supll): 70A

[78] Spencer WF, Linehan WM, Walther MM, et al. Immunotherapy with interleukin-2 and alpha-interferon in patients with metastatic renal cell cancer with in situ primary cancers: a pilot study. *J Urol* 1992; 147(1): 24-30.

[79] Fleischmann JD, Kim B. Interleukin-2 immunotherapy followed by resection of residual renal cell carcinoma. *J Urol* 1991; 145(5): 938-41.

[80] Mani S, Todd MB, Katz K, Poo WJ. Prognostic factors for survival in patients with metastatic renal cancer treated with biological response modifiers. *J Urol* 1995; 154(1): 35-40.

[81] Kankuri M, Pelliniemi TT, Pyrhonen S, Nikkanen V, Helenius H, Salminen E. Feasibility of prolonged use of interferon-alpha in metastatic kidney carcinoma: a phase II study. *Cancer* 2001; 92(4): 761-7.

[82] 82. Tsuda S, Koga S, Nishikido M, et al. Evaluation of bone metastases from renal cell carcinoma. *Hinyokika Kiyo* 2001; 47(3): 155-8.

[83] No authors listed. Interferon-alpha and survival in metastatic renal carcinoma: early results of a randomised controlled trial. Medical Research Council Renal Cancer Collaborators. *Lancet* 1999; 353(9146): 14–7.

[84] Fyfe G, Fisher RI, Rosenberg SA, Sznol M, Parkinson DR, Louie AC. Results of treatment of 255 patients with metastatic renal cell carcinoma who received high-dose recombinant interleukin-2 therapy. *J Clin Oncol* 1995; 13(3): 688–96.

[85] Negrier S, Escudier B, Lasset C, et al. Recombinant human interleukin-2, recombinant human interferon alfa-2a, or both in metastatic renal-cell carcinoma. Groupe Francais d'Immunotherapie. *N Engl J Med* 1998; 338(18): 1272-8.

[86] Wadler S, Wersto R, Weinberg V, Thompson D, Schwartz EL. Interaction of fluorouracil and interferon in human colon cancer cell lines: cytotoxic and cytokinetic effects. *Cancer Res* 1990; 50(18): 5735–9.

[87] Reiter Z, Ozes ON, Blatt LM, Taylor MW. A dual anti-tumor effect of a combination of interferon-alpha or interleukin-2 and 5-fluorouracil on natural killer (NK) cell-mediated cytotoxicity. *Clin Immunol Immunopathol* 1992; 62(1 Pt 1): 103–11.

[88] Bleumer I, Oosterwijk E, De Mulder P, Mulders PFA. Immunotherapy for renal cell carcinoma. *Eur Urol* 2003: 44: 65-75.

[89] Mickisch GH, Garin A, van Poppel H, de Prijck L, Sylvester R. Radical nephrectomy plus interferon-alfa-based immunotherapy compared with interferon alfa alone in metastatic renal-cell carcinoma: a randomised trial. *Lancet* 2001; 358(9286): 966–70.

[90] Bennett RT, Lerner SE, Taub HC, Dutcher JP, Fleischmann J. Cytoreductive surgery for stage IV renal cell carcinoma. *J Urol* 1995; 154(1): 32-4.

[91] Fallick ML, McDermott DF, LaRock D, Long JP, Atkins MB. Nephrectomy before interleukin-2 therapy for patients with metastatic renal cell carcinoma. *J Urol* 1997; 158(5): 1691-5.

[92] Flanigan RC, Salmon SE, Blumenstein BA, et al. Nephrectomy followed by interferon alfa-2b compared with interferon alfa-2b alone for metastatic renal-cell cancer. *N Engl J Med* 2001; 345(23): 1655–9.

[93] Naitoh J, Kaplan A, Dorey F, Figlin R, Belldegrun A. Metastatic renal cell carcinoma with concurrent inferior vena caval invasion: long-term survival after combination therapy with radical nephrectomy, vena caval thrombectomy and postoperative immunotherapy. *J Urol* 1999; 162(1): 46-50.

[94] Sanchez de la Muela P, Zudaire JJ, Robles JE, et al. Renal cell carcinoma: vena caval invasion and prognostic factors. *Eur Urol* 1991; 19(4): 284-90.

[95] Hoeltl W, Pont J, Kosak D, Honetz N, Marberger M. Treatment decision for stage I non-seminomatous germ cell tumours based on the risk factor "vascular invasion". *Br J Urol* 1992; 69(1): 83-7.

[96] Golimbu M, Joshi P, Sperber A, Tessler A, Al-Askari S, Morales P. Renal cell carcinoma: survival and prognostic factors. *Urology* 1986; 27(4): 291-301.

[97] Mrstik C, Salamon J, Weber R, Sto¨germayer F. Microscopic venous infiltration as predictor of relapse in renal cell carcinoma. *J Urol* 1992; 148: 271–4.

[98] Van Poppel H, Vandendriessche H, Boel K, et al. Microscopic vascular invasion is the most relevant prognosticator after radical nephrectomy for clinically nonmetastatic renal cell carcinoma. *J Urol* 1997; 158(1): 45-9.

[99] Sarti L. Total prosthetic transplantation of the inferior vena cava, with venous drainage restoration of one remaining kidney on the graft, successfully performed on a child with Wilm's tumor. *Surgery* 1970; 67(5): 851-5.

[100] Dale WA, Harris J, Terry RB. Polytetrafluoroethylene reconstruction of inferior vena cava. *Surgery* 1984; 95(5): 625-30.

[101] Katz NM, Spence IJ, Wallace RB. Reconstruction of the inferior vena cava with a polytetrafluoroethylene tube graft after resection for hypernephroma of the right kidney. *J Thorac Cardiovasc Surg* 1984; 87(5): 791-7.

[102] Okada Y, Kumada K, Terachi T, Nishimura K, Tomoyoshi T, Yoshida O. Long-term followup of patients with tumor thrombi from renal cell carcinoma and total replacement of the inferior vena cava using an expanded polytetrafluoroethylene tubular graft. *J Urol* 1996; 155(2): 444-6; discussion 447.

[103] Ardekani RG, Hunter JA, Thomson A. Hidden hypernephroma simulating right atrial tumor. *Ann Thorac Surg* 1971; 11(4): 371-5.

[104] Pagano F, Dal Bianco M, Artibani W, Pappagallo G, Prayer Galetti T. Renal cell carcinoma with extension into the inferior vena cava: problems in diagnosis, staging and treatment. *Eur Urol* 1992; 22(3): 200-3.

[105] Marshall FF, Reitz BA. Technique for removal of renal cell carcinoma with suprahepatic vena caval tumor thrombus. *Urol Clin North Am* 1986; 13(3): 551-7.

In: Trends in Kidney Cancer Research
Editor: Kelvin R. Nunez, pp. 159-206

ISBN 1-59454-141-8

Chapter XI

A Critical Review: A New Trial to Overcome the Multidrug Resistance of Renal Cell Carcinoma: From Theoretical Possibility to Therapeutic Benefit?

Ch. Fleck*
Klinikum der Friedrich-Schiller-Universität Jena, Germany

Abstract

Renal cell carcinoma (RCC) is known to be resistant against a couple of cytostatics. This phenomenon, called multidrug resistance (MDR), is explained first of all by an increase in transport of cytostatics out of RCC or by an enhanced cleavage of these substances in the tumour cells. In the past, attention was focussed on both mechanisms to overcome MDR. Unfortunately, the therapeutic benefit was low in most cases. Therefore, a new trial was tested: the possibility to stimulate the uptake of cytostatic drugs into RCC.

The experiments were started on the basis of the following findings: Organic anions like p-aminohippurate (PAH) are transported across the basolateral membrane of the renal proximal tubule, a mechanism indirectly coupled to sodium via Na^+/α-ketoglutarate co-transport. For about two decades it has been known that the renal excretion capacity of PAH can be stimulated by a suitable treatment schedule *in vivo*. The PAH excretion into urine increases, e.g. after T_3 treatment, by about 60%. In further *in vitro* investigations on renal cortical slices it could be demonstrated that PAH accumulation capacity was significantly increased after *in vivo* stimulation with T_3. Both renal transport capacity and the effect of stimulatory pre-treatment on renal function are age dependent: renal

* Corresponding author: Prof. Dr. Christian Fleck, Klinikum der Friedrich-Schiller-Universität Jena; Institut für Pharmakologie und Toxikologie, D-07740 Jena, Germany. Tel.: ++49+3641+938720; Fax: ++49+3641+938702; E-mail: <Christian.Fleck@mti.uni-jena.de>

excretion capacity of 10-day-old rats is immature, however, in young rats the extent of stimulation of renal transport processes is often larger than in adult animals.

The next step was the creation of an *in vitro* model suitable to stimulate the accumulation of PAH in renal cortical slices of immature and adult rats. For this goal, tissue slices were incubated for 24 hours in Williams medium E containing different concentrations of hormones. After this incubation period, slices were placed in PAH containing Cross-Taggart medium and PAH uptake into kidney tissue was measured for two hours. In both age groups, the accumulation capacity after 24 hours incubation reaches about 40 - 60 % of that of acute two hours incubation experiments (slice to medium ratios [$Q_{S/M}$] after two hours of incubation: immature rats: 9.5 $\pm$ 0.4; adults: 11.4 $\pm$ 0.3). After 24 hours incubation with dexamethasone the PAH uptake capacity significantly increases concentration dependently: 10- and 55-day-old rats: 26 and 36 % increase, respectively. It was concluded that 1.) a stimulation of tubular transport capacity can be performed *in vitro*, and 2.) discrepancies between *in vitro* and *in vivo* stimulation exist concerning PAH accumulation in rat renal cortical slices.

Then the *in vitro* accumulation of PAH was investigated in "intact" human renal cortical slices of normal kidney tissue and in tissue slices of human renal cell carcinoma (RCC). In principle, the accumulation capacity is comparable in renal tissue slices of man and rat ($Q_{S/M}$ between 4 and 8). In man, sex differences in accumulation capacity do not exist. But accumulation capacity drops with age. Tissue slices of RCC are unable to accumulate PAH. Surprisingly, in tumours of stage pT1, PAH uptake is lowest, perhaps as a sign of PAH transport out of the cells. There is no difference between peripheral and central parts of RCC. Age and sex are without influence on PAH uptake in RCC tissue slices. Interestingly, the accumulation capacity of "intact" tissue of kidneys infested with RCC also depends on the severity of the tumour (stage, diameter), but not on the formation of metastases.

The aim of the next experimental approach was to test whether or not the accumulation of PAH can be increased in intact human renal cortical slices obtained from tumour-bearing kidneys of patients suffering from RCC. As in rat's renal tissue slices, in intact human kidney tissue PAH uptake capacity increased significantly after 24 hours incubation in dexamethasone-containing medium (56%). The stimulatory effect became significant already after 12 hours incubation. In additionally performed experiments, it was shown that incubation in T_3-containing medium has different effects: In man, T_3 does not influence PAH accumulation capacity of renal cortical slices whereas in rats the PAH accumulation is significantly lower after 24 hours incubation with T_3.

Thereafter, the response of RCC on dexamethasone or T_3 was investigated using tissue slices *ex vivo*. By this approach the PAH accumulation capacity of RCC should be stimulated as a prerequisite for testing the uptake of anti-tumour drugs. RCC samples were incubated for 24 hours in Williams medium E containing dexamethasone or T_3. Thereafter, the slices were placed in PAH containing a Cross-Taggart medium and $Q_{S/M}$ for PAH uptake was measured. As expected, in intact human renal cortical slices, $Q_{S/M}$ was about 3 and increased in dexamethasone-containing medium up to 150%, whereas T_3 did not influence the PAH accumulation. Despite the fact that in RCC the PAH accumulation was completely abolished ($Q_{S/M}$ ~ 1), after administration of dexamethasone the accumulated amount of PAH increased significantly also in RCC tissue up to 190%. T_3 was without effect in RCC, too. The dexamethasone-mediated

stimulation could be differentiated into responder and non-responder. Altogether, moderate stimulation of tubular transport capacity can be shown *ex vivo* in human RCC, too. The response of RCC on dexamethasone was considered as a basis for new therapeutic strategies to overcome MDR in RCC.
The final aim of the study was to test the accumulation of anticancer drugs (methotrexate = MTX, cisplatin = CP, Tomudex®, topotecan) in intact kidney and in RCC. Kidney tissue slices were incubated in Williams medium E containing dexamethasone, T_3, or EGF. Thereafter slices were placed in anticancer drug containing Cross-Taggart medium and the drug uptake into kidney tissue was measured. As described above, in intact kidney the uptake of PAH (= reference substance) increased significantly only after incubation in dexamethasone, but not in T_3 or EGF. On the other hand, only the accumulation of MTX, but not of CP, Tomudex®, and topotecan, was significantly enhanced after pre-treatment both in intact tissue and in RCC. Discrepancies between the effects of dexamethasone and T_3 and/or EGF indicate different modes of action of these substances at the cellular level.
Unfortunately, the uptake of a variety of anticancer drugs cannot be stimulated effectively in RCC. Evidently the transport of these drugs out of the tumour cells or their metabolism within the tumour is more effective than their uptake. Furthermore, the doses necessary to stimulate the uptake of cytostatics is too high and, therefore, side effects on intact cells must be considered. Thus the therapeutic approach of hormonal stimulation of the uptake of cytostatics cannot be recommended as yet.

Keywords: kidney, transport, p-aminohippurate, multidrug resistance, renal cell carcinoma, anticancer drugs, topotecan, raltitrexed, methotrexate, cisplatin, dexamethasone, triiodothyronine, epidermal growth factor

Introduction

Renal Transport of Organic Anions

Tubular secretion is a unidirectional transcellular transport of organic ions from blood into the proximal tubular cell followed by an efflux of the ion into urine (Takeda et al.,, 2000b). This transport is mediated by different carriers at the basolateral and luminal membranes of the proximal tubulus (Sweet et al., 1997, Sekine et al., 1999, 2000, Russel et al., 2002). Organic anions like p-aminohippurate (PAH), endogenous compounds (urate, prostaglandins), and drugs (especially glucuronides) are tertiary actively transported across the basolateral membrane of the renal proximal tubule in exchange for intracellular α-ketoglutarate, a mechanism indirectly coupled to sodium via Na^+/α-ketoglutarate co-transport (Villalobos et al., 1996, Ullrich 1999, Wolff et al., 1997, 2001). Ullrich (1997) identified the general characteristics (minimal size of 4-10 Å, electrophilic moieties like Cl^- and NO_2) of substances transported by dicarboxylate exchangers. Under physiological conditions, the amount of α-ketoglutarate is sufficient for the exchange of organic anions (Pritchard 1995, Gabriels et al., 1999 Bahn et al., 2002). Furthermore, transport steps within the tubular cell (compartmentation, microtubular system, mitochondria) are involved in the secretion of organic anions (Miller et al., 1993, 1996, Miller and Pritchard, 1994, Masereeuw et al., 1994, Cha und Endou, 2001). Finally, in the kidney, endothelins are regulators of hemodynamics. Masereeuw et al. (2000) reported results linking endothelins to the control of xenobiotic transport.

At the luminal membrane, the efflux of PAH across the electrical potential difference into urine is quite the same in most species (Schmitt und Burckhardt, 1993, Miller et al. (1996). An anion carrier found in the human kidney, transports PAH or urate into the lumen in exchange against OH^-, bicarbonate, chloride, lactate, acetoacetate or succinate (Burckhardt et al., 2001). The members of the organic anion transporting polypeptide (oatp) family do not transport PAH at the luminal membrane (Sweet and Pritchard, 1999). Nevertheless, the multispecific organic anion transporters OAT-K1, OAT-K2, and rOAT-K eliminate a couple of endogenous substances (Uwai et al., 1998, Takeuchi et al., 2001, Hasegawa et al., 2002, Wolff und Su 2002). Functional studies on flounder renal organic anion transporter (fROAT) showed that cationic amino acids lysine 394 and arginine 478 are important for the interaction of OAT1 with PAH (Wolff et al., 2001, Burckhardt et al., 2002). The existence of a variety of OAT isoforms in the kidney seems to be essential for the survival of the organism (Kusuhara et al., 1999, Sweet et al., 2001): another can replace the loss of one subspecies. OAT1 transports more than 100 of organic anions like PAH, dicarboxylates, cyclic nucleotides, prostanoides, urate, β-lactamates, non-steroidal antirheumatics, diuretics, and cytostatics (Sekine et al., 1998, Tojo et al., 1999, Kobayashi et al., 2002a, b) OAT3 transports, beside organic anions, also basic substances like cimetidine (Kusuhara et al., 1999, Feng et al., 2001, 2002). Morita et al. (2001) have seen that the affinity of PAH to OAT2 is low compared to OAT1 and OAT3 (Takeda et al., 2000a, b).

The multidrug resistance related protein 1 (MRP1) is an ATP dependent efflux pump for hydrophobic conjugates (Jedlitschky and Keppler, 2002). MRP2 (= human canalicular multispecific organic anion transporter cMOAT) is expressed in human kidney only to a low extent (Harris et al., 2001). MRP2 transports ATP dependently organic anions like PAH (König et al., 1999, van Aubel et al., 2000a, b, Leier et al., 2000). Because of its broad substrate specificity, MRP2 eliminates methotrexate, too (Han et al., 2001). The expression of MRP2 can be enhanced significantly e.g. by dexamethasone (Johnson und Klaassen, 2002). The human multidrug resistance related protein 4 (MRP4) is located in luminal membranes of proximal tubules and transports cAMP, cGMP, and methotrexate (van Aubel et al., 2002). The isoforms MRP3, MRP5, and MRP6 were found in the kidney, but their function remains still unclear (Cha and Endou, 2001). Uchino et al. (2000) reported that human Na^+-dependent phosphate transporter type 1 (NPT1) expressing cells could transport PAH with low affinity. It was postulated that NPT1 consists of a polyspecific organic anion transporter (Burckhardt et al., 2001).

The first organic anion transporter in human kidney was described as human organic anion transporter 1 (hOAT1) (Reid et al., 1998, Lu et al., 1999, Race et al., 1999, Cha et al., 2000, 2001). hOAT1 plays a key role in the elimination of toxic compounds and drugs (Bahn et al., 2000). Many labs differentiated different splice variants of hOAT1-5 (Hosoyamada et al., 1999, Bahn et al., 2000, Cha et al., 2000, 2001, Sun et al., 2001).

Modulation of Basolateral PAH-Transport

Many compounds interact with PAH transport systems in the kidney (Somogyi, 1996, Gabriels et al., 1999). Both an inhibition and an activation of PAH-transport have been described. Beside reduced energy supply (Cross und Taggart, 1950, Stopp and Bräunlich, 1975), e.g. proteinkinase C or H_2O_2, down regulate PAH transport (Uwai et al., 1998,Lu et al., 1999, Takeda et al., 2000a, b). Probenecid, penicillin, furosemide, bumetanide, α-ketoglutarate, glutarate, indomethacin, dipropylxanthine, betamipron, cilastatine, and fluorescein inhibit PAH transport competitively (Gemba et al., 1981, Lu et al., 1999, Wolff et al., 2001, Takeda et al., 2001, Enomoto et al., 2002). Kuze et al. (1999), Apiwattanakul et al. (1999), and Jariyawat et al. (1999) found an inhibition of renal PAH transport after simultaneous administration of indomethacin, sulindac, diclofenac, and carprofen, after ACE inhibitors (captopril and enalapril), cyclosporin A, and anticancer drugs like methotrexate and semustin.

The stimulation of the excretion of organic anions is of distinct clinical relevance (Dzurik et al., 1991). Glutarate increases the PAH uptake *in vitro* (Villalobos et al., 1996). The withdrawal of sodium from the incubation medium depresses the glutarate-induced stimulation (Villalobos et al., 1996, Edwards et al., 1997). Dzurik et al. (1991) show that the administration of amino acids increases *in vitro* the PAH accumulation in renal tissue of rats as a sign of improved housekeeping. In contrast, Fleck and Pertsch (1998) demonstrated *in vivo* that simultaneous administration of PAH and amino acids reduce the PAH excretion as a result of increased energy consumption in the kidney.

For about two decades it is known that the renal excretion capacity of weak organic acids, e.g. PAH, can be stimulated by a suitable treatment schedule *in vivo* (Stopp and Bräunlich, 1975, 1980, Bräunlich et al., 1986). For this purpose, various xenobiotics (penicillin, probenecid, phenol red, PAH), hormones (T_3, dexamethasone and other glucocorticoids, insulin), and epidermal growth factor were used (Fleck and Bräunlich 1995). The stimulatory effect can be shown after 3 days of pre-treatment: the PAH excretion into urine increases e.g. after T_3 treatment by about 60% (Bräunlich 1988). In further *in vitro* investigations on renal cortical slices it was demonstrated that PAH accumulation capacity was significantly increased after *in vivo* stimulation with T_3, whereas after dexamethasone, pre-treatment stimulation did not occur (Bräunlich et al., 1986, Bräunlich 1987). An increase in protein *de novo* synthesis could be one of the reasons for the stimulation of renal PAH transport (Berkhin and Varshavsky 1975). Both renal transport capacity and the effect of stimulatory pre-treatment on renal function are age dependent (Bräunlich 1981): renal excretion capacity of 10-day-old rats is immature, however, in young rats the extent of the stimulation of renal transport processes is often higher than in adult animals (Fleck and Bräunlich 1990). The following reasons could generally be responsible for the stimulation of renal tubular transport capacity: *a)* an increase in *de novo* synthesis of transport proteins (Ortweiler et al., 1987), *b)* an increase in GFR (Bräunlich et al., 1987), *c)* a raise in renal blood flow (Fleck et al., 1981a), *d)* systemic hormone effects, and *e)* metabolic changes after hormone pre-treatment.

Dexamethasone induces a reduction in body weight in rats whereas the kidney weight increases (Rajashree und Puvanakrishnan, 1998). Glucocorticoids are involved in blood pressure regulation and, thus, indirectly in renal function (Villeneuve et al., 2000, Rajashree und Puvanakrishnan, 1998). Renal perfusion and glomerular filtration increase (Aguirre et al., 1999). On the other hand, very high daily doses of glucocorticoids induce renal damage (Chen et al., 1998). In renal tissue, corticoid receptors exist (Fanestil and Parks, 1981), especially in tubular cells (Stonestreet et al., 1984). Glucocorticoids are transported via the contraluminal membrane into the tubular cells and interact with the transport of PAH (Ullrich et al., 1991). In the kidney, corticoids enhance *de novo* synthesis of proteins, e.g. of Na^{+}-K^{+}-ATPase (Klein et al., 1984).

Thyroid hormones regulate growth and development (Shi et al., 2002). Reduced concentrations of T_3 und T_4 are followed by a diminished GFR and RPF (Capasso et al., 1999). The effect of T_3 is mediated by an increase in protein synthesis (Capasso et al., 1987, de Nayer 1987) and by a modification of membrane potassium permeability (Capasso et al., 1999). Voci et al. (2001) assumed that thyroid hormones are responsible for renal organogenesis. Finally, thyroid hormones control postnatal development of renal phosphate transport (Euzet et al., 1996) and Na^{+}-K^{+}-ATPase activity (Klein et al., 1984).

The capacity of PAH carriers can be influenced by a broad variety of hormones (Fleck and Bräunlich, 1995). The stimulation of renal tubular transport of xenobiotics seems to be caused by an increased *de novo* synthesis of carrier proteins (Silva et al., 1976, Bräunlich et al., 1986, Ortweiler et al., 1987, Bräunlich 1987, Penzold and Bräunlich, 1990) This hypothesis was supported by Bahn et al. (2003) reporting an enhanced expression of mRNA encoding OAT1 after dexamethasone or T_3.

For better understanding of the processes involved in stimulation of renal PAH transport at the cellular level and to clarify the discrepancies between the effects of hormone pretreatment *in vivo* on renal PAH excretion and PAH accumulation in renal cortical slices, a new experimental approach has been developed to stimulate the tubular transport of PAH *in vitro* (Fleck 1997). For this reason, renal cortical slices were incubated for 24 hours in a modified Williams medium E under carbogen gassing. Thereafter, slices were placed in a Cross-Taggart-buffer containing PAH, and the uptake of PAH from the medium into the slices can be measured. Under these experimental conditions, the slice to medium ratio for PAH decreases from about 12 to 6, nevertheless also after this long-lasting incubation period the PAH accumulation is an active one, because under nitrogen atmosphere, PAH uptake is completely abolished.

Renal Cell Carcinoma

Two to three percent of all malignant tumours are renal cell carcinoma (RCC). Until now only localised RCC can be removed successfully by radical tumour extirpation. At the time of RCC diagnosis, in 20% metastases occur distant from the primary tumour and in another 20% of RCC, metastases can be found in the local lymph nodes (Hermanek and Schrott 1990). About one half of the patients undergoing radical tumour nephrectomy die as a consequence of their metastases (Skinner et al., 1971). It is a well-known clinical finding that RCC and its metastases are quite insensitive to any kind of cancer chemotherapy (Mickisch 1994a, c). This multidrug resistance (MDR) is reported to be caused by expression of the MDR1 gene and is characterised by a broad-spectrum cross-resistance to many chemotherapeutic agents (Mickisch et al., 1991, Volm et al., 1991, Chapman and Goldstein 1995, van Brussel and Mickisch 1998). Especially metastases of RCC show signs of multidrug resistance (Samuels et al., 1997, Azpodien et al., 1998, Roigas et al., 1998). In most RCC, the MDR1 gene is over expressed (Somogyi, 1996), followed by a fast efflux of anticancer drugs out of the tumour cells (Mickisch et al., 1991, Volm et al., 1991, Naito et al., 1993, Nishiyama et al., 1993, Chapman and Goldstein, 1995, Rohlff and Glatzer 1995, Bosch and Croop 1996). The favourite hypothesis to explain the phenomenon of multidrug resistance is an increase in transport of chemotherapeutics out of the renal carcinoma cell (Nishiyama et al., 1993, Licht et al., 1995, Leier et al., 1996). Therefore, at the present time surgical removal of the RCC is the method of choice (Mickisch, 1994a, b). MDR is a complex phenomenon based on different biochemical events (Efferth et al., 1993). In the past, a couple of therapeutic strategies have been used to overcome MDR. First of all, a blockade of anticancer drug efflux out of RCC was tried. One approach consisted of an inhibition of the MDR1 gene product P-glycoprotein by calcium antagonists, e.g. verapamil (Mickisch et al., 1990, Woodland et al., 2003) or triazinoaminopiperidine derivates (Efferth et al., 1993, Punt et al., 1997). Furthermore, an inhibition of proteinkinase C, responsible for the regulation of P-glycoproteins was used (Efferth und Volm 1992). Immunological strategies such as the use of monoclonal antibodies (Mickisch, 1992, 1993) or tumour vaccination (Gansbacher et al., 1990) had no beneficial effects. Auto-transplantation of MDR1-transfected bone marrow after high-dose chemotherapy is problematical from the ethical point of view (Mickisch, 1992). One method of overcoming this insensitivity is the use of chemosensitizers, which inhibit the function of the MDR1 gene product P-glycoprotein (Broxterman et al., 1989, Effert et al., 1989, Naito et al., 1993). Few attractive candidates, e.g., verapamil (Berlion et al., 1993, Lai et al., 1993, Mickisch et al., 1991), vitamin E (Okada et al., 1987), and tiapamil analogues (Eliason et al., 1995), which should be included in clinical trials, are given in the literature.

Besides these therapeutic strategies, there was almost no information about the accumulation capacity of RCC, i.e., about the active uptake of a chemotherapeutic agent into the renal carcinoma cell independently of its passive diffusion. Although the latter uptake mechanism is of high practical importance for anticancer drugs (Focan 1995), active uptake of these substances cannot be excluded. However, it remains unclear whether active and/or passive uptake of anticancer drugs on the one hand or their active outward transport, on the other hand, dominates in RCC. As shown above, it is possible to stimulate the tubular accumulation capacity. However, these experiments were performed using PAH as the model substance. Without doubt, the PAH uptake into renal cells is quite different from that of chemotherapeutics. Nevertheless, similar findings can also be expected for anticancer drugs. From this point of view, the question arose whether or not the tubular accumulation capacity in human RCC is diminished and, therefore, the uptake of anticancer drugs is too low for effective tumour therapy. As a first step toward clarifying this question, accumulation experiments on normal human renal cortical tissue and on RCC were compared using PAH as the model substance. The final goal of these experiments was the stimulation of the uptake of cytostatics in human kidney tissue to overcome multidrug resistance because it is a major obstacle to effective chemotherapy of RCC (Mickisch and Schroeder 1996, Motzer et al., 1996, Yu et al., 1999).

We were able to show that the accumulation capacity of RCC is significantly reduced (Fleck et al., 1997a). Therefore, stimulation of the uptake of cytostatic drugs could be beneficial in the treatment of renal cancer and its metastases. At first, we found that PAH accumulation in "intact" human renal tissue can be stimulated after incubation of renal cortical slices in dexamethasone-containing medium (Fleck et al., 1998, 2000). On the basis of the results obtained on rat and on intact human kidney tissue, the transport capacity should be stimulated in RCC. The question arose whether or not the accumulation capacity of RCC is under hormonal control and can be enhanced after incubation with dexamethasone or T_3.

Human kidney proximal tubules express the ATP-dependent export pump for anionic conjugates encoded by the MRP2 gene, too. This multidrug resistance protein is localized to the apical brush-border membrane domain of proximal tubules. MRP2, the first cloned ATP-dependent export pump for anionic conjugates detected in human kidney, may be involved in renal excretion of various anionic endogenous substances, xenobiotics, and cytotoxic drugs. This conjugate-transporting ATPase has similar substrate specificity as the multidrug resistance protein MRP1, and may contribute to the multidrug resistance of RCC (Schaub et al., 1999). Therefore, a stimulation of the uptake of cytostatic drugs could be beneficial in the treatment of RCC and its metastases. However, it has to be kept in mind that RCC metastases have altered MDR-1 expression, probably due to altered differentiation compared to the primary tumour. Thus, the drug resistance phenotype of the primary RCC may not reflect that of their metastases (Gamelin et al., 1999).

Finally, a stimulation of the uptake of cytostatic drugs into RCC was tried. This approach is in line with that of Amato et al. (1995) describing the therapeutic benefit of a combination between interferon and dexamethasone for RCC chemotherapy. For this reason, in our experiments the accumulation of methotrexate (MTX), cis-platinum (CP), topotecan, and Tomudex® was characterized in intact kidney and in RCC with and without *ex vivo* treatment with dexamethasone, T_3, and/or EGF.

These anticancer drugs were chosen for the following reasons: The human MDR protein (MRP) gene family contains at least 6 members. Honscha et al. (2000) reported about a methotrexate carrier in the kidney. This result supports the notion that apical membrane bi-directional organic anion transporters participate in epithelial transport of lipophilic organic anions like MTX in the kidney because the uptake of PAH by OAT1 was moderately inhibited by MTX (Uwai et al., 1998). CP induces the renal expression of P-glycoprotein and canalicular multispecific organic anion transporter (cMOAT or Mrp2), two members of the ATP-binding cassette family (Demeule et al., 1999). The thymidilate synthase inhibitor Tomudex® (Toffoli et al., 2000) has been developed to overcome the potential mechanisms of tumour resistance to MTX (Takimoto and Allegra 1995). The MDR of RCC has been related to the expression of P-glycoprotein and effective drug detoxification mechanisms (Hartmann and Bokemeyer 1999). Treatment of RCC with topotecan, a topoisomerase I inhibitor with little substrate affinity for P-glycoprotein, led to induction of apoptosis in all RCC (Ramp et al., 2000).

MATERIAL AND METHODS

Animals

The animal experiments were carried out on Wistar of which rats (Han: WIST) from our institute's own out-bred stock. In 5- to 15-day-old animals both sexes were used, 55-day-old animals were females. At the beginning of the experiments, 2-month-old animals had an average body weight of about 170 g. The litters were reduced to 6 animals. Their dams nursed young animals. Adult rats were fed a standard diet (Altromin 1316) and tap water ad libitum. Animals were housed under standardized conditions in plastic cages with 12/12 hour light-dark cycles, temperature 22 $\pm$ 2 °C, and humidity of 50 $\pm$ 10 %. At the time the accumulation experiment, the rats were anaesthetised with ether, exsanguinated and the kidneys removed and stored on ice. Animal care and treatment were conducted in conformity with institutional guidelines that are in compliance with international laws.

Patients

Between 1994 and 2002, *in vitro* accumulation experiments were performed on human kidney slices. Intact renal cortical tissue (control) of tumour-bearing kidney was obtained from 139 patients undergoing radical tumour nephrectomy in the Department of Urology, Jena. "Intact" kidney tissue means macroscopically inconspicuous material from the tumour-bearing kidney. RCC were classified in groups pT_1 to pT_3 without multifocal localisation. The distance between intact renal tissue and RCC was $\leq$ 4 cm. The patients were 81 men and 58 women with an average age of 63.3 $\pm$ 11.8 years. Tissue samples (about 1 g) of the peripheral and central part of the tumour and of intact kidney tissue were stored in normal saline on ice (4°C) immediately after kidney removal. After transportation (30-60 minutes), slices were prepared as described below. This study was performed in accordance with internationally accepted ethical standards for human experimentation and was approved by the Ethical Review Committee of the Medical Faculty of the University of Jena.

Stimulation of PAH Excretion Capacity in Rats

60 µg/100 g b.m. dexamethasone (Fortecortin° Mono, E. Merck, Darmstadt) was given to rats i. p. for 3 days, once daily. Following this dose, glucocorticoid receptor sites were completely saturated by dexamethasone (Rafestin-Oblin et al., 1986). Dexamethasone was dissolved in normal saline (1 ml/100 g b.wt.). Controls received the solvent only. Clearance experiments were performed 24 h after the last treatment with dexamethasone. Renal excretion of PAH (E. Merck, Darmstadt) was measured after the administration of doses, which can reliably saturate the transport capacity in rats of different ages: 100 (10-day-old) or 200 (55-day-old) mg PAH/100 g b. wt. dissolved in distilled water (2 ml/100 g b. wt.) i.p. (Bräunlich et al., 1983). Animals were placed in metabolic cages for one hour and urine was collected and measured volumetrically.

Accumulation Experiments on Tissue of Hormone-Treated Rats

In experiments on renal cortical slices, the lumina of the tubuli are collapsed (Wedeen and Weiner, 1973) and the basolateral uptake can be measured because intracellular binding of PAH is of minor importance (Splinter and Bräunlich, 1973).

Acute Experiments (2-hours Incubation Time)

Dexamethasone treated and controlled rats were anaesthetized with ether, exsanguinated and the kidneys were removed and stored in normal saline on ice. Renal cortical slices of rats with pool sizes of about 100 mg (1 mm thick) were incubated in Erlenmeyer flasks with PAH (bi-directional shaking, 100 rpm) in 3 ml Cross-Taggart buffer (pH 7.4; 30°C; oxygen gassing (2.5 l/hour/sample); incubation time 120 minutes; concentration of PAH: 30 μM). Following incubation PAH was determined in the supernatant fraction of the homogenate and in the incubation medium. The uptake of PAH was expressed by the ratio between PAH concentration in the tissue and in the medium after the end of incubation (slice to medium ratio = $Q_{S/M}$) according to Stopp and Bräunlich (1975).

Sub-Chronic Experiments (24-hours Incubation Time)

Additional experiments were performed with 2-, 6-, 12-, 24-, and 48-hour-incubation of renal cortical slices (~100 mg) of untreated rats in Erlenmeyer flasks loaded with 10 ml Williams medium E (WME, Bio Whittaker) which was supplemented with glutamine (292 mg/l), insulin (1μM), gentamicin (50 mg/l), and different concentrations of dexamethasone, T_3 (SIGMA, Deisenhofen, Germany), or epidermal growth factor (BACHEM, Bubendorf, Switzerland) under carbogen gassing (95% O_2/5% CO_2; 2.5 l/hour/sample) adjusted to pH 7.4 and 25 °C. Dexamethasone and T_3 were used in concentrations between 10^{-8} and 10^{-9} μM (Fleck et al., 1998, 2000) EGF was added into the incubation medium in a concentration of 1 μg/ml (Norman et al., 1990). Chemicals were commercially available and of analytical grade. Thereafter, slices were placed in Cross-Taggart-buffer (pH 7.4) containing PAH, and the uptake of PAH or of anticancer drug from the medium into the slices was measured in two-hour accumulation experiments as described above (Figure 1).

To differentiate between active and passive processes involved in accumulation, further experiments were performed under nitrogen atmosphere (2.5 l/hour/sample).

Determination Methods

PAH (SIGMA) was determined colorimetrically (Bratton et al., 1939). CP (Jenapharm, Jena, Germany): Pt concentration was measured by flameless atomic absorption spectrometry (AAS; model EA 4, Carl Zeiss, Jena, Germany) (Winnefeld et al., 1992). MTX was isolated with LC-18 columns (Sulpeco, Deisenhofen, Germany) and determined by HPLC with a K 2500 UV-detector (Knauer, Berlin, Germany) (Nürnberg et al., 1989). Topotecan (Hycamtin®; SmithKline Beecham Pharma, München, Germany) was determined with a reversed-phase HPLC technique (HPLC LC10 system, Shimadzu, Japan) (Loos et al., 1996). The separation was achieved using a Hypersil BDS-C18 column (Langerwehe, Germany). The mobile phase consisted of a gradient mixed from ACN (6% to 16%; flow rate: 0.8 ml/min) and 0,01M potassium dihydrogenphosphate containing 0.3% triethylamine.

Raltitrexed (Tomudex®; Zeneca GmbH, Plankstadt, Germany): For the measurement, an RP-HPLC method was adapted (Hilger et al., 1999). Reduced (GSH) and oxidized (GSSG) glutathione was determined in accordance to Kretzschmar et al. (1989) and Hissin and Hilf (1979), respectively, with slight modifications. In brief: three parts of each homogenate were denaturised and diluted with four parts of metaphosphoric acid (25 % w/v) and 9 parts of 0.2 M Na-phosphate EDTA buffer, pH 8.0. After centrifugation at 20.000 g and 4 °C for 30 min, glutathione was measured in the supernatant. Potassium was measured by flame photometry in the same supernatant after further dilution (1: 20) with H_2O.

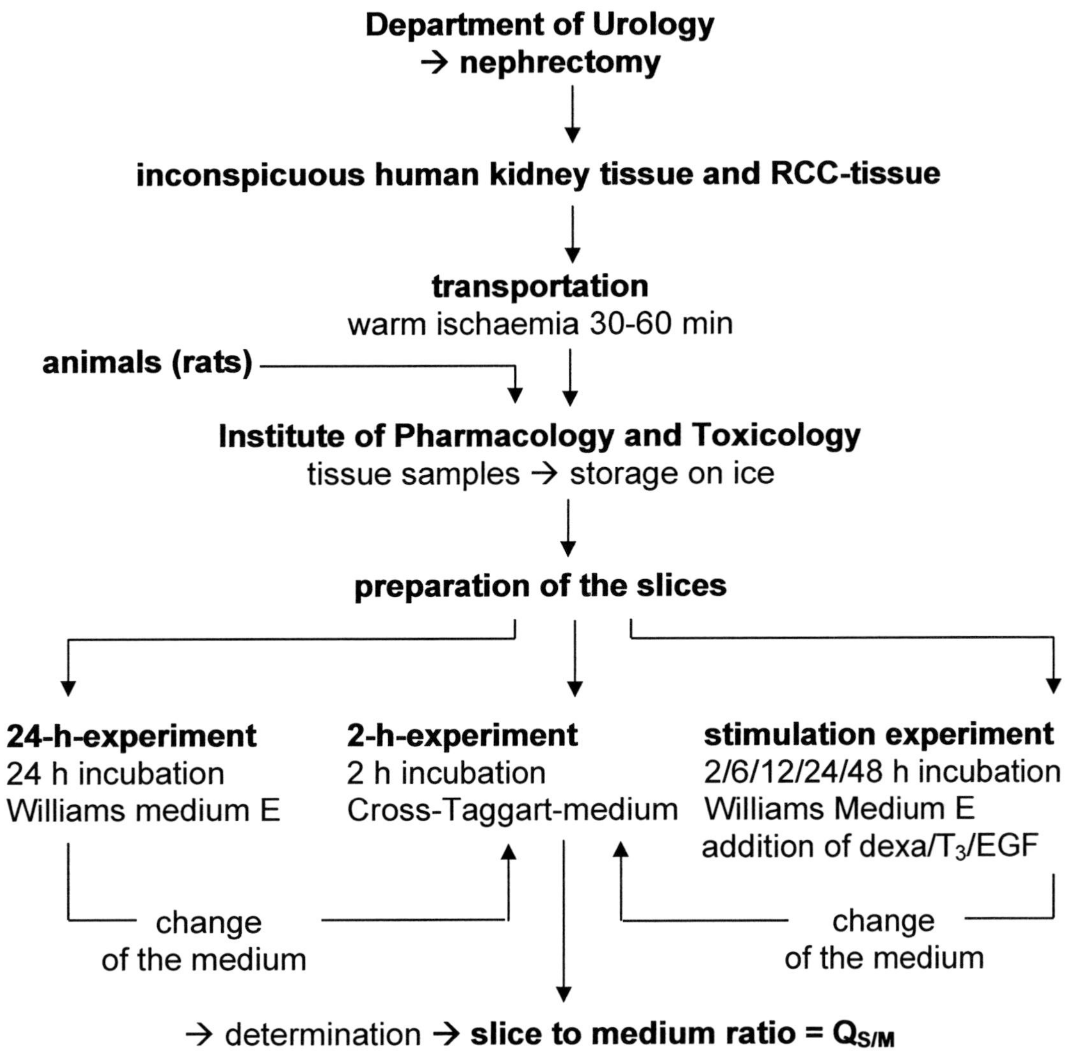

Figure 1. Synopsis of all investigations concerning the stimulation of renal drug transport in rat and man.

Statistics

The results are given as arithmetic means ± SEM of 4 - 6 independent slice preparations. In each patient, 4 slice preparations per one medium concentration were used to minimize methodological variances. In the PAH excretion experiments, n = 6 adult rats were included; in immature rats, the urine of three animals was pooled. Statistically significant differences between various experimental groups were analysed using the Mann-Whitney-test ($p \leq 0.05$).

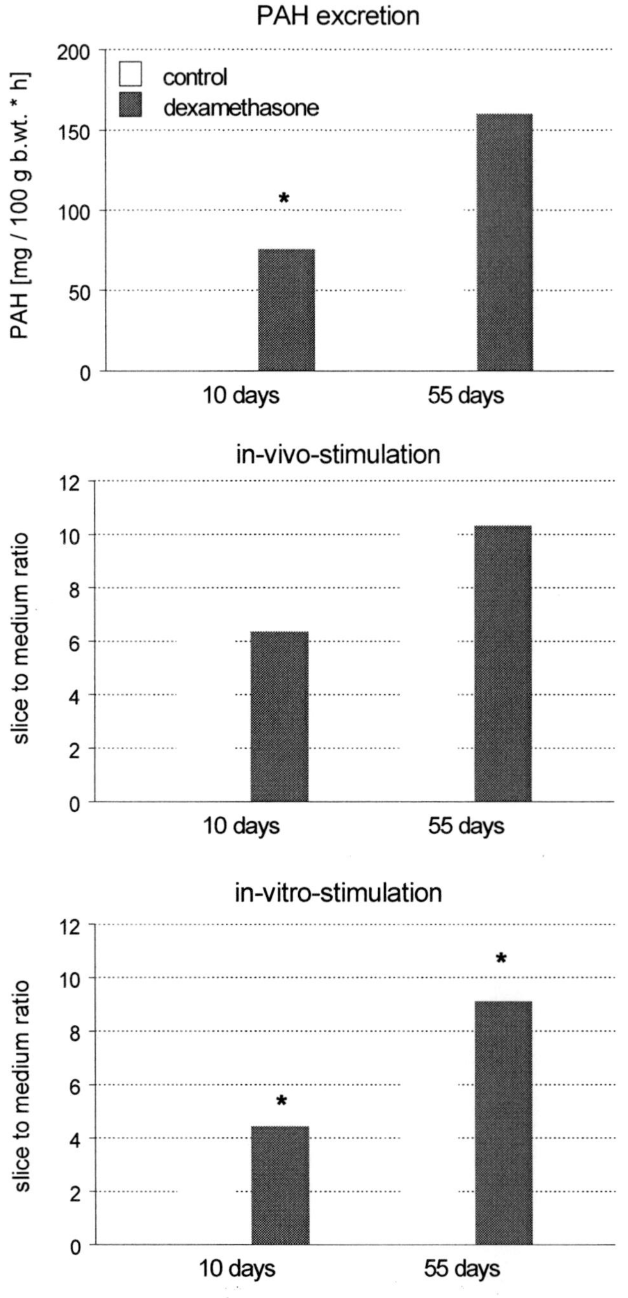

Figure 2. Influence of *in vivo* dexamethasone treatment on urinary PAH excretion and PAH accumulation in renal cortical slices of 10- and 55-day-old rats compared to the effect of a 24 h *in vitro* stimulation (0.5 μM dexamethasone) on PAH accumulation capacity. Arithmetic means ± SEM; n = 4; * - significant dexamethasone effects ($p \leq 0.05$).

RESULTS

In Figure 2, the influence of *in vivo* administration of dexamethasone (60 µg/100 g b.m. for three days, once daily) on renal PAH excretion and PAH accumulation capacity of rat renal cortical slices is compared with the effect of dexamethasone (0.5 µM) administered *in vitro* into the incubation medium on PAH accumulation. In 10-day-old rats, the renal PAH excretion was significantly lower than in adult animals, but it increased significantly after *in vivo* pre-treatment with dexamethasone; in 55-day-old rats this stimulatory effect was not significant. The PAH accumulation capacity of slices was not influenced by *in vivo* pre-treatment with dexamethasone, neither in immature nor in adult rats. However, after 24 hours incubation of renal cortical slices in dexamethasone-containing medium, the PAH *accumulation* was increased significantly in both age groups. This increase was in parallel to the raise in renal PAH *excretion* after *in vivo* pre-treatment with dexamethasone.

To further clarify the *in vitro* effect of dexamethasone, the PAH accumulation in rat renal cortical slices was investigated after 24 hours of incubation in dexamethasone-containing medium. The PAH accumulation in renal cortical slices of adult rats in Williams medium E (Figure 3) reached about two thirds of the values of acute incubation experiments after 24 hours of incubation (11.4 $\pm$ 0.3 *vs.* 7.1 $\pm$ 0.2). Tissue slices of 10-day-old rats tolerated the long-lasting incubation as well, however, the accumulation capacity was diminished to about 40 % (9.5 $\pm$ 0.4 *vs.* 3.7 $\pm$ 0.2). Under a nitrogen atmosphere, the concentration of PAH in slices and in medium was nearly the same ($Q_{S/M} \sim 1$). This indicates that PAH accumulation under oxygen gassing is an active process both after two and 24 hours of incubation time. Despite age differences in two and 24 hours incubation experiments, this experimental approach seems to be qualified for investigation of dexamethasone effects in rats *in vitro*.

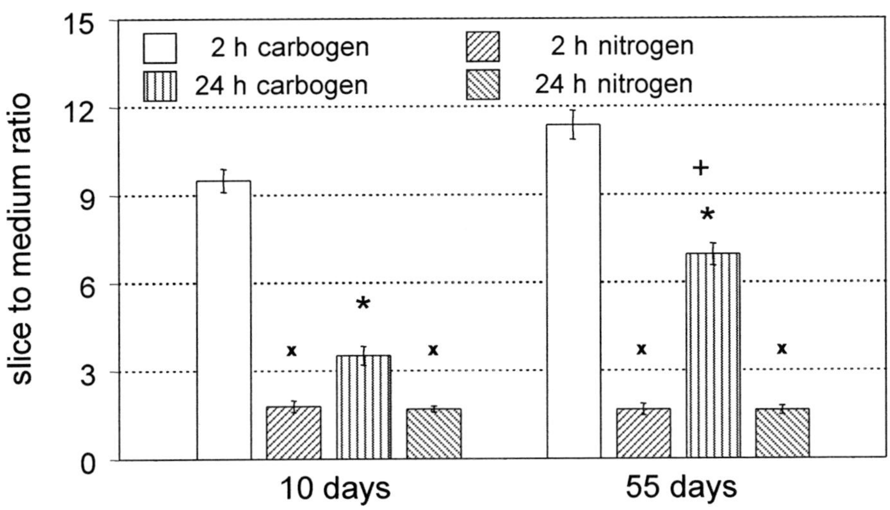

Figure 3. PAH accumulation in renal cortical slices of immature and adult rats under carbogen and nitrogen gassing in dependence on the duration of the incubation. Arithmetic means $\pm$ SEM; n = 4; ^{x} - significant differences between the two gassings, * - significant difference between 2 and 24 hours of incubation; $^{+}$ - significant age differences ($p \leq 0.05$).

As shown in Figure 4, there was no influence of dexamethasone in two hour incubation experiments in a Cross-Taggart medium, neither in immature nor in adult rat renal cortical slices. Age differences of accumulation capacity in control slices were not statistically significant.

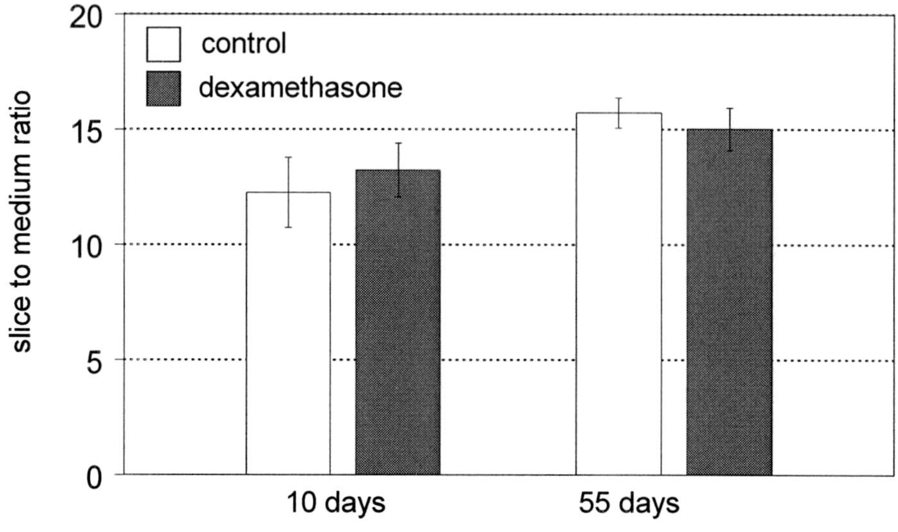

Figure 4. PAH accumulation in renal cortical slices of immature and adult rats during 2 h incubation experiments with and without addition of dexamethasone (0.5 μM) into a Cross-Taggart medium. Arithmetic means ± SEM.

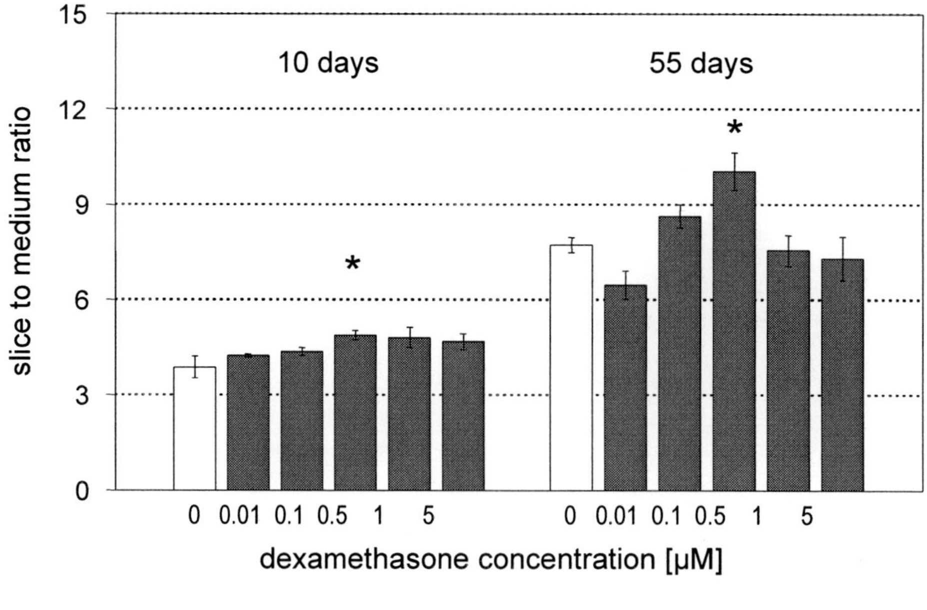

Figure 5. Influence of 24 h incubation in dexamethasone containing Williams medium E on PAH accumulation in renal cortical slices of immature and adult rats. Arithmetic means ± SEM; n = 4; * - significant dexamethasone effects ($p \leq 0.05$).

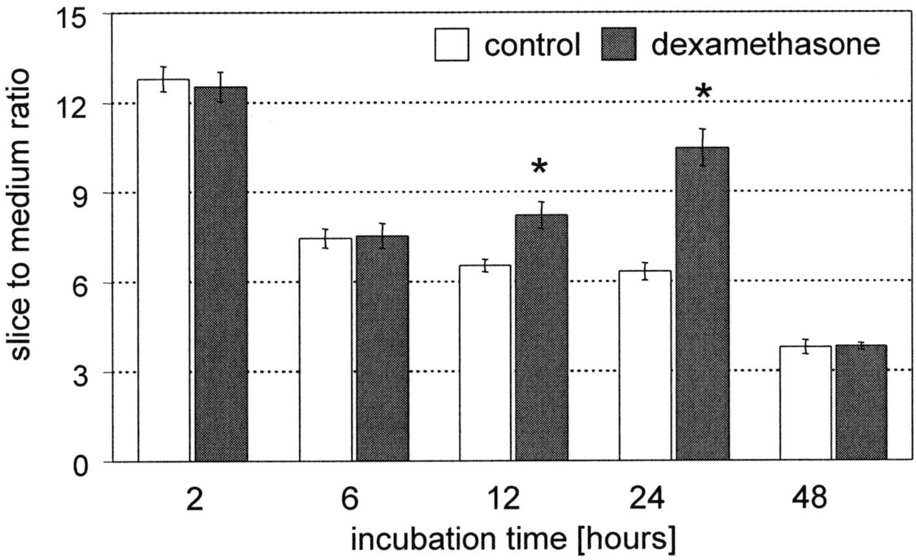

Figure 6. Influence of dexamethasone (0.5 μM) in the incubation medium on PAH accumulation in 55-day-old rat renal cortical slices in dependence on incubation time. Arithmetic means ± SEM; n = 4; * - significant dexamethasone effects ($p \leq 0.05$).

After 24 hours of incubation in dexamethasone containing Williams medium E, the PAH accumulation increased in immature and adult rats by about 26 and 36 %, respectively (Figure 5). This stimulation effect was concentration dependent. An optimal dexamethasone concentration in the medium (0.5 μM) could be found in both age groups.

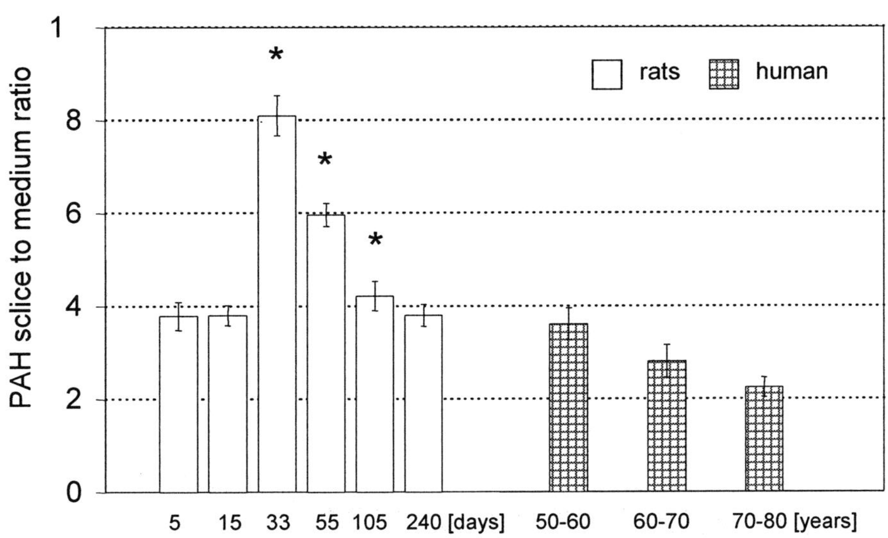

Figure 7. Age course of PAH accumulation capacity in female rats compared to that of humans of both sexes. Arithmetic means ± SEM; n = 6 per group (rats), n = 23 (humans); * - significant differences between consecutive age groups ($p \leq 0.05$).

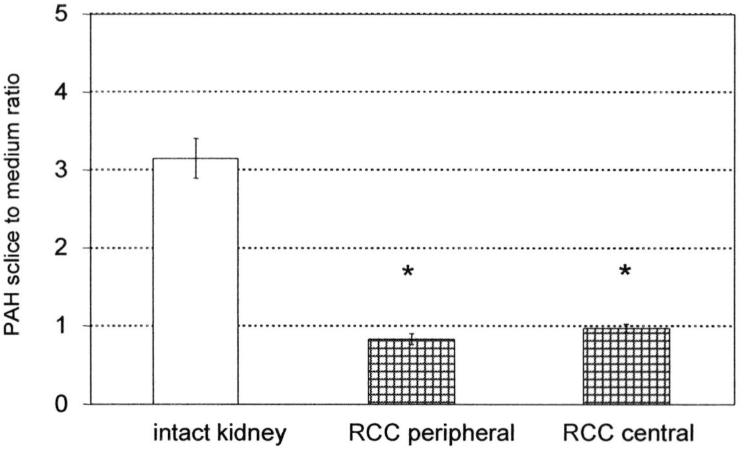

Figure 8. PAH accumulation in "intact" human kidney and in peripheral and central parts of RCC. Arithmetic means ± SEM: n = 23; * - significant reduction in RCC ($p \leq 0.05$).

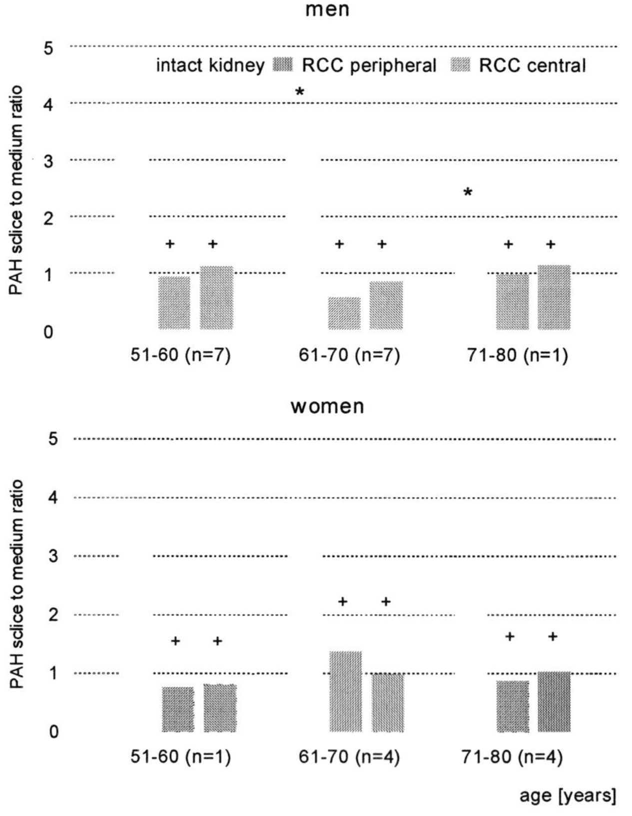

Figure 9. Influence of sex and age on renal PAH accumulation in "intact" human kidney and in peripheral and central parts of renal cell carcinoma (RCC). Arithmetic means ± SEM; + - reductions in RCC; * - significant difference between consecutive age groups ($p \leq 0.05$).

As shown in Figure 6, for adult rats the stimulatory dexamethasone effect was time dependent, too. After two hours (cp. Figure 4) and after six hours of incubation in dexamethasone-containing medium, no stimulation of PAH accumulation occurred. But after 12 and, more pronounced, after 24 hours the reduction in PAH accumulation capacity was avoided and nearly normal values were reached. In these experiments, the maximal dexamethasone effect even reached an increase of 65 %. A longer lasting incubation time (48 hours) was followed by a decrease in PAH uptake in control slices as well as in dexamethasone-treated slices and the stimulatory dexamethasone effect disappeared.

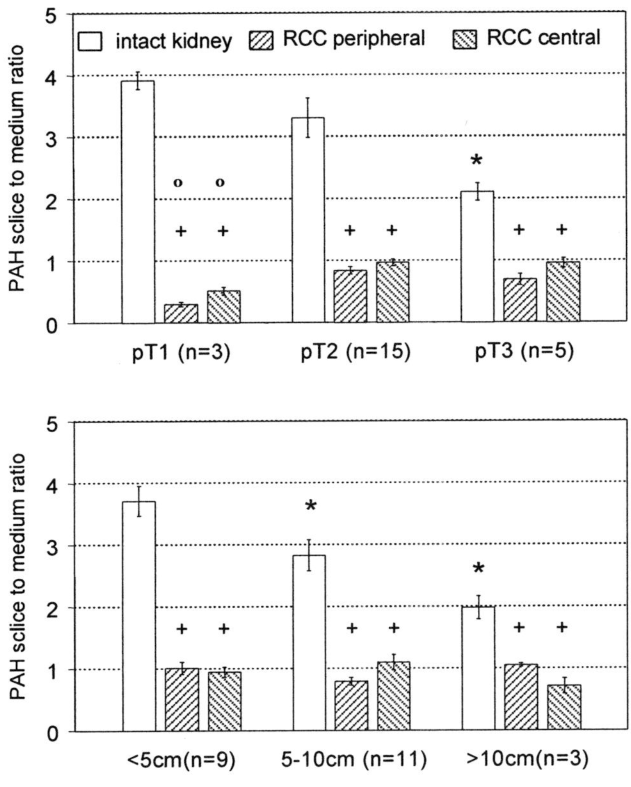

Figure 10. Relation between tumour stage (pT1-3) or tumour diameter and renal PAH accumulation in "intact" human kidney and in peripheral and central parts of renal cell carcinoma (RCC). Arithmetic means ± SEM; n = 23; $^{+}$ - significant reduction in RCC; * - significant difference between consecutive groups of "intact" kidneys; ^{O} – significant difference between pT1 and pT2/pT3 ($p \leq 0.05$).

As shown in Figure 7, the experimental approach used to characterize renal PAH accumulation on rat renal cortical slices can also be used for accumulation experiments on human renal tissue. In rats, the accumulation capacity becomes mature between days 5 and 33 after birth and decreases with increasing age. "Intact" human kidney tissue of our youngest patients (50 to 60 years old) accumulates PAH to the same extent as old rat tissue does. In older patients, accumulation capacity dropped. The slice to medium ratios in humans is between 2.2 and 3.8 and indicate active PAH uptake, which can be completely abolished under nitrogen gassing (not shown).

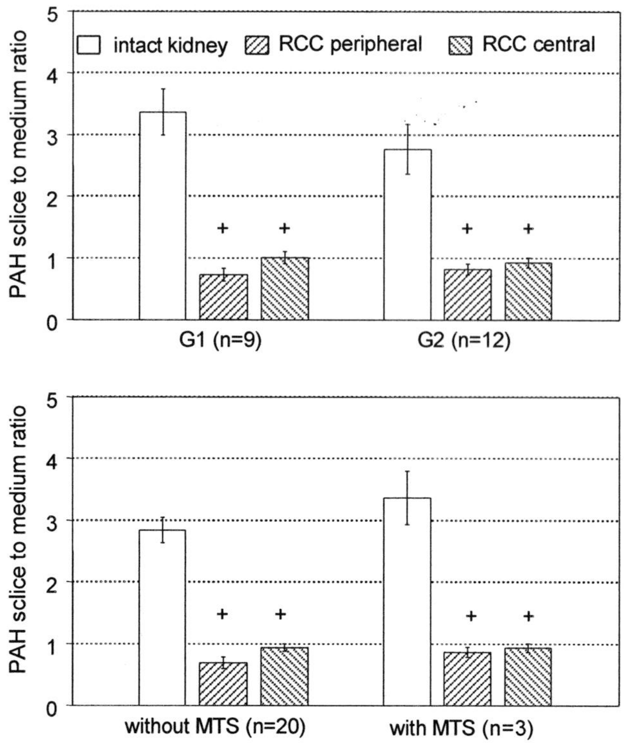

Figure 11. Relation between tumour grading (G1 or G2) or formation of metastases (MTS) and renal PAH accumulation in "intact" human kidney and in peripheral and central parts of RCC. Arithmetic means ± SEM; n = 23; [+] - significant reduction in RCC ($p \leq 0.05$).

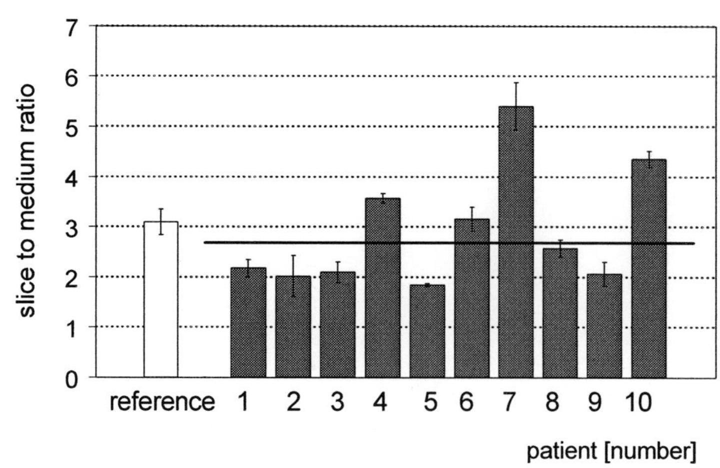

Figure 12. PAH accumulation in "intact" kidney of 10 patients suffering from RCC during 24 h incubation in Williams medium E. Reference: value measured during 2 h incubation in Cross-Taggart medium (n = 25). Arithmetic means ± SEM, 4 samples of each patient per concentration; line - mean value of the 10 patients.

The most important result of this part of our study is given in Figure 8: there is no accumulation of PAH in RCC, neither in the peripheral nor in the central parts of the tumour. Correlations of the slice-to-medium ratios with age and sex are shown in Figure 9. In principle, there are no differences between men and women concerning the age dependence of PAH accumulation in "intact" kidney tissue. The PAH concentration in the RCC is about 1 in all age groups and both sexes, indicating a complete loss of accumulation capacity in the tumour tissue.

Surprisingly, both tumour stage and size of the tumour seem to influence the accumulation capacity of the non-tumour-bearing tissue of the same kidney (Figure 10). The higher the tumour stage, the lower is the PAH accumulation in the "intact" kidney tissue. In stage pT1 RCC, the accumulation of PAH is obviously significantly lower than 1 as a possible sign of active transport of PAH out of the cells. In this group, however, only three samples were measured.

Tumour grading and formation of metastases are not associated with PAH accumulation in either "intact" kidney tissue or RCC (Figure 11).

As described above, in 2 hour PAH accumulation experiments with "intact" human kidney tissue, slice-to medium ratios of 3.12 ± 0.24 could be measured (= reference value in Figure 12). After 24-hour incubation, the PAH accumulation capacity decreased up to 2.68 ± 0.42. However, distinct inter-individual differences between 1.86 and 5.41 could be found.

The addition of dexamethasone of different concentrations into Williams medium E increased the PAH accumulation of intact human renal tissue after 24 hours significantly up to 156% (Figure 13). This stimulatory effect is, like in rats, concentration dependently too but with a maximum at 1 μM.

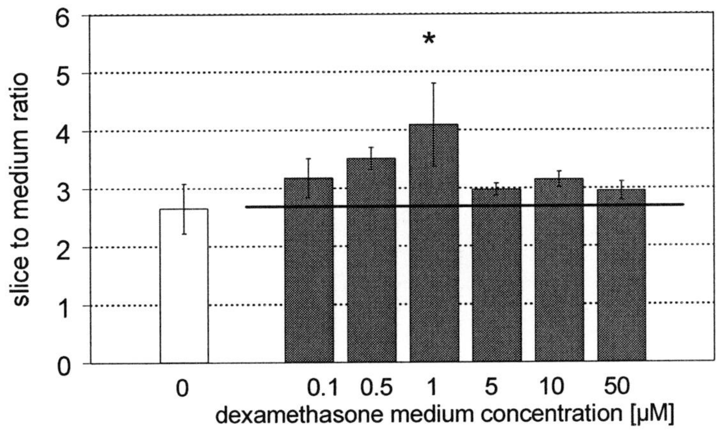

Figure 13. Influence of 24 h incubation in dexamethasone containing Williams medium E on PAH accumulation in renal cortical slices of "intact" kidney of 10 patients suffering from renal cell carcinoma. Arithmetic means ± SEM; n = 4 slice preparations per patient and each concentration; * - significant dexamethasone effect ($p \leq 0.05$); line - mean value of the 10 patients without dexamethasone.

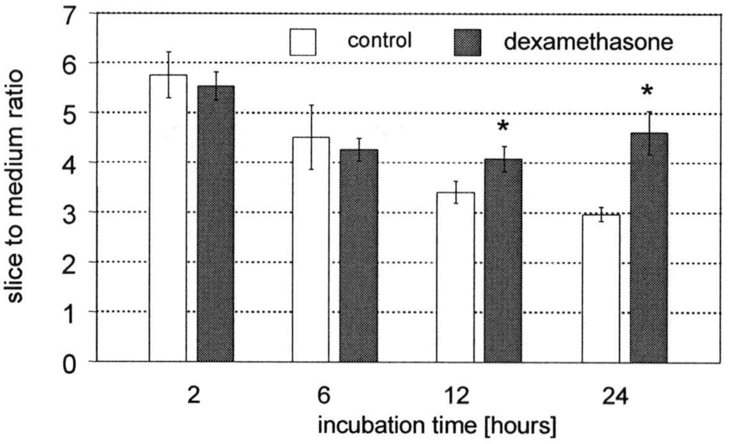

Figure 14. Influence of dexamethasone (1 µM) in the Williams medium E on PAH accumulation in renal cortical slices of "intact" kidney of patients suffering from renal cell carcinoma independent on the incubation time. Arithmetic means ± SEM; n = 3 patients, each 4 samples per time; * - significant dexamethasone effects ($p \leq 0.05$).

In Figure 14, the time dependence of the stimulatory dexamethasone effect is given (cp. Figure 6 for rats). After 2 and 6 hours of incubation in dexamethasone-containing medium, no stimulation of PAH accumulation occurred in "intact" human kidney tissue. But after 12 and, more pronounced, after 24 hours a significant increase in PAH accumulation capacity could be demonstrated.

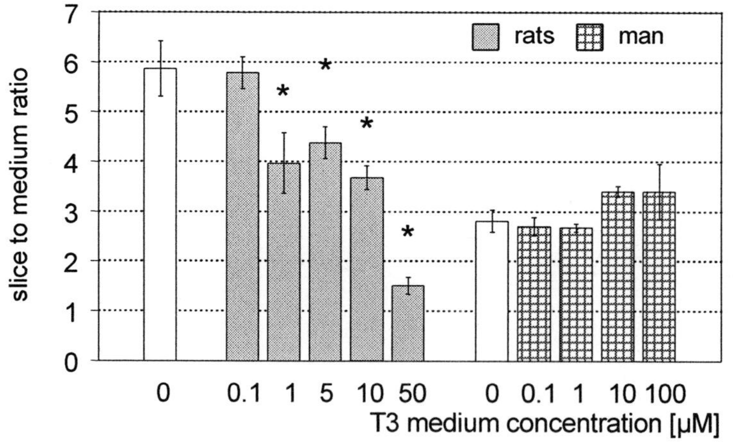

Figure 15. Influence of 24 h incubation in T_3 containing Williams medium E on PAH accumulation in renal cortical slices of adult rats and of "intact" human kidney of 5 patients suffering from renal cell carcinoma. Arithmetic means ± SEM; n = 4 (rats); in each of the 5 patients, 4 slice preparations per concentration were used; * - significant T_3 effect ($p \leq 0.05$).

To further characterize hormone effects on renal PAH accumulation, additional experiments were done using T_3 (Figure 15). After 24-hour incubation of rat's renal cortical slices in T_3 containing Williams medium E, the PAH accumulation dropped concentration dependently down to 20% of controls whereas in man no influence of T_3 could be found.

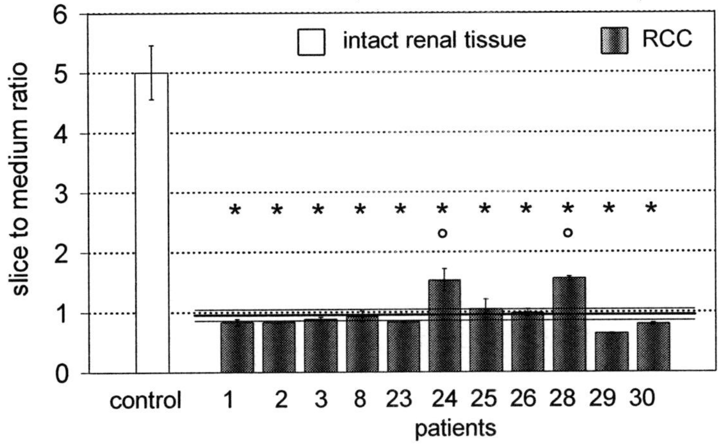

Figure 16. PAH accumulation capacity (2 h incubation) in "intact" human kidney (= control) and in 11 RCC patients (patients can be identified by the numbers at the abscissa). Arithmetic means ± S.E.M.; n = 3-4 samples per patient; * - significant reduction in RCC, ° - significant differences between the single RCC value and RCC mean value (= line) ($p \leq 0.05$).

Table 1. Comparison between the Influence of Dexamethasone (dexa) or T_3 on Potassium Concentration, Reduced (GSH) and Oxidized (GSSG) Glutathione in Rat Kidney (n = 4) and in "Intact" Human Renal Cortical Slices (5 controls) or in 7 RCC after 2- or 24-Hours Incubation under Oxygen Gassing

Treatment	rat			intact			RCC		
	NaCl	**dexa**	**T3**	**NaCl**	**dexa**	**T3**	**NaCl**	**dexa**	**T3**
2-hours-incubation									
potassium	68	76	68	49	62	53	49	53	48
[µmol/g]	± 4	± 4	± 2	± 4	± 4	± 3	± 4	± 3	± 3
GSH	1512	1420	n. d.	1210	1520	1405	948	1184	932
[µmol/g]	± 85	± 62		± 150	± 195	± 120	± 47	± 62	± 34
GSSG	312	230	n. d.	320	290	169	307	267	283
[µmol/g]	± 13	± 9		± 35	± 25	± 65	± 94	± 74	± 74
24-hours-incubation									
potassium	66	63	58	36	53	42	44	48	43
[µmol/g]	± 11	± 2	± 2	± 4	± 7	± 4	± 5	± 2	± 3
GSH	1180	1172	n. d.	725	710	860	984	731	846
[µmol/g]	± 24	± 30		± 30	± 60	± 40	± 51	± 103	± 39
GSSG	155	159	n. d.	150	185	182	131	182	131
[µmol/g]	± 3	± 5		± 10	± 15	± 44	± 36	± 14	± 24

Note: Arithmetic means ± S.E.M.; n = 3-4 patients or 6 rats; n.d. – not determined.

In the 2-hour-accumulation experiments, the human tissue slices were in good condition: both potassium concentrations and GSH or GSSG content were in the normal range (Table 1). As shown in Figure 16, in these experiment on freshly prepared "intact" human kidney PAH is accumulated very effectively ($Q_{S/M} = 5.03 \pm 0.41$; cp. figure 12: 3.12 ± 0.24). On the other hand, in RCC the PAH uptake is completely abolished ($Q_{S/M} \leq 1$). Only in patients No. 24 and No. 28, PAH accumulation could be shown ($Q_{S/M} \sim 1.5$).

After 24-hour-incubation in Williams medium E, the markers for the survival of the slices (intracellular concentrations of K^+, GSH, GSSG) are distinctly deteriorated (e.g. reduction in GSH and GSSG by about 50%, see Table 1). Nevertheless "intact" human kidney tissue accumulates PAH by a factor of ~3 (Figure 17). This significant reduction in PAH accumulation capacity is comparable to that given in Figure 12, but it does not disturb the further interpretation of these experiments because the enrichment of PAH is high enough for further experimental approaches. Interestingly, in RCC the PAH uptake seems to be slightly enhanced compared to the acute experiments performed immediately after kidney removal ($Q_{S/M}$: 1.2 *vs.* 0.98; compare mean values in figures 16 and 17). However, this moderate increase in PAH accumulation is of minor importance; nevertheless, the accumulation capacity of 4 of 22 RCC tissue samples is in the same range as that of "intact" kidney tissue.

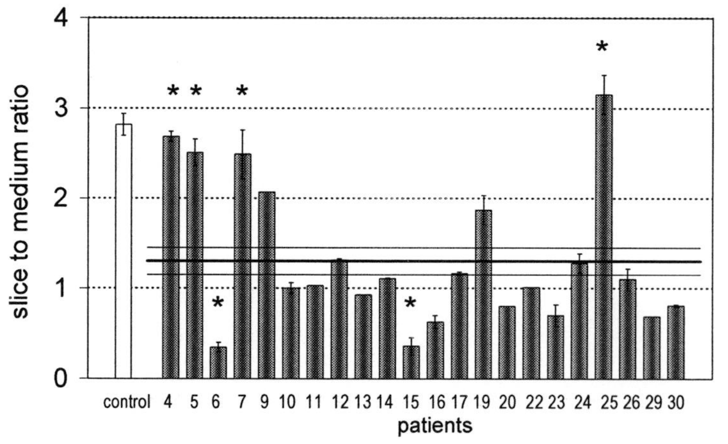

Figure 17. PAH accumulation after 24 h incubation of "intact" human kidney (mean value of 9 patients = control) and of RCC (22 patients can be identified by the numbers at the abscissa). Arithmetic means $\pm$ S.E.M.; n = 3-4 samples per patient; * - significant differences between single RCC value and RCC mean value (= line) ($p \leq 0.05$).

The main question of this part of our study was to clarify the possibility of stimulating the PAH uptake in RCC by 24-hour-incubation in hormone-containing Williams medium E. Also under these experimental conditions, the general parameters characterizing the slice survival after 24-hour incubation were not distinctly changed (Table 1). As shown above, the PAH accumulation in both rat's and man's "intact" kidney tissue can be stimulated 1.5-fold after incubation in a dexamethasone- containing medium, whereas T_3 was without effect (see Figure 20). But concerning the responsiveness of RCC against dexamethasone, the 13 patients investigated can be divided into 6 ”dexamethasone-responders“ and 7 “non-responders” (Figure 18). The average of stimulation effect after dexamethasone reaches about 190 ± 32 % in the group of responders. The reasons for these different reactions after dexamethasone incubation could be dependent on the tumour stage and histology.

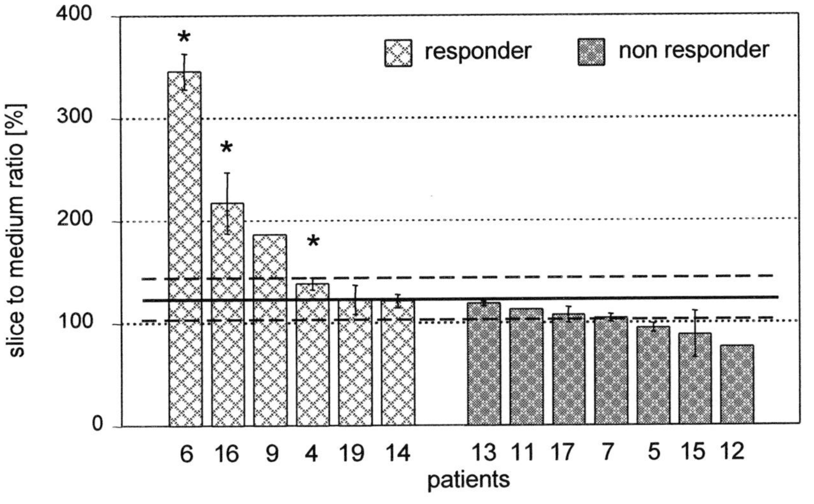

Figure 18. Influence of dexamethasone on PAH accumulation in RCC after 24 h incubation in dexamethasone containing Williams medium E. The patients were classified into “responders” and “non-responders” to dexamethasone. Arithmetic means ± S.E.M.; n = 3-4 samples per patient; continuous lines = mean ± S.E.M.; * - significant differences between RCC and controls (= 100 %) ($p \leq 0.05$).

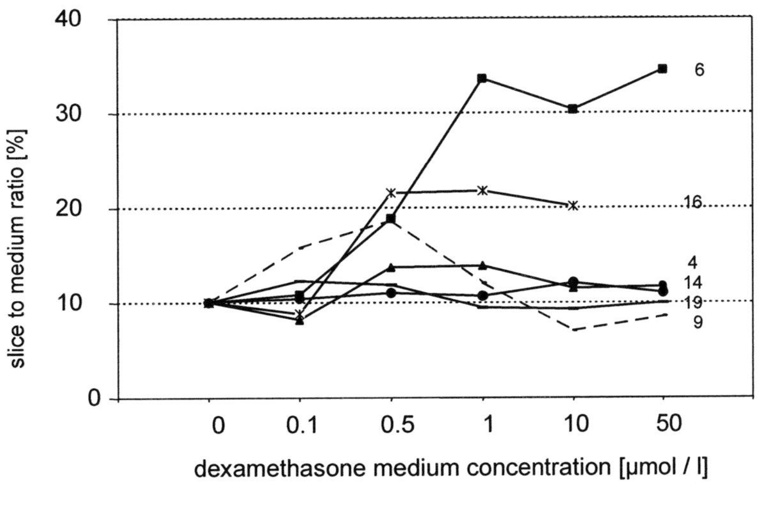

Figure 19. Dose dependence of the dexamethasone effect on the PAH accumulation after 24 h incubation in dexamethasone containing Williams medium E (WE) of the 6 “dexamethasone responders” (patient’s number see figure 18). Extent of stimulation is given in % of slices incubated in WE alone. Arithmetic means ± S.E.M.; n = 3-4 samples per patient and concentration.

A further specificity of the reaction of RCC tissue slices after dexamethasone incubation consists of its concentration dependency (Figure 19): The "responder" reacted maximally at different dexamethasone medium concentrations, most pronounced between concentrations of 0.5 and 1 μM. Only in patient No. 9 is a further increase in dexamethasone medium concentration above1 μM followed by a reduced PAH accumulation capacity.

For characterization of the energy dependence of hormone effects, experiments were performed under oxygen or nitrogen gassing (Figure 20). In principle, without oxygen supply no active PAH accumulation occurs. Thus the stimulatory effect of incubation of intact human kidney tissue and RCC tissue in dexamethasone containing medium is doubtless an energy consuming process whereas in the absence of oxygen equilibrium between tissue slices and medium occurs ($Q_{S/M} \sim 1$).

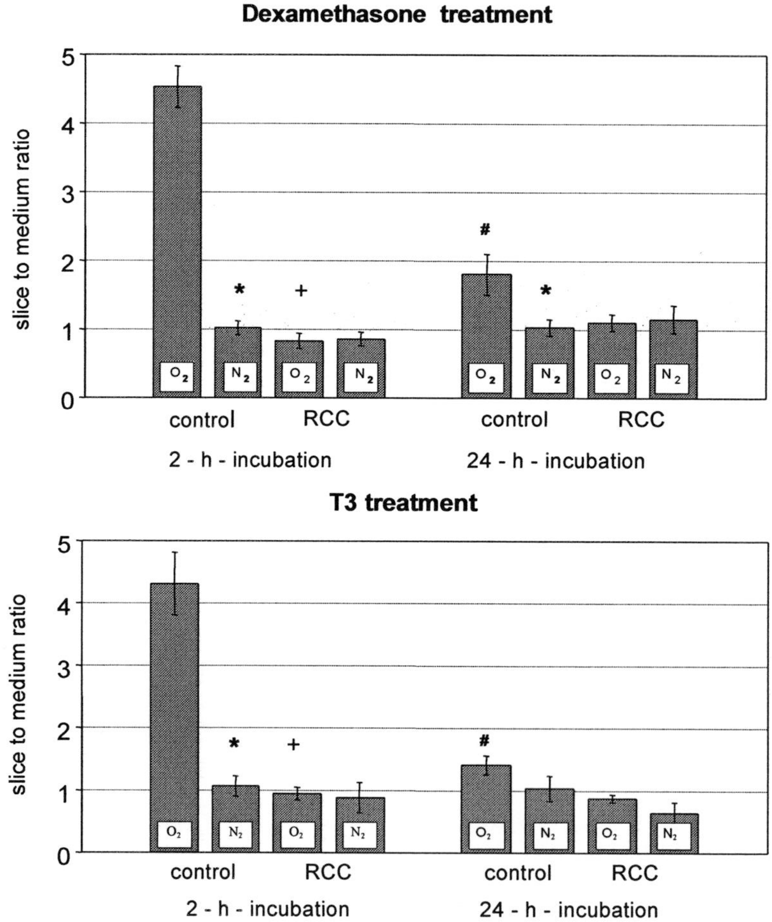

Figure 20. Comparison between the influence of dexamethasone or T_3 on PAH accumulation after 2 or 24 h incubation of "intact" human kidney (controls) or of RCC under oxygen or nitrogen gassing. Arithmetic means $\pm$ S.E.M.; n = 3-4 samples per patient; 12 controls and RCC were investigated (8 x dexamethasone, 4 x T_3); * - significant influence of nitrogen; $^+$ - significant differences between controls and RCC, $^\#$ - significant influence of 24 h hormone pre-treatment ($p \leq 0.05$).

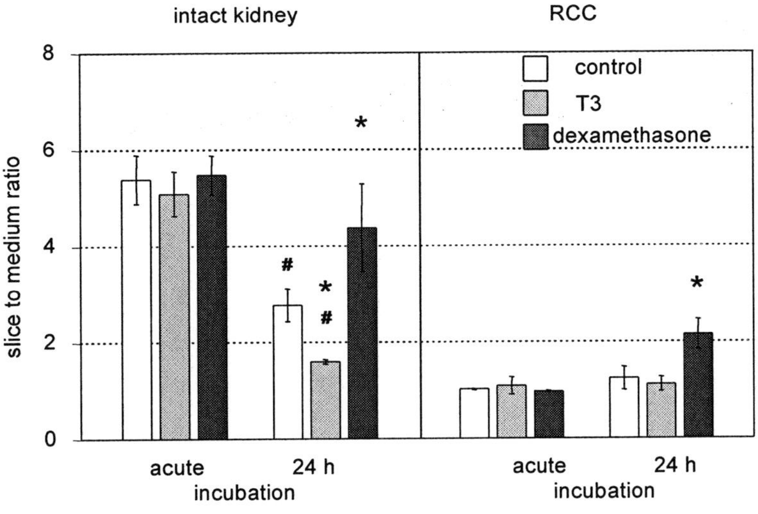

Figure 21. Influence of dexamethasone or T_3 (2 and 24 h incubation) on PAH accumulation in "intact" human kidney and in RCC. Arithmetic means $\pm$ S.E.M.; n = 6 patients, 3-4 measurements per patient; * - significant hormone effect; # - significant difference between 2 and 24 h incubation ($p \leq 0.05$).

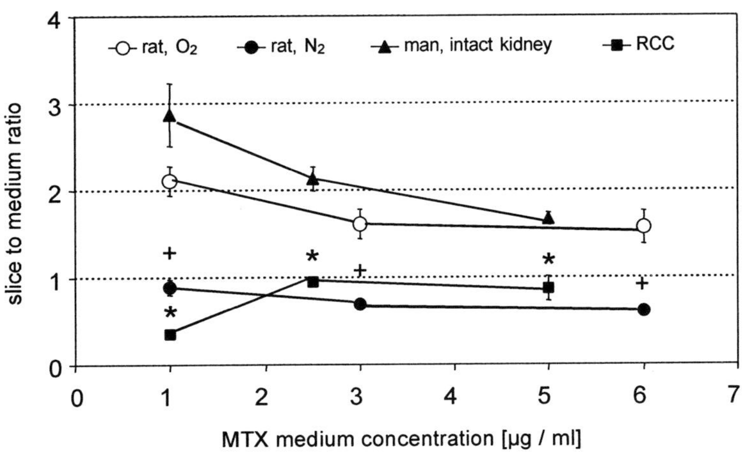

Figure 22. Concentration and energy dependence (O_2- or N_2-gassing) of MTX accumulation in rat and "intact" human kidney and in RCC during 2 h incubation. Arithmetic means $\pm$ S.E.M.; n = 6; * - significant difference between "intact" human kidney and RCC ($p \leq 0.05$); + - significant difference between oxygen and nitrogen ($p \leq 0.05$).

The addition of dexamethasone into the incubation medium increased the PAH accumulation in renal tissue of rats and in "intact" human kidney (Figure 21, left) as a sign of *ex vivo* stimulation. The optimal dexamethasone concentration was between 0.5 and 1.0 µM in the incubation WE medium. 2-hour incubation with dexamethasone or T_3 was without effect on PAH accumulation, both in intact kidney and in RCC, whereas after 24 hours a significant increase in PAH accumulation capacity could be demonstrated. In "intact" human renal tissue, the PAH accumulation capacity dropped after 24-hour incubation and can be increased by dexamethasone up to 156 %. On the other hand, T_3 decreased PAH uptake in intact human kidney. In RCC, PAH uptake can be stimulated significantly after 24 hours of dexamethasone incubation by about 90 %, while T_3 is without effect on PAH accumulation (Figure 21, right). For presentation of the data given in figure 21, only "dexamethasone responders" were chosen.

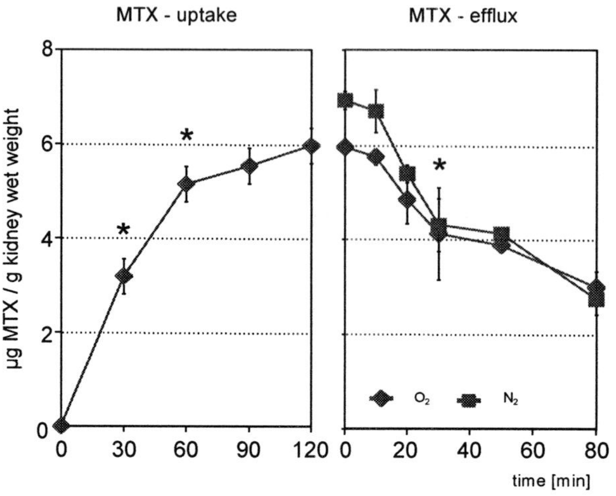

Figure 23. Time dependence of MTX (10 µg/ml) uptake and MTX efflux under O_2 and N_2 incubation in rat kidney. Arithmetic means ± S.E.M.; n = 4 per time; * - significant differences between two subsequent times ($p \leq 0.05$).

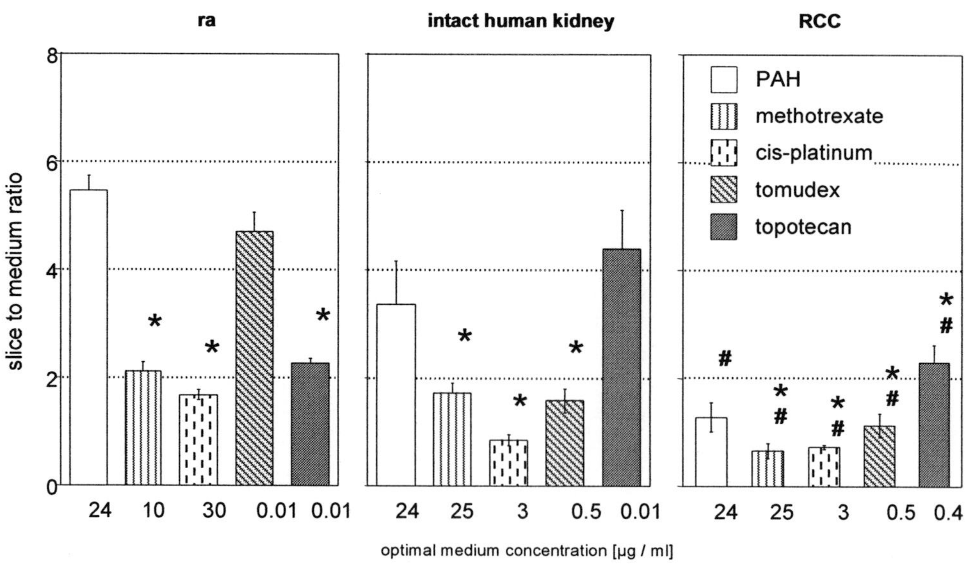

Figure 24. Comparison between rat and "intact" human kidney and RCC concerning the maximal accumulation of PAH, MTX, CP, Tomudex®, and topotecan (2 h incubation). The optimal medium concentration is given at the bottom of the columns. Arithmetic means ± S.E.M.; n = 6 rats or 3-6 patients with 3-4 measurements per patient; * - significantly different from PAH ($p \leq 0.05$); # - significant difference between "intact" human kidney and RCC ($p \leq 0.05$).

In the last part of this study, the renal handling of anticancer drugs was investigated. Compared to PAH, the accumulation of MTX is significantly lower, especially in rat's and "intact" human kidney, and the concentration dependency is of minor importance (Figure 22). Evidently this indicates, first of, all a passive influx of the lipophilic MTX into kidney tissue. The difference between "intact" human kidney and RCC shown for PAH could be confirmed for MTX as well. RCC is unable to enrich MTX. Therefore, the passive uptake shown for "intact" human kidney is not as effective compared to the efflux of MTX in RCC cells if one assumes nearly similar passive enrichment in "intact" kidney and in RCC. Finally, in rat kidney it was shown that MTX uptake is not only a passive, but an oxygen consuming process, too.

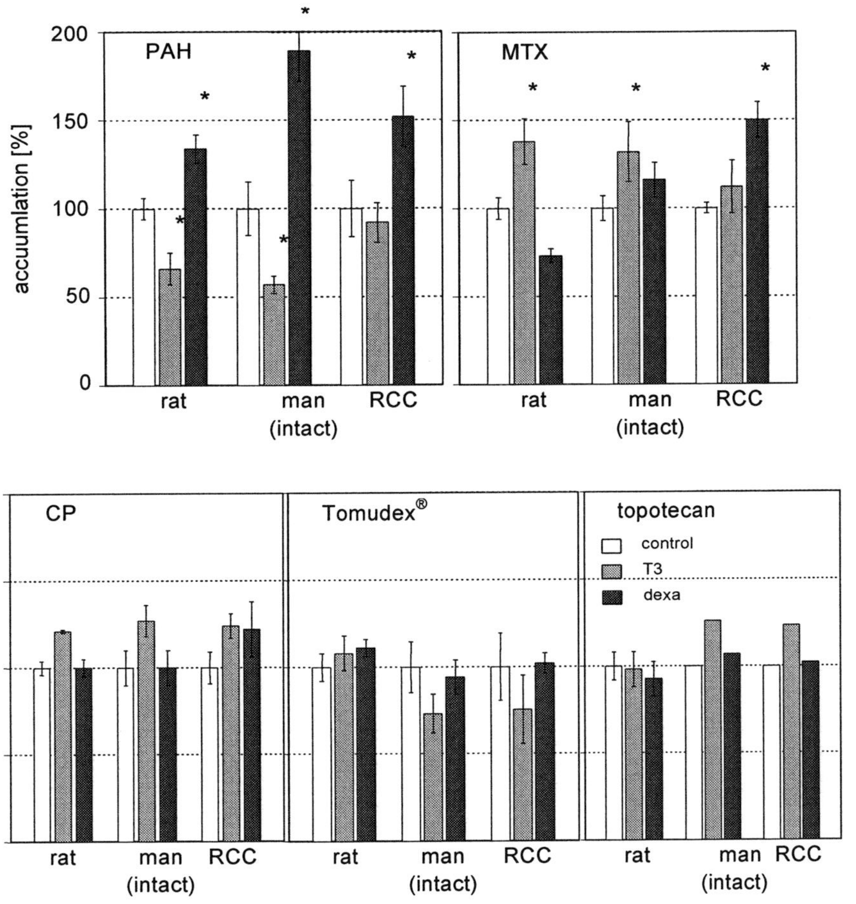

Figure 25. Effects of dexamethasone (dexa.) or T_3 on accumulation of PAH, MTX, CP, Tomudex®, and topotecan in rat and "intact" human kidney and in RCC. Maximal changes after 24 h incubation are given in % of corresponding controls (= 100 %). Arithmetic means ± S.E.M.; n = 6 patients, 3-4 measurements per patient; * - significant hormone effect ($p \leq 0.05$).

The uptake of MTX in rat kidney reaches a steady state after about 2 hours (Figure 23). The efflux of MTX is not energy consuming. That means there is evidently no active transport out of the renal cortical slices of rats. Unfortunately, comparable experiments were not performed on "intact" human kidney and on RCC.

The maximal 2-hour-incubation of anticancer drugs is concentration dependent and distinctly lower compared to PAH in rat and "intact" human renal tissue and in RCC (Figure 24). In general, anticancer drug accumulation is significantly lower in RCC in relation to "intact" renal tissue. However, the uptake of topotecan is more effective in "intact" human kidney compared to rat. On the other hand, the maximal accumulation of Tomudex® is quite comparable to that of PAH in rat, but not in man.

In principle, the maximal accumulation capacity for anticancer drugs can be stimulated in rat and "intact" human kidney tissue (Figure 25). However, in contrast to PAH, in the case of MTX, T_3 is effective in "intact" human kidney whereas dexamethasone is not. On the other hand, in RCC the accumulation of MTX is slightly enhanced only after dexamethasone. In contrast to PAH and MTX, there is no stimulation effect of both dexamethasone and T_3 on the accumulation of CP, Tomudex®, and topotecan into intact kidney, neither in rat's nor in "intact" human kidney and RCC.

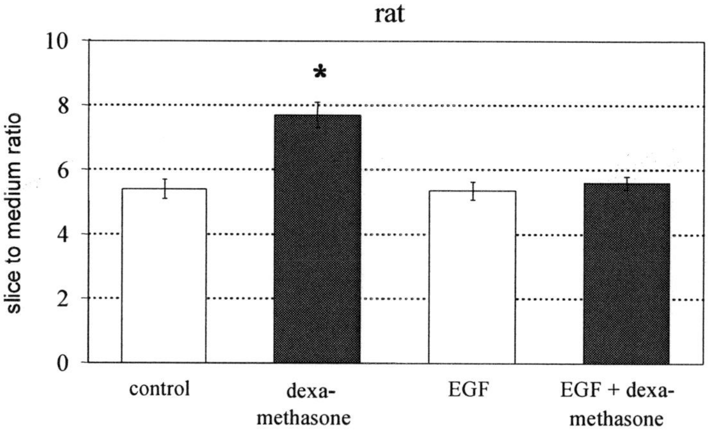

Figure 26. Accumulation of PAH in rat kidney after 24 h incubation in WE medium E containing EGF (1µg/ml) or dexamethasone (10^{-8} M) alone and EGF in combination with dexamethasone. Arithmetic means $\pm$ S.E.M.; n = 6. * - significant hormone effect ($p \leq 0.05$).

Based on the hypothesis that the cellular EGF effect is mediated by dexamethasone (Rogers et al., 1995), combination studies were done in rat kidney tissue. EGF alone seems to be without effects on renal transport capacity (Figure 26). After additional incubation of rat renal cortical slices in dexamethasone plus EGF, the stimulatory effect of dexamethasone on PAH uptake completely disappeared. Because of lack of EGF effect in rats, respective experiments on human tissue were not performed.

Discussion

PAH Handling in Renal Cortical Slices

For various reasons it is necessary to prove drug effects in *in vitro* models (exclusion of the influences of the nervous system and of hormones, characterization of effects on the cellular level, restrictions by the animal protection law, and financial reasons) (Parrish et al., 1995). Therefore, we have established an *in vitro* incubation system to estimate the handling of drugs in renal cortical slices. It was shown that under our experimental conditions the survival of the slices seems to be sufficient (GSH and potassium concentration, PAH accumulation capacity). This experimental approach is suitable for experiments on renal cortical slices of immature and adult rats despite age differences in renal PAH accumulation which exist (Stopp and Bräunlich 1975, Agarwal and Rao 1994). After 24-hour-incubation in PAH-free Williams medium E, the PAH uptake is distinctly reduced compared to acute experiments on freshly prepared renal cortical slices. Nevertheless $Q_{S/M}$-values reach about 40 and 60% in 10- and 55-day-old rats, respectively. This reflects the immature renal PAH transport capacity in 10-day-old rats measured *in vivo* (Bräunlich 1981). The PAH uptake after 24-hour-incubation was an active one because under nitrogen atmosphere, PAH uptake was abolished.

The first question to be answered using this new approach was to clarify the discrepancy between the effects of a pre-treatment with dexamethasone *in vivo* on renal PAH excretion and PAH accumulation in renal cortical slices (Bräunlich et al., 1992a). Such differences between *in vivo* and *in vitro* effects have been reported e.g. for hydroxysuccimide: although this substance exerts direct effects on renal function *in vitro*, it is not a nephrotoxicant *in vivo* (Rankin et al., 1995). Glucocorticoids have been reported to increase renal transport of organic anions like PAH (Bräunlich et al., 1993b) and to protect against e.g. cisplatin-induced nephrotoxicity (Uozumi et al., 1995). It could be confirmed that *in vivo* pre-treatment with dexamethasone increases the renal excretion of PAH distinctly in immature rats, whereas this effect is not significant in adult animals. This is in accordance with Bräunlich and Pils (1992b). On the other hand, there is no effect of *in vivo* pre-treatment with dexamethasone on *in vitro* accumulation of PAH. This lack of effect of *in vivo* pre-treatment with dexamethasone on *in vitro* PAH accumulation has been explained in previous experiments by an increase in kidney weight resulting in an increase in total transported PAH amounts *in vivo*, whereas per 1 g kidney weight there was no increase in PAH uptake capacity (Bräunlich et al., 1993a). In the present study, we administered dexamethasone directly in contact with the renal cortical slices so that pharmacokinetic interferences can be excluded. The *in vitro* stimulation of kidney tissue with dexamethasone was followed by a significant increase in PAH accumulation capacity both in immature and in adult animals. In principle, these findings are in parallel with our results after *in vivo* pre-treatment with dexamethasone. It can be concluded that both *in vivo* and *in vitro* stimulation with dexamethasone increase renal PAH transport capacity.

At the beginning of our study, it was not decided whether or not dexamethasone improves only the incubation condition. However, in following experiments the dexamethasone effects on protein synthesis, which means an increase of mRNA encoding

OAT1, *de-novo* synthesis could be proved unambiguously using the PCR technique (Bahn et al., 2003).

This first part of our study showed that it is possible to use the experimental approach for accumulation experiments established for rats on human renal tissue as well. A comparable method was reported by Fisher et al. (1994) using human kidney cortical slices for nephrotoxicity testing.

PAH Transport in "Intact" Human Kidney and in RCC

The most impressive difference between the PAH accumulation capacity of rats and humans is the maximal extent of intracellular PAH enrichment: in rats it is about twice as high as in humans. Organ functions of laboratory animals are generally at a higher level than those of humans (Klinger et al., 1983). Therefore, it remains to be clarified whether it is justified to compare adult rats with elderly men concerning their renal accumulation capacity. It should be taken into consideration that the Cross-Taggart buffer used for experiments on rat kidney might not be optimal for human renal tissue. In the past, it was verified that both Cross-Taggart medium and William medium E are suitable for experiments on human tissue, too (results not shown).

However, kidney removal in accordance with Robsen et al. (1969), the preparation of tissue samples, and the transportation of the samples from the clinic to the laboratory were time consuming. Therefore an ischemic period of about one hour could not be avoided in patients. Previously it has been shown for ischemic rat kidney tissue that the accumulation capacity for PAH is diminished dependent on the duration of ischemia (Fleck et al., 1993).

As reported above, in rats the well-known age course of PAH accumulation capacity could be reproduced: it becomes mature at 1 month of life and decreases thereafter with increasing age. Also in "intact" human kidney the PAH accumulation is inversely correlated with age, although investigations were performed only on tissue samples of relatively elderly patients. This finding is in good accordance with the literature (Palmer and Levi 1996). Sex differences of accumulation capacity reported for e.g. rats – males can accumulate PAH better than females (Bräunlich et al., 1993a), evidently do not exist in older humans. Buist et al. (2002) found in adult male rats a higher content of OAT1-mRNA compared to female rats. Because OAT1 is responsible first of all for PAH transport (Uwai et al., 1998 Hasegawa et al., 2002) these findings explain the sex differences.

Surprisingly, the PAH accumulation capacity of "intact" human kidney is correlated with the pT status of RCC in the same kidney, i. e., the invasive growth of the RCC obviously depresses the surrounding renal tissue before its infiltration occurs, but the definitive reason for decreased PAH transport in non-cancerous tissue of tumour-bearing kidney is not as yet clear.

As could be expected, the accumulation capacity of RCC tissue is completely abolished when slice-to-medium ratio of PAH reaches about 1, both in central and in peripheral parts of the tumour. This might reflect at least two phenomena:

- RCC is completely undifferentiated and, therefore, unable to accumulate PAH actively. Obviously this effect occurs relatively early during the development of the RCC. As shown in Figure 11, at later times there are no further differences regarding tumour grade and metastatic status.
- Additional transport mechanisms are possibly expressed in RCC, transporting PAH out of the cell. Such a bi-directional transport has been shown previously for phenol red in renal tissue of healthy rats in a dose-dependent manner (Fleck et al., 1987). This efflux might be performed by the mechanisms responsible for the phenomenon of multidrug resistance, although the latter have been described for anticancer drugs only (Gottesman et al., 1995). This hypothesis is supported by the fact that in tumour stage 1 RCC the slice-to-medium ratios of PAH are below 0.5. This can be explained, first of all, by increased transport of PAH out of the cell, because a reduced passive influx of PAH followed by ratios lower than 1 is less probable. Altogether, there are no further differences in the accumulation capacity of RCC tissue if this parameter is correlated to tumour grading, size, and age of the patients. Thus the measured reduction of PAH accumulation capacity in RCC occurs relatively early in the course of tumour growth and remains constant at later times. However, the influence of age on the parameters mentioned cannot be decided definitively in our experiments because of the relatively low number of observations.

Stimulation of PAH Transport in "Intact" Human Kidney

A very interesting result of this study was to prove the possibility of stimulating *in vitro* the renal tubular transport capacity in "intact" human kidney, too. In the rat, an optimal dexamethasone concentration of 0.5 μM could be found whereas in man, 1.0 μM was optimal. Age differences concerning the stimulatory dexamethasone effect found in rats are of minor importance for men, because in RCC patients the average age was between 55 and 70 years, thus the influence of age could not be detected. Until now, only a few results exist in the literature describing a stimulation of renal tubular secretion capacity in man; e.g. the repeated administration of sulfamerazine stimulating the renal excretion of PAH in man (Traeger et al., 1976). *In vitro* investigations of the accumulation capacity of human kidney after stimulatory treatment *in vivo* have not been described in the literature before.

The general possibility of stimulating the renal uptake of drugs like PAH could be the first evidence of overcoming the multidrug resistance of RCC against cytostatics like 5-fluorouracil, leucovorin, zidovudine, or methotrexate (Efferth et al., 1995, Sharfman et al., 1995). MDR represents a major problem in the successful therapy of neoplastic diseases. Although P-glycoprotein is expressed in many cell lines and occurs in human tumours, its expression is not a universal feature of MDR, suggesting that other mechanisms are operating, too (Bellamy 1996). The enhanced export of glutathione xenobiotic conjugates is coupled to the multidrug resistance associated gene product MRP1 (Bosch and Croop 1996, Jedlitschky et al., 1996) and could be antagonized by an increased uptake of these xenobiotics. Other export routes out of the RCC cell could even be diminished as shown for cholesterol transport: the reduced release of free cholesterol from RCC cells may, in part, be responsible for the accumulation of cholesterol in human renal cancer (Clayman et al., 1987). Many approaches to counteract MDR have been published in the literature. Well-qualified candidates seem to be calcium channel blockers like verapamil (Mickisch et al., 1991) and dexverapamil with reduced cardiac toxicity (Motzer et al., 1995). In a study of Amato et al. (1995) it was shown that the co-administration of dexamethasone improves the tolerance of intermittent high-dose interferon. Perhaps this strategy might be combined with the stimulation of the uptake of anticancer drugs by dexamethasone to obtain benefits in RCC therapy?

Despite this optimistic interpretation of our results, a few critical points must be considered:

- Dexamethasone is a substrate to the MDR1 gene product (Schinkel et al., 1995). Therefore, it cannot be ruled out that *in vitro* dexamethasone pre-treatment does not stimulate uptake but simply interferes with the known transport proteins evacuating PAH from the plasma that has been diffused into the cell passively. Nevertheless, the effectivity of dexamethasone to stimulate renal PAH excretion after *in vivo* pre-treatment in rats, indicates the practicability of this approach in patients, too.
- Anticancer chemotherapy is focussed on progressed RCC and on their metastases. It remains to be seen whether metastases are susceptible in the same way, as does the original RCC. Furthermore, the administration of high-dose dexamethasone could attack healthy cells in the organism as well. Therefore, the effect of anticancer drugs could be enhanced also in intact tissues. Nothing is known about the sensitivity of intact cells compared to RCC and its metastases against dexamethasone. Finally, general side effects of high-dose dexamethasone therapy should be kept in mind.
- A last aspect consists of the different effects of dexamethasone in comparison to T_3. We interpret the lack of T3 effect on renal PAH accumulation in human kidney tissue and the significant reduction of PAH accumulation in rat renal cortical slices as follows: T_3 has a catabolic effect and, therefore the so-called housekeeping of the tubular cells increases. In rats, this metabolic stimulus is responsible for enhanced energy consumption and the PAH uptake is diminished as shown previously for renal amino acid reabsorption (Fleck et al., 1997b). Perhaps this phenomenon is of minor importance in human kidney tissue and the T_3 effect on transport capacity could be masked in man.

Stimulation of PAH Transport in RCC

Evidently, the reactivity of RCC on dexamethasone is not uniform: “responders” and “non-responders” can be differentiated. A correlation between accumulation capacity and tumour stage cannot be calculated because of the small number of patients. However, the extent of dexamethasone effect seems to be more pronounced in RCC compared to intact human kidney tissue.

But as shown above, the PAH transport capacity of RCC disappeared nearly completely. Therefore it remains uncertain, whether or not later stages of RCC are under hormonal control. In other words, a response on dexamethasone can be expected, first of all, in the early stages of RCC. This assumption is supported by Tobe and co-workers (1995). They reported that a comparison of MDR1 levels between histological types revealed that there was significantly more MDR1 in clear cell tumours than in oncocytomas. However, the mean MDR1 level of the more undifferentiated clear cell tumours was significantly lower than the mean MDR1 level of the adjacent normal kidney. MDR1 levels in early stages of clear cell tumours were lower than in tumours that had spread into perinephric tissue or had metastasized. In conclusion, MDR1 expression decreases in the more undifferentiated tumours, but still remains at levels high enough to be drug resistant. Higher MDR1 expression in the invasive tumours compared with non-invasive tumours suggests that MDR1 expression and invasiveness may be linked. MDR-1 expression seems to correlate with the differentiation of the RCC and thus its value as an objective measure of the degree of differentiation should be further explored (Hofmockel et al., 1997).

If it were possible to increase the uptake of drugs into RCC under *in vivo* conditions, it might be possible to enhance the concentration of anticancer drugs in RCC and its metastases and, therefore, to improve the effectivity of chemotherapy. Without doubt, this is only one side of the coin: the enhanced uptake of anticancer drugs could be followed by an increase in its efflux out of the tumour cell. Therefore, the results presented in this paper may reflect the sum of two different phenomena: dexamethasone could both increase PAH uptake into RCC and it could accelerate the efflux out of the RCC. Unfortunately, these two aspects could not be differentiated by our experimental approach. Furthermore, MDR can be either intrinsic or acquired and it can be caused by several mechanisms. The so-called classical MDR has been mainly held responsible for the MDR phenotype for urologic malignancies. However, several other MDR pathways have also been identified. MDR can be caused by membrane-bound MRP, the detoxifying glutathione metabolism, the antiapoptotic protein BCL2, and changes in levels or activity of the topoisomerase enzymes (van Brussels and Mickisch 1998).

A second unsolved problem consists of chemical differences between PAH (weak organic acid) and most anticancer drugs. It has to be also taken into consideration that in the cases of anticancer drugs, hormones other than dexamethasone, e. g. T_3 or EGF could enhance the enrichment of these compounds in RCC because they could both increase the uptake and reduce the efflux of anticancer drugs out of RCC (Efferth et al., 1995, Sharfman et al., 1995).

The following restrictions should be considered concerning the interpretation of the PAH results:

- The accumulation capacity of both "intact" renal tissue and RCC can be stimulated *ex vivo*. Evidently the stimulation phenomenon, measured after incubation with dexamethasone, is the consequence of an increased *de-novo* synthesis of carrier proteins as shown for rat kidney (Bahn et al., 2003). On the other hand, the stimulation of PAH transport could result from a better nutritional state of the renal cortical slices indicated by the general parameters intracellular K^+ and glutathione (see table 1).
- Dexamethasone is a substrate to the MDR1 gene product (Schinkel et al., 1995). Therefore, it cannot be excluded that *ex vivo* dexamethasone interferes with the

transport proteins evacuating PAH from the tubular cell (Ullrich 1999). Nevertheless, dexamethasone-mediated stimulation of PAH accumulation indicates an overwhelming of increased PAH uptake compared to its efflux.

- Anticancer chemotherapy is focussed, first of all, on RCC metastases. It has been reported previously that cellular expression of p-glycoprotein, which mediates MDR, is associated with enhanced tumour dissemination, i.e., metastases are more susceptible to anticancer drug therapy (Meyer et al., 1999). Beside this, the administration of high-dose dexamethasone could disturb the general metabolic status in the organism. Therefore, the effect of anticancer drugs could be enhanced also in intact tissues.

Transport of Anticancer Drugs in "Intact" Renal Tissue and in RCC and its Stimulation

In principle, *ex vivo* experiments are qualified to characterise the renal accumulation capacity of anticancer drugs in human kidney (Fleck et al., 2002). Nevertheless, the transporters responsible for active uptake of anticancer drugs are different from those mediating PAH transport. The extent of the passive influx of the highly lipophilic cytostatics cannot be predicted. Discrepancies between the effects of dexamethasone and T_3 and/or EGF indicate different modes of action of these substances concerning the cellular handling of anticancer drugs. Obviously, the transport of cytostatics out of the kidney cells is more effective than their uptake, also after stimulation of the latter.

As mentioned in the introduction, organic anions like PAH are secreted into urine via OATs (Uchino et al., 2000). PAH was investigated by Leier et al. (2000) to be also a substrate for the apical MDR protein MRP2, for MDR 1 or MDR 3 (Moran et al., 1997), or lipoprotein receptor-related protein (Liu et al., 2000), which are known to transport anticancer drugs. Along this line, Hohage et al. (2000) showed a different type of stimulation: calcium channel blockers increase the transport of organic anions across the basolateral membrane of proximal tubules, probably by activation of proteinkinase C (You et al., 2000). The ATP-dependent export pump for anionic conjugates and amphiphilic anions was cloned and localized to the apical membrane of proximal tubules in human and rat kidney. PAH is a good substrate for the ATP-dependent export pump MRP2. The localization and function of MRP2 indicate that this unidirectional transport protein contributes to the secretion of PAH and other amphiphilic anions into the lumen of kidney proximal tubules. MRP2 has similar substrate specificity as the multidrug resistance protein MRP1, and may contribute to the multidrug resistance of RCC (Schaub et al., 1999). Altogether it seems more or less to be justified to compare renal PAH transport with those of anticancer drugs. Organic ion transporters in the kidney proximal tubule play an essential role in eliminating a wide range of organic ions including anticancer drugs and their metabolites (You et al., 2000). MDR is explained first of all by an increase in transport of cytostatics out of RCC (Leier et al., 1996). However, RCC metastases have altered MDR 1 expression compared to the primary tumour. Thus, the drug resistance phenotype of primary RCC may not reflect that of its metastases (Gamelin et al., 1999). An investigation of the stimulation of anticancer drug transport in

RCC is a first step in this direction. Later, results obtained on RCC have to be proven with anticancer drugs used in the chemotherapy of RCC metastases.

The final goal of the experiments was to stimulate the uptake of cytostatics into human kidney, especially into RCC. MDR 1 expression decreases in the more undifferentiated tumours, but still remains at levels high enough to be drug resistant. Higher MDR 1 expression in invasive tumours compared with non-invasive tumours suggests that MDR 1 expression and invasiveness may be linked (Hofmockel et al., 1997).

If it were possible to increase the uptake of anticancer drugs into RCC under *ex vivo* conditions, it might be possible to enhance the uptake of these drugs *in vivo* to improve the effectivity of the chemotherapy. However, an increased efflux out of the tumour cell could follow the enhanced intracellular concentration of anticancer drugs. Therefore, the results described in this review, both for PAH and cytostatics, may reflect the sum of increased drug uptake into RCC and accelerated efflux out of the cells.

The PAH accumulation capacity of "intact" human kidney tissue and of RCC can be stimulated *ex vivo*. Own PCR data show that PAH carrier synthesis seems to be enhanced by dexamethasone (Bahn et al., 2003). If these findings could be reproduced for anticancer drug transporters, the effect of hormones on the accumulation of these substances might be clarified.

A last aspect has to be kept in mind: the administration of high-dose dexamethasone or other hormones/drugs could disturb the metabolism in the organism. Therefore, the effect of anticancer drugs would be enhanced, but side effects of high-dose hormone therapy have to be taken into consideration.

Altogether, RCC is a disease known to demonstrate a high degree of intrinsic chemotherapy drug resistance, and this has been shown to be related to intrinsic over expression of p-glycoprotein (Samuels et al., 1997). The addition of high doses of dexamethasone or T_3 was not able to modulate this resistance in RCC. Therefore, the stimulation of renal tubular accumulation capacity is no suitable therapeutic strategy to overcome MDR in RCC. Nevertheless, combination therapy seems to be the method of choice: The combination of various drugs – cytostatics plus e.g. hormones or different anticancer drugs, (Punt et al., 1997, Naito et al., 1998), significantly increased the life span of mice inoculated with drug-resistant tumour cells without any significant side effects, whereas chemotherapy with the anticancer agent alone did not increase the life span at all.

ABBREVIATIONS

cMOAT	canalicular multispecific organic anion transporter
CP	cisplatin
dexa.	dexamethasone
EGF	epidermal growth factor
fROAT	flounder renal organic anion transporter
GFR	glomerular filtration rate
GSH	reduced glutathione
GSSG	oxidized glutathione

hOAT	human organic anion transporter
MDR	multidrug resistance
mOAT	mouse organic anion transporter
MRP	multidrug resistance related protein
MTX	methotrexate
NPT	human Na^+-dependent phosphate transporter
OAT	organic anion transporter
OAT-K	kidney specific organic anion transporter
oatp	organic anion transporting polypeptide
OCT	organic cation transporter
OCTN	organic cation transporter novel type/carnitine transporter
PAH	p-aminohippurate
$Q_{S/M}$	slice-to-medium ratio
RCC	renal cell carcinoma
rOAT	rat organic anion transporter
RT-PCR	reverse transcriptase polymerase chain reaction
T_3	triiodothyronine
T_4	thyroxine
TDX	Tomudex®, (raltitrexed)
TPT	topotecan
WE	Williams medium E

REFERENCES

Agarwal AK, Rao SS (1994) Susceptibility of ageing kidney to quinidine. *Pharmacol Res 29*: 145-154.

Aguirre JA, Ibarra FR, Barontini M, Arrizurieta EE and Armando I (1999) Effect of glucocorticoids on renal dopamine production. *Eur J Pharmacol 370*: 271-278.

Amato R, Meyers C, Ellerhorst J, Finn L, Kilbourn R, Sella A, Logothetis C (1995) A phase I trial of intermittent high-dose alpha-interferon and dexamethasone in metastatic renal cell carcinoma. *Ann Oncol 6*: 911-914.

Apiwattanakul N, Sekine T, Chairoungdua A, Kanai Y, Nakajima N, Sophasan S, Endou H (1999) Transport properties of nonsteroidal anti-inflammatory drugs by organic anion transporter 1 expressed in Xenopus laevis oozytes. *Mol Pharmacol 55*: 847-854.

Azpodien J, Buer J, Probst-Kepper M, Övermann K (1998) Immunchemotherapie des fortgeschrittenen Nierenzellkarzinoms. In: Nierenzellkarzinom – Renal Cell Carcinoma. Eds.: Schnorr, D, Loening, SA, Blackwell Berlin – Wien, pp. 160-168.

Bahn A, Prawitt D, Buttler D, Reid G, Enklaar T, Wolff NA, Ebbinghaus C, Hillemann A, Schulten HJ, Gunawan B, Fuzesi L, Zabel B, Burckhardt G (2000) Genomic structure and *in vivo* expression of the human organic anion transporter 1 (hOAT1) gene. *Biochem Biophys Res Commun 275*: 623-630.

Bahn A, Knabe M, Hagos Y, Rodiger M, Godehardt S, Graber Neufeld DS, Evans K K, Burckhardt G, Wright SH (2002) Interaction of the metal chelator 2,3-dimercapto-1-

propanesulfonate with the rabbit multispecific organic anion transporter 1 (rbOAT1). *Mol Pharmacol 62*: 1128-1136.

Bahn A, Hauß A, Appenroth D, Ebbinghaus D, Steinmetzer P, Burckhardt G, Fleck C (2003) RT-PCR-based evidence for the *in vivo* stimulation of renal tubular p-aminohippurate (PAH) transport by triiodthyronine (T3) or dexamethasone (DEXA) in kidney tissue of immature and adult rats. *Exp Toxic Pathol Exp Toxic Pathol 54*: 367-373.

Bellamy WT (1996) P-glycoproteins and multidrug resistance. *Ann Rev Pharm Toxicol 36*: 161-183.

Berkhin EB, Varshavsky BY (1975) Substrate induction of tubular secretion of organic compounds in the kidney. *Proc Acad Sci USSR 220*: 1463-1466.

Berlion M, Arvelo F, Leonce S, Bourgeois Y, Rigaudy P, Bizzari JP, Poupon MF (1993) Antitumor activity of the new vinca-alkaloid S 12363 alone or in combination with verapamil on a human multidrug resistant renal carcinoma xenograft. *In Vivo 7*: 399-405.

Bosch I, Croop J (1996) P-glycoprotein multidrug resistance and cancer. Biochim Biophys Acta - Rev on Cancer 1288: F37-F54.

Bratton AC, Marshall EK, Babbitt D, Hendrickson AR (1939) A new coupling component for sulfanilamide determinations. *J Biol Chem 128*: 537-550.

Bräunlich H (1981) Excretion of drugs during postnatal development. *Pharmac Ther 12*: 299-320.

Bräunlich H (1987) Transport of p-aminohippurate in renal cortical slices of rats of different ages following treatment with thyroid hormones. *Biomed Biochim Acta 46*: 251-257.

Bräunlich H (1988) Hormonal control of postnatal development of renal tubular transport of weak organic acids. *Pediatr Nephrol 2*: 151-155.

Bräunlich H, Pils W (1992) Synergistic effect of triiodothyronine and dexamethasone on renal tubular transport of p-aminohippurate in rats of different ages. *Dev Pharmacol Ther 19*: 50-56.

Bräunlich H, Fleck C, Bajanowski T, Miosge W (1983) Dosisabhängigkeit und Altersabhängigkeit des renalen tubulären Transportes von p-Aminohippursäure (PAH) bei Ratten nach Injektion von Einzeldosen. *Pharmazie 38*: 483-485.

Bräunlich H, Köhler A, Schmidt I (1986) Acceleration of p-aminohippurate excretion in immature rats by dexamethasone treatment. *Med Biol 64*: 267-270.

Bräunlich H, Jahn F, Bartha J (1987) Hemodynamic parameters and renal blood flow following stimulation of renal tubular transport processes by treatment with thyroid hormones. *Pharmazie 42*: 846-848.

Bräunlich H, Rassbach H, Vogelsang S (1992) Stimulation of renal tubular transport of p-aminohippurate in rats of different ages by treatment with adrenocortical steroids. *Dev Pharmacol Ther 19*: 1-5.

Bräunlich H, Meinig T, Grosch U (1993a) Postnatal development of sex differences in renal tubular transport of p-aminohippurate (PAH) in rats. Exp *Toxicol Pathol 45*: 309-313.

Bräunlich H, Rössler S, Gerhardt C (1993b) Influence of sympathetic nervous system on dexamethasone-stimulated renal tubular transport of p-aminohippurate in young rats. *Dev Pharmacol Ther 20*: 86-92.

Broxterman HJ, Pinedo HM, Kuiper CM, van der Hoeven JJ, de Lange P, Quak JJ, Scheper RJ, Keizer HG, Schuurhuis GJ, Lankelma J (1989) Immunohistochemical detection of P-glycoprotein in human tumor cells with a low degree of drug resistance. *Int J Cancer 43*: 340-343.

Buist SCN, Cherrington NJ, Choudhuri S, Hartley DP, Klaassen CD (2002) Gender-specific and developmental influences on the expression of rat organic anion transporters. *J Pharmacol Exp Ther 301*: 145-151.

Burckhardt G, Wolff NA (2000) Structure of renal organic anion and cation transporters. *Am J Physiol Renal Physiol 278*: F853-F866.

Burckhardt G, Bahn A, Wolff NA (2001) Molecular physiology of renal p-aminohippurate secretion. *News Physiol Sci 16*: 114-118.

Burckhardt G, Wolff NA, Bahn A (2002) Molecular characterization of the renal organic anion transporter 1. *Cell Biochem Biophys 36*: 169-174.

Cano A, Baum M, Moe OW (1999) Thyroid hormone stimulates the renal Na/H exchanger NHE3 by transcriptional activation. *Am J Physiol 276*: C102-C108.

Capasso G, De Santo NG, Kinne R (1987) Thyroid hormones and renal transport: Cellular and biochemical aspects. *Kidney Int 32*: 443-451.

Capasso G, de Tommaso G, Pica A, Anastasio P, Capasso J, Kinne R and de Santo NG (1999) Effects of thyroid hormones on heart and kidney functions. *Min Electrol Metab 25*: 56-64.

Cha SH, Endou H (2001) Molecular aspects of organic ion transporters in the kidney. *Kor J Physiol Pharmacol 5*: 107-122.

Cha SH, Sekine T, Kusuhara H, Yu E, Kim JY, Kim DK, Sugiyama Y, Kanai Y, Endou H (2000) Molecular cloning and characterization of multispecific organic anion transporter 4 expressed in the placenta. *J Biol Chem 275*: 4507-4512.

Cha SH, Sekine T, Fukushima JI, Kanai Y, Kobayashi Y, Goya T, Endou H (2001) Identification and characterization of human organic anion transporter 3 expressing predominantly in the kidney. *Mol Pharmacol 59*: 1277-1286.

Chapman AE, Goldstein LJ (1995) Multiple drug resistance: Biologic basis and clinical significance in renal-cell carcinoma. *Sem Oncol 22*: 17-28.

Chen A, Sheu LF, Ho YS, Lin YF, Chou WY, Wang JY, Lee WH (1998) Administration of dexamethasone induces proteinuria of glomerular origin in mice. *Am J Kidney Dis 31*: 443-452.

Clayman RV, Figenshau RS, Prigge WF, Forstrom L, Gebhard RL (1987) Transport of circulating serum cholesterol by human renal cell carcinoma. *J Urol 137*: 1262-1265.

Cross RJ, Taggart JV (1950) Renal tubular transport. Accumulation of p-aminohippurate by rabbit kidney slices. *Am J Physiol 161*: 181-190.

De Nayer P (1987) Thyroid hormon action at the cellular level. *Hormone Res 26*: 48-57.

Demeule M, Brossard M, Beliveau, R (1999) Cisplatin induces renal expression of P-glycoprotein and canalicular multispecific organic anion transporter. *Am J Physiol 277*: F832-F840.

Dzurik R, Gerykova M, Spustova V (1991) P-aminohippurate accumulation in kidney cortex slices: stimulation by dicarboxylates, amino acids and their oxoanalogues. *Physiol Res 40*: 339-344.

Edwards RM, Stack E, Trizna W (1997) Alpha-Ketoglutarate transport in rat renal brush-border and basolateral membrane vesicles. *J Pharmacol Exp Ther 281*: 1059-1064.

Efferth T, Volm M (1992) Expression of protein kinase C in human renal cell carcinoma cells with inherent resistance to doxorubicin. *Anticancer Res 12*: 2209-2212.

Efferth T, Lohrke H, Volm M (1989) Reciprocal correlation between expression of P-glycoprotein and accumulation of rhodamine 123 in human tumors. *Anticancer Res 9*: 1633-1637.

Efferth T, Dunn TA, Berlion M, Langenbahn H, Pommerenke EW, Volm M (1993) Reversal of inherent multidrug-resistance in primary human renal cell carcinoma cell cultures by S9788. *Anticancer Res 13*: 905-908.

Efferth T, Fabry U, Osieka R (1995) Is there a realistic chance for the clinical modulation of multidrug resistance? *Onkol 18*: 258-260.

Eliason IF. Ramuz H, Yoshikubo T, Ishikawa T, Yamamoto T, Tsuruo T (1995) Novel dithiane analogues of tiapamil with high activity to overcome multidrug resistance in vitro. *Biochem Pharmacol 30*: 187-196.

Enomoto A, Takeda M, Shimoda M, Narikawa S, Kobayashi Y, Kobayashi Y, Yamamoto T, Sekine T, Cha SH, Niwa T, Endou H (2002) Interaction of human organic anion transporters 2 and 4 with organic anion transport inhibitors. *J Pharmacol Exp Ther 301*: 797-802.

Euzet S, Lelievre-Pegorier M, Merlet-Benichou C (1996) Effect of 3,5,3'-triiodothyronine on maturation of rat renal phosphate transport: kinetic characteristics and phosphate transporter messenger ribonucleic acid and protein abundance. *Endocrinol 137*: 3522-3530.

Fanestil DD, Parks CS (1981) Steroid hormones and the kidney. *Ann Rev Physiol 43*: 637-649.

Feng B, Dresser MJ, Shu Y, Johns SJ, Giacomini KM (2001) Arginine 454 and lysine 370 are essential for the anion specificity of the organic anion transporter, rOAT3. *Biochem 40*: 5511-5520.

Feng B, Shu Y, Giacomini KM (2002) Role of aromatic transmembrane residues of the organic anion transporter, rOAT3, in substrate recognition. *Biochem 41*: 8941-8947.

Fisher RL, Sanuik JT, Gandolfi AJ, Brendel K (1994) Toxicity of cisplatin and mercuric chloride in human kidney cortical slices. *Hum Exp Toxicol 13*: 517-523.

Fleck, C (1997) In vitro stimulation of renal tubular p-aminohippurate transport by dexamethasone in kidney tissue of immature and adult rats. *Exp Toxic Pathol 49*: 87-92.

Fleck C, Bräunlich H (1990) Age dependent differences in stimulation and compensation of renal and biliary transport processes. *Arzneim Forsch - Drug Res 40*: 1047-1053.

Fleck C, Bräunlich H (1995) Renal handling of drugs and amino acids after impairment of kidney or liver function - influences of maturity and protective treatment. *Pharmac Ther 67*: 53-77.

Fleck, C, Bartha, J, Kersten, L, Hably, C, Bräunlich, H (1981a) Renal blood flow after stimulation of p-aminohippurate transport. *Arch Int Pharmacodyn Ther 252*: 133-138.

Fleck C, Bräunlich H, Stopp M (1981b) Stimulation des renalen Fremdstofftransportes nach unilateraler Nephrektomie. *Acta biol med germ 40*: 1053-1060.

Fleck C, Pertsch J (1998) Epidermal growth factor (EGF) increases the renal transport of amino acid in amino acid loaded rats. *Amino Acids 15*: 307-320.

Fleck C, Kunze C, Bräunlich H (1987) Relation between renal and hepatic excretion of drugs: V. Factors influencing accumulation of phenol red in kidney and liver tissue from rats of different ages. *Exp Pathol 32*: 99-110.

Fleck C, Haubold D, Hillmann T, Möckel H, Möckel M, Bräunlich H (1993) Evaluation of methods indicating higher susceptibility of immature rats to renal ischemia. *Exp Toxicol Pathol 45*: 155-160.

Fleck C, Göckeritz S, Schubert J (1997a) Tubular PAH transport capacity in human kidney tissue and in renal cell carcinoma: correlation with various clinical and morphological parameters of the tumor. *Urol Res 25*: 167-171.

Fleck C, Aurich M, Schwertfeger M (1997b) Stimulation of renal amino acid reabsorption after treatment with triiodothyronine or dexamethasone in amino acid loaded rats. *Amino Acids 12*: 265-279.

Fleck C, Kratochwil E, Winterstein K, Göckeritz S, Schubert J (1998) *In vitro* stimulation of renal tubular p-aminohippurate transport by dexamethasone in rat kidneys and in intact kidney tissue of patients suffering from renal cell carcinoma. *Urol Res 26*: 143-148.

Fleck C, Bachner B, Göckeritz S, Karge E, Strohm U, Schubert J (2000) Ex vivo stimulation of renal tubular p-aminohippurate transport by dexamethasone and triiodothyronine in human renal cell carcinoma. *Urol Res 28*: 383-390.

Fleck C, Hilger R, Jurkutat S, Karge E, Merkel U, Schimske A, Schubert J (2002) Ex vivo stimulation of renal transport of the cytostatic drugs methotrexate, cisplatin, topotecan (Hycamtin) and raltitrexed (Tomudex) by dexamethasone, T3 and EGF in intact human and rat kidney tissue and in human renal cell carcinoma. *Urol Res 30*: 256-262.

Focan C (1995) Circadian rhythms and cancer chemotherapy. *Pharmacol Ther 67*: 1-52.

Foulkes EC, Blanck S (1990) Site of uptake of nonfiltered amino acids in rabbit kidney. *Proc Soc Exp Biol Med 193*: 56-60.

Gabriels G, Werners A, Mauss S, Greven J (1999) Evidence for differential regulation of renal proximal tubular p-aminohippurate and sodium-dependent dicarboxylate transport. *J Pharmacol Exp Ther 290*: 710-715.

Gamelin E, Mertins SD, Regis JT, Mickley L, Abati A, Worrell RA, Linehan WM, Bates SE (1999) Intrinsic drug resistance in primary and metastatic renal cell carcinoma. *J Urol 162*: 217-224.

Gansbacher B, Zier K, Daniels B, Cronin K, Banneriji Rk, Balboa E (1990) Interleukin-2 gene transfer into tumor cells abrogates tumorigenicity and induces protective immunity. *J Exp Med 172*: 1217-1224.

Gemba M, Taniguchi M, Matsushima Y (1981) Effect of bumetanide on p-aminohippurate transport in renal cortical slices. *J Pharmacobiodyn 4*: 162-166.

Gottesman MM, Hrycyna CA, Schoenlein PV, German UA, Pastan I (1995) Genetic analysis of the multidrug transporter. *Am Rev Genetics 29*: 607 649.

Han YH, Kato Y, Haramura M, Ohta M, Matsuoka H, Sugiyama Y (2001) Physicochemical parameters responsible for the affinity of methotrexate analogs for rat canalicular multispecific organic anion transporter (cMOAT/MRP2). *Pharm Res 18*: 579-586.

Harris MJ, Kuwano M, Webb M, Board PG (2001) Identification of the apical membrane-targeting signal of the multidrug resistance-associated protein 2 (MRP2/MOAT). *J Biol Chem 276*: 20876-20881.

Hartmann JT, Bokemeyer C (1999) Chemotherapy for renal cell carcinoma. *Anticancer Res 19*: 1541-1543.

Hasegawa M, Kusuhara H, Sugiyama D, Ito K, Ueda S, Endou H, Sugiyama Y (2002) Functional involvement of rat organic anion transporter 3 (rOat3; Slc22a8) in the renal uptake of organic anions. *J Pharmacol Exp Ther 300*: 746-753.

Hermanek P, Schrott KM (1990) Evaluation of the new tumor, nodes and metastases classification of renal cell carcinoma. *J Urol 144*: 238-242.

Hilger RA, Heinrichs D, Mayer S, Harstrick A, Scheulen ME, Seeber S (1999) Influence of tomudex on the pharmacokinetics of 5-FU and its metabolism: a phase I trial. In: *Proc 90th Ann Meeting Amer Assoc Cancer Res 40*: 550.

Hissin PJ, Hilf R (1976) A fluorimetric method for determination of oxidized and reduced glutathione in tissues. *Anal Biochem 74*: 214-226.

Hofmockel G, Bassukas ID, Wittmann A, Dammrich J (1997) Is the expression of multidrug resistance gene product a prognostic indicator for the clinical outcome of patients with renal cancer? *Brit J Urol 80*: 11-17.

Hohage H, Steinmetz M, Mergelsberg U, Lohr M, Greven, J (2000) Regulation of the renal basolateral transport system for organic anions by calcium channel blockers. *Pharmacol Res 41*: 25-30.

Honscha W, Dotsch KU, Thomsen N, Petzinger E (2000) Cloning and functional characterization of the bile acid-sensitive methotrexate carrier from rat liver cells. *Hepatol 31*: 1296-1304.

Hosoyamada M, Sekine T, Kanai Y, Endou H (1999) Molecular cloning and functional expression of a multispecific organic anion transporter from human kidney. *Am J Physiol 276*: F122-F128.

Jariyawat S, Sekine T, Takeda M, Apiwattanakul N, Kanai Y, Sophasan S, Endou H (1999) The interaction and transport of ß-lactam antibiotics with the cloned rat renal organic anion transporter 1. *J Pharmacol Exp Ther 290*: 672-677.

Jedlitschky G, Keppler D (2002) Transport of leukotriene C4 and structurally related conjugates. *Vitam Horm 64*: 153-184..

Jedlitschky G, Leier I, Buchholz U, Barnouin K, Kurz G, Keppler D (1996) Transport of glutathione, glucuronate, and sulfate conjugates by the MRP gene-encoded conjugate export pump. *Cancer Res 56*: 988-994.

Johnson DR, Klaassen CD (2002) Regulation of rat multidrug resistance protein 2 by classes of prototypical microsomal enzyme inducers that activate distinct transcription pathways. *Toxicol Sci 67*: 182-189.

Klein LE, Hisao P, Bartolomei M, Lo CS (1984) Regulation of rat renal (Na^+-K^+)-adenosine triphosphatase activity by triiodthyronine and corticosterone. *Endocrinol 115*: 1038-1042.

Klinger W, Müller D, Kleeberg U, Barth A (1983) Extrapolation von Tierversuchen auf Reaktionen beim Menschen. *Pharmazie 8*:621-623.

Kobayashi Y, Ohshiro N, Shibusawa A, Sasaki T, Tokuyama S, Sekine T, Endou H, Yamamoto T (2002a) Isolation, characterization and differential gene expression of multispecific organic anion transporter 2 in mice. *Mol Pharmacol 62*: 7-14.

Kobayashi Y, Hirokawa N, Ohshiro N, Sekine T, Sasaki T, Tokuyama S, Endou H, Yamamoto T (2002b) Differential gene expression of organic anion transporters in male and female rats. *Biochem Biophys Res Commun 290*: 482-487.

König J, Nies AT, Cui Y, Leier I, Keppler D (1999) Conjugate export pumps of the multidrug resistance protein (MRP) family: localization, substrate specifity and MRP2-mediated drug resistance. *Biochim Biophys Acta 1461*: 377-394.

Kretzschmar M, Franke H, Zimmermann T, Dargel R, Klinger W (1989) Glutathione synthesis and export in experimental liver cirrhosis induced by thioacetamide: Relations to ultrastructural changes. *Exp Pathol 36*: 113-122.

Kusuhara H, Sekine T, Utsunomiya Tate N, Tsuda M, Kojima R, Cha S H, Sugiyama Y, Kanai Y, Endou H (1999) Molecular cloning and characterization of a new multispecific organic anion transporter from rat brain. *J Biol Chem 274*: 13675-13680.

Kuze K, Graves P, Leahy A, Wilson P, Stuhlmann H, You G (1999) Heterologous expression and functional characterization of a mouse renal organic anion transporter in mammalian cells. *J Biol Chem 274*: 1519-1524.

Lai T, Collins CM, Hall P,. Morgan AP, Smith PJ, Stonebridge BR, Svmes MO (1993) Verapamil enhances doxorubicin activity in cultured human renal carcinoma cells. *Eur J Cancer 29A*: 378-383.

Leier I, Jedlitschky G, Buchholz U, Center M, Cole SP, Deeley RG, Keppler D (1996) ATP-dependent glutathione disulphide transport mediated by the MRP gene-encoded conjugate export pump. *Biochem J 314*: 433-437.

Leier I, Hummel-Eisenbeiss J, Cui Y, Keppler D (2000) ATP-dependent para-aminohippurate transport by apical multidrug resistance protein MRP2. *Kidney Int 57*: 1636-1642.

Licht T, Gottesman, MM, Pastan I (1995) Transfer of the MDR 1 (multidrug resistance) gene: Protection of hematopoetic cells from cytotoxic chemotherapy, and selection of transduced cells in vivo. *Cytokin Mol Ther 1*: 11-20.

Liu CX, Musco S, Lisitsina NM, Forgacs E, Minna JD, Lisitsyn NA (2000) LRP-DIT, a putative endocytic receptor gene, is frequently inactivated in non-small cell lung cancer cell lines. *Cancer Res 60*: 1961-1967.

Loos WJ, Stoter G, Verweij J, Schellens JHM (1996) Sensitive high-performance liquid chromatographic fluorescence assay for the quantitation of topotecan (SKF 104864-A) and its lactone ring-opened product (hydroxy-acid) in human plasma and urine. *J Chromatogr B 678*: 309-315.

Lu R, Chan BS, Schuster VL (1999) Cloning of the human kidney PAH transporter: narrow substrate specificity and regulation by protein kinase C. *Am J Physiol 276*: F295-F303.

Masereeuw R, van den Bergh EJ, Bindels RJM, Russel FGM (1994) Characterization of fluorescin transport in isolated proximal tubular cells of the rat: Evidence for mitochondrial accumulation. *J Pharmacol Exp Ther 269*: 1261-1267.

Masereeuw R, Terlouw SA, van Aubel RA, Russel FG, Miller DS (2000) Endothelin B receptor-mediated regulation of ATP-driven drug secretion in renal proximal tubule. *Mol Pharmacol 57*: 59-67.

Meyer N; Duensing S, Anastassiou G, Brevis-Nunez F, Grosse J, Ganser A, Azpodien J (1999) Altered expression of beta 1 integrins in renal carcinoma cell lines exposed to vinblastine. *Anticancer Res 19*: 1509-1512.

Mickisch GH (1992) Gentherapeutische Strategien für die Onkologie - Ein urologischer Standpunkt. *Akta Urol 23*: 206-215.

Mickisch GH (1993) Immunologische Ansätze zur Überwindung von Chemoresistenz. *Akta Urol 24*: 87-94.

Mickisch GH (1994a) Chemoresistance of renal cell carcinoma: 1986-94. *World J Urol* 12: 214-223.

Mickisch GH (1994b) Therapie des Nierenzellkarzinoms - Eine Aktualisierung notwendig? *Akta Urol 25*: 77-83.

Mickisch GH (1994c) Multidrug resistance of renal cell carcinoma: From laboratory curiosity to clinical reality. *Akta Urol 25*: 327-337.

Mickisch GH, Kössig J, Keilhauer G, Schlick E, Tschada R and Alken P (1990) Effects of calcium antagonists in multidrug resistant primary human renal cell carcinomas. *Cancer Res 50*: 3670-3674.

Mickisch GH, Merlino GT, Alken PM, Gottesman MM, Pastan I (1991) New potent verapamil derivatives that reverse multidrug resistance in human renal carcinoma cells and in transgenic mice expressing the human MDR1 gene. *J Urol 146*: 447-453.

Mickisch GH, Schroeder FH (1996) Multidrug resistance in renal cell carcinoma: Eight years of experience. In: Luciani L, Debryne FMJ, Schalken AJ (eds.): Basic research in urologic oncology, Karger, Basel, pp. 161-177.

Miller DS, Pritchard JB (1994) Nocodazole inhibition of organic anion secretion in teleost renal proximal tubules. *Am J Physiol 267*: R695-R704.

Miller DS, Stewart DE, Pritchard JB (1993) Intracellular compartmentation of organic anions within renal cells. *Am J Physiol 264*: R882-R890.

Miller DS, Letcher S, Barnes DM (1996) Fluorescence imaging study of organic anion transport from renal proximal tubule cell to lumen. *Am J Physiol 271*: F508-F520.

Moran E, Larkin A, Doherty G, Kelehan P, Kennedy S, Clynes M (1997) A new mdr-1 encoded P-170 specific monoclonal antibody: (6/1C) on paraffin wax embedded tissue without pretreatment of sections. *J Clin Pathol 50*: 465-471.

Morita N, Kusuhara H, Sekine T, Endou H, Sugiyama Y (2001) Functional characterization of rat organic anion transporter 2 in LLC-PK1 cells. *J Pharmacol Exp Ther 298*: 1179-84.

Motzer RJ, Lyn P, Fischer P, Lianes P, Ngo RL, Cordoncardo C, Obrien JP (1995) Phase I/II trial of dexverapamil plus vinblastine for patients with advanced renal cell carcinoma. *J Clin Oncol 13*: 1958-1965.

Motzer RJ, Bander NH, Nanus DM (1996) Renal cell carcinoma. *New Engl J Med 335*: 865-875.

Naito S, Sakamoto N, Kotoh S, Goto K, Matsumoto T, Kumazawa J (1993) Expression of P-glycoprotein and multidrug resistance in renal cell carcinoma. *Eur Urol 24*: 156-160.

Naito S; Koike K, Ono M, Machida T, Tasaka S, Kiue A, Koga H, Kumazawa J (1998) Development of novel reversal agents, imidazothiazole derivatives, targeting MDR1- and MRP-mediated multidrug resistance. *Oncol Res 10*: 123-132.

Nishiyama K, Shirahama T, Yoshimura A, Sumizawa T, Furukawa T, Ichikawa-Haraguchi M, Akiyama S, Ohi Y (1993) Expression of the multidrug transporter, P-glycoprotein, in renal and transitional cell carcinomas. *Cancer 71*: 3611-3619.

Norman J, Tsau YK, Bacay A, Fine LG (1990) Epidermal growth factor accelerates functional recovery from ischaemic acute tubular necrosis in the rat: role of the epidermal growth factor receptor. *Clin Sci 78*: 445-450.

Nürnberg B, Kohlbrenner M, Faulkner R, Fürst DE (1989) Rapid quantitation of methotrexate and its metabolites in human serum, urine and bile, using solid-phase extraction and high-performance liquid chromatography. *J Chromatogr 24*: 476-482.

Okada S, Hamazaki S, Ebina Y, Li JL, Midorikawa O (1987) Nephrotoxicity and its prevention by vitamin E in ferric nitrilotriacetate-promoted lipid peroxidation. *Biochim Biophys Acta 922*: 28-33.

Ortweiler W, Jahn F, Bräunlich H (1987) Increase of 14C-leucine uptake following stimulation of renal tubular transport processes. *Biomed Biochim Acta 46*: 271-276.

Palmer BF, Levi M (1996) Effect of aging on renal function and disease. In: Brenner BM (ed) The kidney, 5th Ed. WB Saunders, Philadelphia, pp. 2274-2298.

Parrish AR, Gandolfi AJ, Brendel K (1995) Minireview: Precision cut tissue slices: Applications in Pharmacology and toxicology. *Life Sci 57*: 1887-1901.

Pasino DA, Miura K, Goldstein RS, Hook JB (1985) Cephaloridine nephrotoxicity: strain and sex differences in mice. *Fundam Appl Toxicol 5*: 1153-1160.

Penzold K, Braunlich H (1990) Insulin stimulates postnatal development of renal tubular transport of p-aminohippurate. *Biomed Biochim Acta 49*: 1227-1230.

Pritchard JB (1995) Intracellular alpha-ketoglutarate controls the efficacy of renal organic anion transport. *J Pharmacol Exp Ther 274*: 1278-1284.

Punt CJ, Voest EE, Tueni E, Van Oosterom AT, Backx A, De Mulder PH, Hecquet B, Lucas C, Gerard B, Bleiberg H (1997) Phase IB study of doxorubicin in combination with the multidrug resistance reversing agent S9788 in advanced colorectal and renal cell cancer. *Br J Cancer 76*: 1376-1381.

Race JE, Grassl SM, Williams WJ, Holtzman EJ (1999) Molecular cloning and characterization of two novel human renal organic anion transporters (hOAT1 and hOAT3). *Biochem Biophys Res Commun 255*: 508-514.

Rafestin-Oblin ME, Lombes M, Lustenberger P, Blanchardic P, Michaud A, Claire M (1986) Affinity of corticosteroids for mineralcorticoid and glucocorticoid receptors of the rabbit kidney: Effect of steroid substitution. *J Steroid Biochem 25*: 527- 534.

Rajashree S, Puvanakrishnan R (1998) Dexamethasone induced alterations in enzymatic and nonenzymatic antioxidant status in heart and kidney of rats. *Mol Cell Biochem 181*: 77-85.

Ramp U, Dejosez M, Mahotka C, Czarnotta B, Kalinski T, Wenzel M, Lorenz I, Müller M, Krammer P, Gabbert HE, Gerharz CD (2000) Deficient activation of CD95 (APO-1/Fas)-mediated apoptosis: a potential factor of multidrug resistance in human renal cell carcinoma. *Brit J Cancer 82*: 1851-1859.

Rankin GO, Shih HC, Hong SK, Nicoll DW, Anestis DK, Ball JG, Brown PI, Valentovic WA (1995) Role of chloride groups in the nephrotoxic potential of N-(3,5-dichlorophenyl)-2-hydroxysuccinimide, an oxidative metabolite of N-(3,5-dichlorophenyl)succinimide. *Toxicol Lett 78*: 49-56.

Reid G, Wolff NA, Dautzenberg FM, Burckhardt G (1998) Cloning of a human renal p-aminohippurate transporter, hROAT1. *Kidney Blood Press Res 21*: 233-237.

Robsen CJ, Churchill BM, Anderson W (1969) The results of radical nephrectomy for renal cell carcinoma. *J Urol 101*: 297-301.

Rogers SA, Miller SB, Hammerman MR (1995) Triiodothyronine stimulates renal epidermal growth factor expression in adult rat. *Am J Physiol 268*: F218-F234.

Rohlff C, Glatzer RI (1995) Regulation of multidrug resistance through the cAMP and EGF signalling pathways. *Cellular Signalling 7*: 431-443.

Roigas J, Deger S, Schröder J, Schnorr D (1998) Chemoimmuntherapie des metastasierenden Nierenzellkarzinoms an der Klinik für Urologie der Charité – Erfahrungen und Ergebnisse. In. Nierenzellkarzinom – Renal Cell Carcinoma. Eds.: Schnorr, D, Loening, SA, Blackwell Berlin – Wien, pp. 138-143.

Russel FGM, Masereeuw R, van Aubel RAMH (2002) Molecular aspects of renal anionic drug transport. *Ann Rev Physiol 64*: 563-594.

Samuels BL, Hollis DR, Rosner GL, Trump DL, Shapiro CL, Vogelzang NJ, Schilsky RL (1997) Modulation of vinblastine resistance in metastatic renal cell carcinoma with cyclosporine A or tamoxifen: a cancer and leukemia group B study. *Clin Cancer Res 3*: 1977-1984.

Schaub TP, Kartenbeck J, König J, Spring H, Dorsam J, Staehler G, Storkel S, Thon WF, Keppler D (1999) Expression of the MRP2 gene-encoded conjugate export pump in human kidney proximal tubules and in renal cell carcinoma. *J Am Soc Nephrol 10*: 1159-1169.

Schinkel AH, Wagenaar E, van Deemter L, Mol CA, Borst P (1995) Absence of the mdr1a P-glycoprotein in mice affects tissue distribution and pharmacokinetics of dexamethasone, digoxin, and cyclosporin A. *J Clin Invest 96*: 1698-1705.

Schmitt C, Burckhardt G (1993) p-Aminohippurate/2-oxoglutarate exchange in bovine renal brush-border and basolateral membrane vesicles. *Eur J Physiol 423*: 280-290.

Sekine T, Cha SH, Endou H (2000) The multispecific organic anion transporter (OAT) family. *Eur J Physiol 440*: 337-350.

Sekine T, Cha SH, Tsuda M, Apiwattanakul N, Nakajima N, Kanai Y, Endou H (1998) Identification of multispecific organic anion transporter 2 expressed predominantly in the liver. *FEBS Lett 429*: 179-182.

Sekine T, Seok HC, Yoshikatsu K, Endou H (1999) Molecular biology of multispecific organic anion transporter family (OAT family). *Clin Exp Nephrol 3*: 237-243.

Sekine T, Watanabe N, Hosoyamada M, Kanai Y, Endou H (1997) Expression cloning and characterization of a novel multispecific organic anion transporter. *J Biol Chem 272*: 18526-18529.

Sharfman WH, Urba WJ, Smith JW, Janik JE, Curti, BD, Gause BL, Holmlund JT, Steis RG, Beauchamp AE, Longo DL (1995) Phase I/II trial of 5-fluorouracil, leucovorin, zidovudine and dipyridamole for patients with metastatic colorectal cancer, renal cell carcinoma and malignant melanoma. *Int J Oncol 6*: 579-583.

Shi YB, Ritchie JWA, Taylor PM (2002) Complex regulation of thyroid hormone action: multiple opportunities for pharmacological intervention. *Pharmacol Ther 94*: 235-251.

Silva P, Torretti J, Hayslett JP, Epstein FH (1976) Relation between Na-K-ATPase activity and respiratory rate in the rat kidney. *Am J Physiol 230*: 1432-1438.

Skinner DG, Calvin RB, Vermillion CD, Pfister RC, Leadbetter WF (1971) Diagnosis and management of renal cell carcinoma. A clinical and pathologic study of 309 cases. *Cancer 28*:1165-1177.

Somogyi A (1996) Renal transport of drugs: specificity and molecular mechanisms. *Clin Exp Pharmacol Physiol 23*: 986-989.

Splinter FK, Bräunlich H (1973) Binding of p-aminohippuric acids, hydrochlorothiazide and cyclopenthiazide serum proteins in rats of various ages. *Acta Biol Med Germ 31*: 621-625.

Stonestreet BS, Hansen NB, Laptook AR, Oh W (1984) Glucocorticoid accelerates renal functional maturation in fetal lamb. *Early Hum Dev 8*: 331-341.

Stopp M (1982) Postnatale Entwicklung und Stimulation des renalen tubulären Transportes von p-Aminohippursäure. Promotion B, Medizinische Fakultät, Universität Jena.

Stopp M, Bräunlich H (1975) Die Akkumulation von p-Aminohippursäure und Zyklopenthiazid in Nierenrindenschnitten verschieden alter Ratten und ihre Abhängigkeit von der Energiebereitstellung. *Acta biol med germ 34*: 89-98.

Stopp M, Bräunlich H (1980) In vitro analysis of drug-induced stimulation of renal tubular p-aminohippurate (PAH) transport in rats. *Biochem Pharmacol 29*: 983-986.

Sun W, Wu RR, van Poelje PD, Erion MD (2001) Isolation of a family of organic anion transporters from human liver and kidney. *Biochem Biophys Res Commun 283*: 417-422.

Sweet DH, Pritchard JB (1999) The molecular biology of renal organic anion and organic cation transporters. *Cell Biochem Biophys 31*: 89-118.

Sweet DH, Bush KT, Nigam SK (2001) The organic anion transporter family: from physiology to ontogeny and the clinic. *Am J Physiol Renal Physiol 281*: F197-F205.

Sweet DH, Wolff NA, Pritchard JB (1997) Expression cloning and characterization of ROAT1. The basolateral organic anion transporter in rat kidney. *J Biol Chem 272*: 30088-30095.

Takeda M, Sekine T, Endou H (2000a) Regulation by protein kinase C of organic anion transport driven by rat organic anion transporter 3 (rOAT3). *Life Sciences 67*: 1087-1093.

Takeda M, Hosoyamada M, Cha SH, Sekine T, Endou H (2000b) Hydrogen peroxide downregulates human organic anion transporters in the basolateral membrane of the proximal tubule. *Life Sciences 68*: 679-687.

Takeda M, Narikawa S, Hosoyamada M, Cha SH, Sekine T, Endou H (2001) Characterization of organic anion transport inhibitors using cells stably expressing human organic anion transporters. *Eur J Pharmacol 419*: 113-120.

Takeuchi A, Masuda S, Saito H, Abe T, Inui K (2001) Multispecific substrate recognition of kidney-specific organic anion transporters OAT-K1 and OAT-K2. *J Pharmacol Exp Ther 299*: 261-267.

Takimoto CH, Allegra CJ (1995) New antifolates in clinical development. *Oncol Huntingt 9*: 649-656.

Tobe SW, Noble-Topham SE, Andrulis IL, Hartwick RW, Skorecki KL, Warner E (1995) Expression of the multiple drug resistance gene in human renal cell carcinoma depends on tumor histology, grade, and stage. *Clin Cancer Res 1*: 1611-1615.

Toffoli G, Corona G, Tolusso B, Sartor F, Sorio R, Mini E, Boiocchi M (2000) Resistance to methotrexate in SKOV-3 cell lines after chronic exposure to carbamazepine is associated with a decreased expression of folate receptor. *Int J Cancer 85*: 683-690.

Tojo A, Sekine T, Nakajima N, Hosoyamada M, Kanai Y, Kimura K, Endou H (1999) Immunhistochemical localization of multispecific renal organic anion transporter 1 in rat kidney. *J Am Soc Nephrol 10*: 464-471.

Traeger A, Bräunlich H, Bräunlich I, Geyer A, Hoppe H, Kubens S, Stein G (1976) Untersuchungen zur Kinetik von p-Aminohippursäure und von Sulfamerazin nach wiederholter Applikation von Sulfamerazin bei Schulkindern, Erwachsenen und Greisen. *Dtsch Gesundh-Wsn 31*: 2250-2253.

Uchino H, Tamai I, Yamashita K, Minemoto Y, Sai Y, Yabuuchi H, Miyamoto K, Takeda E, Tsuji (2000) A p-aminohippuric acid transport at renal apical membrane mediated by human inorganic phosphate transporter NPT1. *Biochem Biophys Res Comm 270*: 254-259.

Ullrich KJ (1997) Renal transporters for organic anions and organic cations, structure requirements for substrates. *J Membr Biol 158*: 95-107.

Ullrich KJ (1999) Affinity of drugs to the different renal transporters for organic anions and organic cations. In situ K_i values. In: Amidon, GL, Sadée, W (eds.): Membrane transporters as drug targets, Kluwer Academic / Plenum Publishers New York, Boston, Dordrecht, London, Moscow, pp. 159-179.

Ullrich KJ, Rumrich G, Papavassiliou F, Hierholzer K (1991) Contraluminal p-aminohippurate transport in the proximal tubule of the rat kidney. VIII. Transport of corticosteroids. *Eur J Physiol 418*: 371-382.

Uozumi J, Koikawa Y, Yasumasu T, Ueda T, Kumazawa J (1995) The effect of methylprednisolone on cisplatin-induced nephrotoxicity in rat renal cortical slices. *Res Exp Med Berl 195*: 231-235.

Uwai Y, Okuda M, Takami K, Hashimoto Y, Inui K (1998) Functional characterization of the rat multispecific organic anion transporter OAT1 mediating basolateral uptake of anionic drugs in the kidney. *FEBS Lett 438*: 321-324.

van Aubel RAMH, Masereeuw R, Russel FGM (2000a) Molecular pharmacology of renal organic anion transporters. *Am J Physiol Renal Physiol 279*: F216-F232.

van Aubel RAMH, Peters JG, Masereeuw R, van Os CH, Russel FGM (2000b) Multidrug resistance protein mrp2 mediates ATP-dependent transport of classic renal organic anion p-aminohippurate. *Am J Physiol Renal Physiol 279*: F713-F717.

van Aubel RAMH, Smeets PHE, Peters JGP, Bindels RJM, Russel FGM (2002) The MRP4/ABCC4 gene encodes a novel apical organic anion transporter in human kidney proximal tubules: putative efflux pump for urinary cAMP and cGMP. *J Am Soc Nephrol 13*: 595-603.

Van Brussel JP, Mickisch GH (1998) Circumvention of multidrug resistance in genitourinary tumors. *Int J Urol 5*: 1-15.

Villalobos AR, Dunnick CA, Pritchard JB (1996) Mechanisms mediating basolateral transport of 2,4-dichlorophenoxyacetic acid in rat kidney. *J Pharmacol Exp Ther 278*: 582-589.

Villeneuve A, Gignac S, Provencher PH (2000) Glucocorticoids decrease endothelin-A- and -B-receptor expression in the kidney. *J Card Pharmacol 36*: S238-S240.

Voci A, Demori, Bottazzi C and Fugassa E (2001) Regulation of renal growth and IGFBP-4 expression by triiodothyronine during rat development. *Horm Metab Res 33*: 256-262.

Volm M, Pommerenke EW, Efferth T, Lohrke H, Mattern J (1991) Circumvention of multi-drug resistance in human kidney and kidney carcinoma in vitro. *Cancer 67*: 2484-2489.

Wedeen RP, Weiner B (1973) The distribution of p-aminohippuric acid in rat kidney slices. II. Depth of uptake. *Kidney Int 3*: 214-221.

Winnefeld K, Schröter H, Strech S.: Mitteilungen aus dem Applikationslabor Carl Zeiss Jena GmbH, AAS 6/92 (1992).

Wolff MW, Su TZ (2002) Cloning and tissue-specific expression of spliced variants of the rat organic anion transporter (rOAT-K). *DNA Seq 13*: 15-25.

Wolff NA, Werner A, Burkhardt S, Burckhardt G (1997) Expression cloning and characterization of a renal organic anion transporter from winter flounder. *FEBS Lett 417*: 287-291.

Wolff NA, Grunwald B, Friedrich B, Lang F, Godehardt S, Burckhardt G (2001) Cationic amino acids involved in dicarboxylate binding of the flounder renal organic anion transporter. *J Am Soc Nephrol 12*: 2012-2018.

Woodland C, Koren G, Wainer IW Batist G Ito S (2003) Verapamil metabolites: potential P-glycoprotein-mediated multidrug resistance reversal agents. *Can J Physiol Pharmacol 81*: 800-805.

You G, Kuze K, Kohanski RA, Amsler K, Henderson S (2000) Regulation of mOAT-mediated organic anion transport by okadaic acid and protein kinase C in LLC-PK (1) cells. *J Biol Chem 275*: 10278-10284.

Yu DS, Sun GH, Ma CP, Chang SY (1999) Cocktail modulator mixtures for overcoming multidrug resistance in renal cell carcinoma. *Urology 54*: 377-381.

In: Trends in Kidney Cancer Research
Editor: Kelvin R. Nunez, pp. 207-222

ISBN 1-59454-141-8

Chapter XII

SURVIVING AS INDICATOR OF DIAGNOSIS AND PROGRESSION IN TRANSITIONAL CELL CARCINOMA

Kuniaki Nakanishi*
Department of Pathology, National Defense Medical College, Tokorozawa, Japan

ABSTRACT

The members of the IAP family, including survivin, have recently emerged as modulators of an evolutionarily conserved step in apoptosis. Survivin is present during embryonic and fetal development, but is generally down-regulated in normal adult tissues. However, it becomes reexpressed in a variety of cancers. During tumorigenesis, survivin expression is inversely correlated with apoptosis inhibition and positively correlated with proliferation and angiogenesis. This article reviews the relationships between survivin expression and diagnosis, progression, or prognosis in transitional cell carcinoma (TCC). A regards survivin expression in normal samples, no survivin is detected in urine or in transitional cells in the urinary bladder and upper urinary tract. As regards diagnosis, survivin expression has been detected with high sensitivity in urine samples, using ELISA; therefore, this noninvasive test is well suited to bladder cancer, and a disease with high rates of recurrence. However, the relevance of survivin expression to the progression or prognosis of TCC remains controversial.

Key words: survivin, transitional cell carcinoma.

---

* Corresponding author: Kuniaki Nakanishi MD, Department of Pathology, National Defense Medical College, Tokorozawa 359-8513, Japan. Phone: +81-42-995-1626; Fax: +81-42-991-1612; e-mail: nknsknak@ndmc.ac.jp

INTRODUCTION

More than 55,000 new cases of bladder cancer were expected to be diagnosed in the USA in 2002 (1), and this disease is responsible for approximately 12,000 deaths per year in the USA. Transitional cells are the origin of at least 90% of bladder carcinomas. Approximately 80% of cases are superficial and papillary at the time of first presentation. Recurrences are frequent, and approximately 10-15% of recurrences will progress to muscle-invasive disease. Moreover, approximately 20% of bladder carcinomas are found to invade muscle at the time of initial presentation. Approximately 5% of patients will have de novo metastatic disease, at the time of diagnosis and an additional 50% of those who are diagnosed originally with muscle-invasive disease will develop a recurrence. In recent years, many diagnostic and prognostic factors in cancer have been described, including programmed cell death (apoptosis).

A disruption of the regulation of cell proliferation, which normally occurs via apoptosis, contributes to the development of a variety of cancers both by aberrantly extending cell viability and by favoring the accumulation of transforming mutations (2). Contributions to the regulatory process are known to be made by proteins that either promote or counteract apoptotic cell death. Several proteins that inhibit apoptosis have been identified: these include such bcl-2 family members as bcl-2 and bcl-xL, as well as inhibitors of apoptosis, or IAPs. IAP proteins have recently emerged as modulators of an evolutionarily conserved step in apoptosis, which may potentially involve direct inhibition of terminal effector caspase-3, -7, and -9 (3-5). Survivin, a recently described member of the IAP family (6), has been found to be expressed during embryonic and fetal development (7). Furthermore, although it is generally down-regulated and of low detectability in normal adult tissues, it becomes prominently reexpressed in a variety of cancers (8-41). Survivin, unlike with other members of the IAP family, is characteristic of a protein that inhibits apoptosis and regulates cell division (38-41).

The last few years have seen the publication of several reviews of the actions of IAPs (including survivin) and of the mechanisms by which they modulate apoptosis (4,5,38-41). This article reviews the possible relationship between survivin expression and the clinical and pathologic features of cancers to try to clarify its clinical significance, especially whether assessing survivin expression can help to predict biologic behavior and clinical outcome in transitional cell carcinoma (TCC).

STRUCTURE OF SURVIVIN

Survivin was discovered in 1997 by hybridization screening of a human genomic library using the cDNA of the effector cell protease receptor-1 (EPR-1) (6). The human *survivin* gene consists of 15kb on the telomeric position of chromosome 17, and is localized to band q25, approximately 3% of the distance from the telomere (42). The human *survivin* gene contains of four exons and three introns, and its coding strand contains an open reading frame (ORF) of 426 nucleotides complementary to EPR-1 (6). There are a TATA-less promoter and GC-rich regions of canonical CpG islands upstream of this ORF (6,43,44). The interactions between EPR-1 and survivin transcripts form a potential gene-regulation mechanism by "natural" antisense expression (45,46).

The human *survivin* gene encodes a protein of 142 amino acids, with a molecular weight of approximately 16.5kDa (6). The human survivin proteins are encoded by primary transcripts of 1.9kb and a second band of 3.4kb that can be detected in fetal kidney and liver by the use of a survivin-specific single-strand probe. The second band may represent a partially processed RNA or an alternatively spliced form of survivin. The organization of the survivin protein is unique (as compared with those of other IAPs). Survivin contains only one copy of a baculovirus *iap* repeat (BIR), which is typically repeated two or three times in mammalian IAPs and is essential for any apoptosis inhibitor, but no zink-binding domain (known as the RING finger motif) (5). The structure of the survivin protein is closely linked to its function as an inhibitor of apoptosis.

Antiapoptosis Function of Survivin

Survivin is a characteristic protein that inhibits apoptosis and regulates cell division (5,39-42,47,48). It plays an important role in the suppression of apoptosis by either directly or indirectly inhibiting the activity of caspases, which are a family of cysteine proteases that induce apoptosis, although a role for survivin as a direct inhibitor of caspases remains controversial. In apoptosis, two major pathways are known: the mitochondrial pathway and the death-receptor pathway (4,5,38-41). The first pathway begins when cytochrome c is released by mitochondria into the cytosol. The cytochrome c binds to apoptosis protease activating factor-1 (Apaf-1), resulting in a promotion of the catalytic activation of caspase-9 in the present of dATP or ATP. The second pathway involves activation of caspase-8 via death receptors, such as the fibroblast-associated (Fas) and tumor necrosis factor (TNF) families of receptors. The activation of an initiator caspase, such as caspase-8 or caspase-9, can activate downstream effector caspases such as caspase-3 (this can probably also be done by caspase-6 and caspase-7).

In the case of the first pathway, evidence of an indirect regulation of caspase activity by survivin has been obtained using a mutagenetic technique (49). Loss of phosphorylation at threonine 34 (T34) in mutant survivin, in which T34 is mutated to nonphosphorylatable alanine (T34A), results in dissociation of the survivin-caspase-9 complex on the mitotic apparatus.Hence, survivin phosphorylation at threonine 34 (T34) is necessary for the association of survivin with processed caspase-9. Furthermore, it is well known that several IAP family members suppress apoptosis by direct inhibition of caspases (50). Thus, X-chromosome-linked IAP (XIAP), which contains three BIR domains, directly inhibits at least three members of the caspase family of cell-death proteases: namely, caspase-3 and caspase-7 (51), each via a linker region between the first two BIR domains (50), and caspase-9, via its third BIR domain (BIR3). Comparison of the structure of survivin with that of XIAP reveals that the BIR domain of survivin appears to be closely related in three-dimensional structure to the BIR3 of XIAP. Thus, survivin is thought to bind caspase-9 (49). Recently, hepatitis B X-interacting protein (HBXIP) has been reported to operate as a cofactor for survivin, allowing it to bind and suppress activation of pro-caspase-9, thereby selectively suppressing apoptosis (52).In addition, survivin binds a second mitochondrial-derived activator of caspases; namely, (Smac)/ direct IAP binding protein with low pl (DIABLO), which can promote apoptosis by binding to and suppressing the inhibitory effects of the IAP proteins (53,54). Smac/ DIABLO is released from mitochondria into the cytosol along with cytochrome c in the mitochondrial apoptosis pathway.

In addition, it is well known that p53 is associated with both the mitochondrial pathway and the death-receptor pathway, and that the bcl-2 family is associated with the mitochondrial pathway (55-57). p53 is located on chromosome 17p13.1 and encodes a 53-kDa nuclear phosphoprotein with DNA-binding properties (55). Furthermore, p53 is a tumor-suppressor molecule involved in the growth arrest and apoptosis of various types of cells (56). The B cell lymphoma/leukaemia-2 (*bcl-2*) gene was first discovered at the breakpoint of t(14:18) in a follicular non-Hodgkin's B-cell lymphoma (57). The bcl-2 family of proteins includes both inhibitors [such as bcl-2 and long isoform (bcl-X_L)] and promoters [such as bcl-2-associated X protein (bax)] of apoptosis. In the mitochondrial pathway, upstream stimuli such as activation of p53 induce expression of pro-apoptotic bcl-2 family proteins, such as bax, into the pores in the outer mitochondrial membrane. Anti-apoptotic proteins such as bcl-2 and bcl-X_L inhibit the membrane-permeabilizing effects of bax, while other downstream effector caspases, such as caspase-9, are not activated, and apoptosis is thereby inhibited. In another p53 pathway, p53 stimulates apoptosis directly by up-regulation of receptors such as Fas (55,56).

A role for survivin in cell division is suggested by its protein structure. The amino terminal portion of survivin consists of three α-helices (residues 14-21, 31-41, 68-80) and 3 β-sheets (residues 43-45, 55-58, 61-64). Those structures closely resemble the BIR-containing proteins from yeast and *C. elegans*, which are involved in cytokinesis (47). Removal of the c-terminal helix prevents survivin from localizing to microtubules (48). Thus, during the cell cycle, survivin is expressed in the G2/M phase. Survivin is first detected on centromeres at prophase/metaphase, is present in the spindle midzone during anaphase/telophase, but is no longer detected by the end of telophase (48). Disruption of the survivin-microtubule interactions that occur at the beginning of mitosis results in increased caspase-3 activity with loss of the anti-apoptotic function of survivin (48). Another report has indicated that survivin is localized to kinetochores until metaphase, then to the spindle midzone in anaphase, and in the cleavage plane during telophase and cytokinesis (58). These localization patterns resemble those of the inner centromere protein (INCENP) (59), which is known as a chromosomal passenger protein. Chromosomal passenger proteins are carried on the chromosomes to the center of the cell at metaphase, in the plane of the future cleavage furrow, and are important for cytokinesis and chromosome movement during cell division. On the basis of its localization during the cell cycle, survivin has been postulated to be a chromosomal passenger protein (58).

Survivin Expression in Normal Tissues

Although survivin expression is not found in most tissues in normal adults, as mentioned above, human survivin expression has been reported in a few normal adult tissues, including placenta (60), colonic mucosa (61), endometrium (62), thymus (6), and keratinocytes of the basal layer of the skin (63). In a Northern blotting analysis, some normal adult tissues exhibited in low levels of survivin (6). This pattern of survivin expression contrasted with the broad distribution of IAPs in normal adult tissues (3-5), although it should be said that even in the case of the IAPs, levels of expression differed among tissues. In detail, in the placental tissues survivin has been detected in syncytiotrophoblasts, villous cytotrophoblast cells, and extravillous cytotrophoblast cells in cell columns in the first trimester, as well as in the chorionic membrane in tissues at term (60). In the normal colonic mucosa, survivin expression is mostly restricted to the base of the colonic crypts (61). In a study of the endometrium, survivin mRNA was detected in all samples (9 of 9) of endometrium taken during the secretory phase, but in only 4 out of 7 samples taken during the proliferative phase, and not at all in the atrophic endometrium [using the reverse transcription-polymerase chain reaction (RT-PCR)] (62). By immunohistochemistry, survivin is found to be expressed most strongly in the nuclei of glandular epithelial cells during the late secretory phase, but it is not expressed in glandular epithelial cells in the proliferative phase.

In fetal tissues, survivin is present in large amounts. In 10- to 21-week-old human fetuses, survivin has been observed to be prominent in the proximal tubules of the kidney, the acinar tubules of the lung at the canalicular stage, pancreatic endocrine islets, endometrial glands, epidermis, thymic medulla, spinal cord neurons, and the axial mesenchymal space surrounding the somites (using immunohistochemistry) (7). In the skin, survivin staining is prominent in the basal layer of the interdigital space (7). Survivin mRNA is detected at the bottom of early crypts of fetal intestine by *in situ* hybridization (7). By Western blotting, survivin is detected as a single band of ~ 16.5kd in tissue extracts of fetal gastrointestinal tract, liver, heart, lung, and kidney (6,7). During development in the mouse, survivin is diffusely expressed in the brain at E11.5, but has decreased to undetectable levels by E15-21, consistent with there being a developmental pattern (7). Similar results concerning survivin expression at E14.5 in mouse lung and intestine have been reported (7).

With regard to survivin expression in normal transitional cells of the urinary tract, Smith et al (34), using Western blot and RT-PCR, found that none of 16 healthy volunteers had detectable survivin in urine samples. Furthermore, three other investigators found that normal transitional cells of the bladder or upper urinary tract cantained no detectable survivin (using immunohistochemistry) (30-32,34).

Survivin Expression in Cancer

Numerous reports have examined the role of survivin in cancer. Several studies found that while survivin expression was not apparent in the normal cells of any organs, it was expressed in all the most common cancers (by immunohistochemistry, Western blotting, and RT-PCR) (6,8-37). By immunohistochemistry, survivin expression was seen to be restricted to the cytoplasm and/or nuclei of tumor cells. However, no survivin immunoreactivity was observed in infiltrating lymphocytes or other stroma cells. Survivin immunohistochemical expression has been described in 96% of lung (6,9), 82.7% of oral (11), 80% of esophageal (13), 34.5-88.0% of gastric (14-16), 53.2-100% of colonic (6,16-19), 88% of pancreatic

(6,20,21), 70.7% of breast (6,22), and 73.5% of ovarian (27) carcinomas, as well as in 47% of neuroblastoma (24) and 60% of hematopoietic malignancies, including large cell non-Hodgkin's lymphoma (6,25). Survivin has also been detected in 85.5-100% of lung (8-10), 70.6% of esophageal (12), 68% of gastric (15), 63.5% of colonic (18), 76.9% of pancreatic (20,21), and 31.1% of hepatocellular (23) cancinomas by RT-PCR, and in 58.3% of gastric (15) carcinomas and 100% of soft tissue sarcomas (26) by Western blotting and/or ELISA. Thus, the percentage of survivin-positive cases in several tumors varies from about 31% to 100% of tumor tissues (6,9-28). In the lung, survivin mRNA/GAPDH mRNA has been demonstrated in all normal tissues and carcinomas using semiquantitative RT-PCR, although in normal tissues it was at very low levels (9,10).

In general, the presence of survivin may be a useful diagnostic marker in certain malignancies, and moreover in certain carcinomas it may be an indicator both of a more aggressive progression (such as advanced stage), and of a poorer prognosis (such as decreased overall and disease-free survivals and an increased recurrence rate) than those associated with carcinomas without survivin expression. Furthermore, with regard to its value as a prognostic marker, several studies of, for example, non-small-cell lung carcinoma (8), oral squamous cell carcinoma (11), esophageal squamous cell carcinoma (12), gastric adenocarcinoma (16), colorectal adenocarcinoma (18,19), neuroblastoma (24), diffuse large B-cell lymphoma (25), and soft tissue sarcoma (26) have demonstrated the prognostic impact of survivin. In esophageal (13), pancreatic (21), and breast (22) carcinomas, however, the presence of survivin has been found to show no association with patients survival (using immunohistochemistry). With regard to its value as a diagnostic marker for tumors, serum survivin levels were detected in 8.2% to 21.6% of 51 lung and 49 colorectal cancer patients (using ELISA), thus indicating that it might be an attractive novel marker for the diagnosis of these cancers (28,29).

In addition, correlations between survivin and bcl-2 or p53 have been examined in a variety of tumors. In the case of bcl-2, immunohistochemical expression has been confirmed not only in tumor cells, but also in normal mucosal cells and infiltrating lymphocytes. Several investigators have revealed a close relationship between immunoreactivity for bcl-2 and clinicopathologic findings in a variety of tumors (64-68), and have suggested that bcl-2 expression may be an indication of a favorable prognosis. In the case of p53 immunostaining, it is generally accepted that the accumulated p53 represents a mutated type because inactivation of p53 predisposes to a dysregulated proliferation and aberrantly prolonged survival of mutated cells. The presence of p53 mutations has been shown to affect prognosis in some cancers (69). However, the correlations between survivin and bcl-2 or p53 in carcinomas remain controversial. In gastric carcinomas, survivin expression has been found to correlate with immunoreactivity for both bcl-2 and p53 (14). Those authors suggested that p53 may negatively regulate survivin expression via a mechanism that can potentially be disrupted by cancer-associated mutations of p53 (since, as mentioned above, it is generally agreed that the accumulated p53 represents the mutated type). In contrast, survivin expression has been found to correlate with immunoreactivity for bcl-2, but not with p53 expression, in colorectal and breast carcinomas (17,22), whereas it correlates with immunoreactivity for p53, but not with bcl-2 expression, in pancreatic and ovarian adenocarcinomas (21,27).

Analyses of the relationship between survivin expression and tumor-cell apoptosis (using the mean apoptotic index) have revealed a significant inverse correlation between these two factors in gastric (14), colorectal (17), and breast (22) cancers. In other words, the mean apoptotic index was significantly lower in survivin-positive tumors than in survivin-negative ones.

SURVIVIN EXPRESSION IN TRANSITIONAL CELL CARCINOMA

As regards survivin expression in TCC of the urinary tract, we know of only six published reports: 3 on the urinary bladder, 1 on the upper urinary tract, and 2 on urine (Table 1, 30-37). The existence of a relationship between survivin expression and clinicopathologic findings or prognosis is controversial, to judge from published reports. By immunohistochemistry, survivin expression has been found to be restricted to the cytoplasm and/or nuclei of tumor cells (30,32-34). The reported percentage of survivin-positive cases has varied from about 18% to 78% of cancer tissues (30,32,34). Afew years ago, in a study of TCC of the urinary bladder by immunohistochemistry, Swana et al (30), who examined the primary tumors of 36 patients with localized bladder cancer (25 men and 11 women; average age, 66 years; range, 51 to 78), reported detecting survivin expression in 78% of tumors, and in an even higher proportion of high-grade tumors (15 of 16 grade II and III tumors). Furthermore, they found that the time to first recurrence was significantly shorter in patients with survivin-positive grade I tumors than in those with survivin-negative grade I tumors. Lehner et al (32), who examined healthy transitional cell epithelium, in 14 cases of TCC in situ and 45 TCCs (grades 1-3, 15 of each) of the urinary bladder, detected nuclear staining for survivin in 47% of 59 TCC cases (26 of 45 TCCs and 2 of 14 TCC in situ) and cytoplasmic staining in 71% (34 of 45 TCCs and 8 of 14 TCC in situ). Furthermore, the association of nuclear staining with TCC was statistically significant in both healthy bladder mucosa and TCC in situ, and patients with TCC and a nuclear pattern of survivin localization had a greater period of disease-free survival (27.2 months) than patients with a TCC that showed no nuclear staining for survivin (9.9 months). Nuclear localization of survivin is a marker for TCC, but is rarely present in premalignant or benign bladder mucosal specimens. In contrast, in TCC of the upper urinary tract we found (31) that survivin is expressed in the cytoplasm of tumor cells and is present in only 12.7% of 126 patients requiring surgical resection of the upper urinary tract, and we failed to find a relationship between survivin expression and clinicopathologic factors or disease-free survival. In TCC, survivin expression may be lower in the upper urinary tract than in the urinary bladder. We cannot be sure of the reason for these discrepancies (relating to survivin expression in the nuclei and/or cytoplasm of tumor cells, the incidence of survivin expression, and the relationship between survivin expression and clinicopathologic findings or survival) among the above three reports. However, the three studies differ in the sites examined (two reports on the urinary bladder vs. 1 report on the upper urinary tract), in the number of cases investigated (36 cases, 59 cases, 126 cases), in the antibodies used [a rabbit polyclonal antibody against different recombinant survivins prepared in Yale University School of Medicine, a rabbit polyclonal antibody against

Table 1 Expression of Survivin in Tissues and Urine in Cases of Transitional Cell Carcinoma

Site	Detection	Expression of survivin	Positive surviving expression: breakdown by stage and grade	Survival	Reference
Tumor					
Bladder	IH	28/36	Grade: 13/20 in low grade, 15/16 in high grade	35.5 ± 16.3 for survivin (-) vs. 11.5 ± 6.2 for survivin (+) for disease-free survival (months) ($p<0.05$)	30
Upper urinary tract	IH	16/126	Grade: 11/77 in low grade, 5/49 in high grade Stage: 10/49 in stage 0, 0/20 in stage I or II, 6/56 in stage III or IV	Not a prognostic factor in disease-free and overall survivals (log rank test: 0.31 and 0.37, respectively)	31
Bladder	IH	28/59 (nuclear staining) 42/59 (cytoplasmic staining)	Grade: Nuclear and cytoplasmic staining (2/14 & 8/14 of in situ, 8/15 &10/15 in grade I, 8/15 & 11/15 in grade II, 10/15 & 13/15 in grade III, respectively) Stage: Nuclear and cytoplasmic staining (12/22 & 15/22 in stage 0, 6/13 & 11/13 in stage I, 5/6 & 6/6 in stage 2, 2/3 & 1/3 in stage 3, 1/1 & 1/1 in stage 4, respectively)	Nuclear staining: median 10 months for survivin (+) vs. median 8.5 months for survivin (-) for disease-free survival (not significant)	32
Bladder	RT-PCR	9/30	Grade: 1/21 in low grade, 8/9 in high grade		33

Table 1 Expression of Survivin in Tissues and Urine in Cases of Transitional Cell Carcinoma (Continued)

Site	Detection	Expression of survivin	Positive surviving expression: breakdown by stage and grade	Survival	Reference
Urine					
Bladder	RT-PCR	31/31 (new or recurrent bladder cancer) 3/33 (treated bladder cancer)	Grade: 0/0 in grade I, 13/13 (mean survivin score, 1.3) in grade II, 7/7 (1.5) in grade III, 6/6 (2.2) in grade IV Stage: 6/6 (mean survivin score, 2.5) of in situ, 4/4 (1.0) in stage 0, 12/12 (1.6) in stage I, 6/6 (1.7) in stage II or III, 3/3 (1.7) in stage not determined		34
Bladder	WB	25/27* treatments (0.8±1.3 ng/ml urine before treatment)	Grade (before treatment): 0/1 (0 ng/ml urine) in grade 1, 6/11 (0.5±0.7 ng/ml urine) in grade II, 8/10 (0.6±0.9 ng/ml urine) in grade III, 3/4 (2.6±2.1 ng/ml urine) in grade IV Grade (after treatment): 0/1 (0 ng/ml urine) in grade 1, 5/11 (0.4±0.7 ng/ml urine) in grade II, 6/10 (0.4±0.4 ng/ml urine) in grade III, 3/4 (11.6±19.6 ng/ml urine) in grade IV Stage (before treatment): 6/7 (1.8±2.0 ng/ml urine) of in situ, 5/11 (0.3±0.5) in stage 0, 6/8 (0.8±0.8 ng/ml urine) in stage I Stage (after treatment): 5/7 (6.9±15.1 ng/ml urine) of in situ, 5/12 (0.4±0.7) in stage 0, 4/8 (0.4±0.5 ng/ml urine) in stage I Before treatment: recurrent (n=9, 1.5±1.8 ng/ml urine), remission (n=15, 0.3±3.9 ng/ml urine) After treatment: recurrent (n=9, 5.7±13.2 ng/ml urine), remission (n=15, 0.1±3.9 ng/ml urine)	Survivin 1 mo after last treatment: greater than 0.1 ng/ml urine (recurrence 8/12 and 10/11 after 1 mo and 1 year, respectively), 0.1 or less ng/ml urine (recurrence 0/14 and 2/14 after 1 mo and 1 year, respectively)	35

IH, immunohistochemistry; RT-PCR, reverse transcription-polymerase chain reaction; WB, Western blotting

* negative values were less than 0.1ng/ml urine.

different recombinant survivins prepared as peptide sequence ($A^3PTLPPAWQPFLKDHRI^{19}$), and a commercially available rabbit polyclonal antibody], in the methods used (one immunostaining method, a different immunostaining method, and the streptavidin-biotin complex method), and in additional techniques (pressure-cooking pretreatment, autoclave pretreatment). Furthermore, discrepancies may have arisen as a result of the different ways in which immunoreactivity was quantified.

As regards RT-PCR, two reports have been published. Schultz et al (36), who examined survivin mRNA expression in 32 urothelial cell carcinomas using real-time quantitative PCR, detected survivin mRNA in all bladder tumor tissues, and they obtained median values for survivin mRNA (normalized to the transcript levels of the housekeeping gene cyclophilin) of 0.26 for superficial tumors ($n = 17$) and 0.78 for invasive tumors ($n = 15$). A significant relationship with increasing pathologic stage ($p < 0.001$) and another with grade ($p < 0.001$) were observed by those workers. Although survivin mRNA expression does not relate to disease progression or the patient-survival period, patients with superficial bladder tumors and normalized survivin values over 0.26 had an increased risk of recurrence (log-rank test: $p = 0.018$). Therefore, the above authers suggested that a quantitative assessment of survivin mRNA can identify invasive and high-grade urothelial cell carcinomas, and may be useful as an indicator of an early recurrence of superficial tumors. Furthermore, Gazzaniga et al (33), who examined both normal and tumoral bladder tissues using RT-PCR, noted survivin expression in 9/30 (30%). When the dependence between gene expression and the relapse-free time of patients was evaluated, survivin showed no statistically significant ability to predict relapses. Therefore, those workers suggested that survivin expression cannot be used to identify patients with a high risk of relapse.

With regard to the diagnosis of bladder cancer by urine cytology, three reports have been published (34-36). Smith et al (34), who examined survivin in the urine of healthy volunteers ($n = 17$) and in that of patients with nonneoplastic urinary tract disease ($n = 30$), genitourinary cancer ($n = 30$), new-onset or recurrent bladder cancer ($n = 46$), or treated bladder cancer ($n = 35$) by a novel detection system, Western blot, and RT-PCR, detected survivin in the urine samples of all 46 patients with new or recurrent bladder cancer [using the novel detection system (31 of 31) or RT-PCR (15 of 15)], but not in the urine samples of 32 of 35 patients treated for bladder cancer and having negative cystoscopy results. None of the healthy volunteers or patients with prostate, kidney, vaginal, or cervical cancer had detectable survivin in their urine samples. Among the 30 patients with nonneoplastic urinary tract disease, survivin was detected in 3 patients in whom bladder abnormalities were noted using cystoscopy and in 1 patient with an increased prostate-specific antigen level. The patients with low-grade bladder cancer had significantly lower urine survivin levels than patients with carcinoma in situ. Therefore, those authors suggested that a highly sensitive and specific determination of urine survivin might provide a simple, noninvasive diagnostic test to identify patients with new or recurrent bladder cancer. Sharp et al (37) demonstrated that survivin is highly expressed in bladder cancer. Survivin was detected in the whole urine of patients with TCC using a simple antibody-based test. The sensitivity of survivin-testing for new or recurrent bladder cancer was 100%, while the specificity for other neoplastic and non-neoplastic genitourinary disease was 95%. They suggested that the high sensitivity of this simple, noninvasive test is well suited to bladder cancer, a disease with high rates of recurrence. Very-recently, Hausladen et al (35) examined urine survivin in patients with TCC who received intravesical instillation of bacillus Calmette-Guerin or mitomycin C, and suggested that it may predict recurrence. In the urine from 25 subjects (who received 27 such intravesical treatments) collected prior to, during, and after treatment, urinary survivin levels were higher in subjects in whom TCC recurred following treatment than in those who achieved remission. Actually, survivin levels increased several fold during the treatment, but the highest survivin levels were measured in subjects with recurrence. Median post-treatment survivin values were zero in those who achieved remission and 1.0 ng/ml urine in subjects in whom TCC recurred. The presence of urinary survivin at 1 month after completion of the treatment predicted TCC recurrence with 100% sensitivity and 78% specificity. The specificity to predict TCC recurrence increased to 92% after 1 year. No TCC recurred for 1 year in 12 of the 14 subjects with a posttreatment survivin level of 0.1 ng or less per ml urine. Further, 3 of the 4 subjects who were surviving-positive, but in remission, at 1 month after the completion of treatment had recurrent TCC within 1 year. Subjects who exhibited urinary survivin after the completion of intravesical instillation treatment had a high likelihood of TCC recurrence. On the basis of these data, this noninvasive test may be a useful tool for the detection of bladder cancer, a disease with high rates of recurrence.

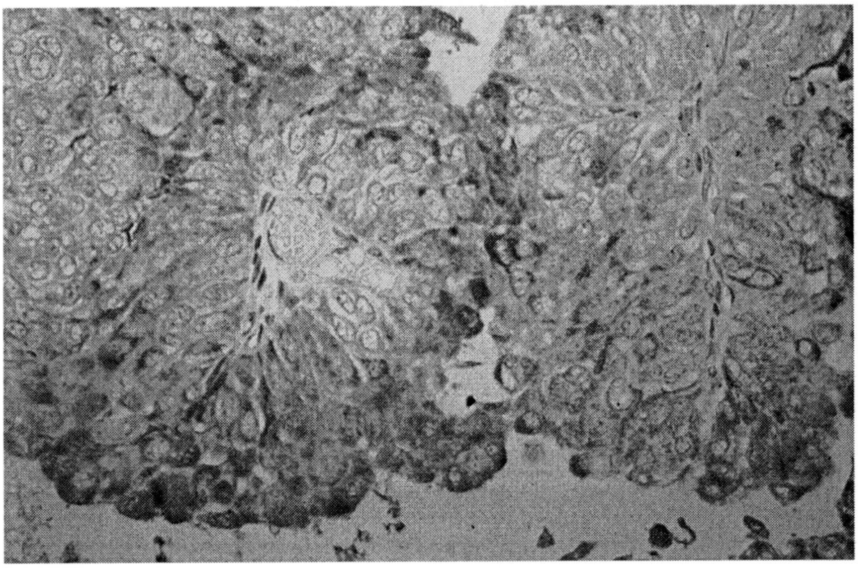

Figure 1 Survivin expression in transitional cell carcinoma of the upper urinary tract.

Concerning the relationships between survivin expression and p53, bcl-2, and apoptotic index, two reports have been published. Swana et al (30) found that immunostaining for bcl-2 or p53 was not correlated with disease-recurrence in 36 patients with localized bladder cancer. All the tumors had a low apoptotic index (0.8 to 1 percent) on the basis of an assessment of internucleosomal DNA fragmentation. Moreover, in our recent study of TCC-UUT we could not find a relationship between survivin expression and either bcl-2 oncoprotein expression or p53 oncoprotein expression (using immunohistochemistry) (31). In a RT-PCR study, Gazzaniga et al noted that a BCL-2/BAX ratio >1 was found in 53% and a

BCL-2/BAX expression ratio <1 in 46.6% of 30 superficial TCC bladder tissues (33). When they evaluated the dependence between each gene expression and the relapse-free time of the patients, a high BCL-2/BAX ratio reached statistical significance in its ability to predict relapses.

Conclusions

This article has reviewed the relationships between survivin expression and diagnosis, progression, or prognosis in transitional cell carcinoma. As regards survivin expression in normal samples, no survivin is detected in urine or transitional cells of the urinary bladder and upper urinary tract. As regards diagnosis, survivin expression can be detected with high sensitivity in urine samples using ELISA: therefore, this noninvasive test is well suited to bladder cancer, a disease with high rates of recurrence. However, the relevance of survivin expression to the progression and prognosis of TCC remains controversial.

Acknowledgments

The author is indebted to Dr. R. Timms for correcting the English.

References

[1] Jemal A, Murray T, Samuels A, Ghafoor A, Ward E, Thun MJ. Cancer statistics, 2003. *CA Cancer J Clin*. 2003;53:5-26.

[2] Thompson CB. Apoptosis in the pathogenesis and treatment of disease. *Science* 1995;267:1456-62.

[3] LaCasse EC, Baird S, Korneluk RG, MacKenzie AE. The inhibitors of apoptosis (IAPs) and their emerging role in cancer. *Oncogene*. 1998;17:3247-59.

[4] Verhagen AM, Coulson EJ, Vaux DL. Inhibitor of apoptosis proteins and their relatives: IAPs and other BIRPs. *Genome Biol*. 2001;2: 1-10.

[5] Deveraux QL, Reed JC. IAP family proteins -- suppressors of apoptosis. *Genes Dev.* 1999;13:239-52.

[6] Ambrosini G, Adida C, Altieri DC. A novel anti-apoptosis gene, *survivin*, expressed in cancer and lymphoma. *Nature Med* 1997;3:917-21.

[7] Adida C, Crotty PL, McGrath J, Berrebi D, Diebold J, Altieri DC. Developmentally regulated expression of the novel cancer anti-apoptosis gene *survivin* in human and mouse differentiation. *Am J Pathol* 1998;152:43-9.

[8] Monzo M, Rosell R, Felip E, Astudillo J, Sanchez JJ, Maestre J, Martin C, Font A, Barnadas A, Abad A. A novel anti-apoptosis gene: re-expression of survivin messenger RNA as a prognosis marker in non-small-cell lung cancers. *J Clin Oncol*. 1999;17:2100-4.

[9] Falleni M, Pellegrini C, Marchetti A, Oprandi B, Buttitta F, Barassi F, Santambrogio L, Coggi G, Bosari S. Survivin gene expression in early-stage non-small cell lung cancer. *J Pathol.* 2003;200:620-6.

[10] Hofmann HS, Simm A, Hammer A, Silber RE, Bartling B. Expression of inhibitors of apoptosis (IAP) proteins in non-small cell human lung cancer. *J Cancer Res Clin Oncol.* 2002;128:554-60.

[11] Muzio LL, Pannone G, Staibano S, Mignogna MD, Rubini C, Mariggio MA, Procaccini M, Ferrari F, Rosa GD, Altieri DC. Survivin expression in oral squamous cell carcinoma. *Br J Cancer.* 2003;89:2244-8.

[12] Kato J, Kuwabara Y, Mitani M, Shinoda N, Sato A, Toyama T, Mitsui A, Nishiwaki T, Moriyama S, Kudo J, Fujii Y. Expression of survivin in esophageal cancer: correlation with the prognosis and response to chemotherapy. *Int J Cancer* 2001;95:92-5.

[13] Grabowski P, Kuhnel T, Muhr-Wilkenshoff F, Heine B, Stein H, Hopfner M, Germer CT, Scherubl H. Prognostic value of nuclear survivin expression in oesophageal squamous cell carcinoma. *Br J Cancer.* 2003;88:115-9.

[14] Lu CD, Altieri DC, Tanigawa N. Expression of a novel antiapoptosis gene, survivin, correlated with tumor cell apoptosis and p53 accumulation in gastric carcinomas. *Cancer Res.* 1998;58:1808-12.

[15] Yu J, Leung WK, Ebert MP, Ng EK, Go MY, Wang HB, Chung SC, Malfertheiner P, Sung JJ. Increased expression of survivin in gastric cancer patients and in first degree relatives. *Br J Cancer.* 2002;87:91-7.

[16] Okada E, Murai Y, Matsui K, Isizawa S, Cheng C, Masuda M, Takano Y. Survivin expression in tumor cell nuclei is predictive of a favorable prognosis in gastric cancer patients. *Cancer Lett.* 2001;163:109-16.

[17] Kawasaki H, Altieri DC, Lu CD, Toyoda M, Tenjo T, Tanigawa N. Inhibition of apoptosis by survivin predicts shorter survival rates in colorectal cancer. *Cancer Res.* 1998;58:5071-4.

[18] Sarela AI, Scott N, Ramsdale J, Markham AF, Guillou PJ. Immunohistochemical detection of the anti-apoptosis protein, survivin, predicts survival after curative resection of stage II colorectal carcinomas. *Ann Surg Oncol.* 2001;8:305-10.

[19] Sarela AI, Macadam RC, Farmery SM, Markham AF, Guillou PJ. Expression of the antiapoptosis gene, survivin, predicts death from recurrent colorectal carcinoma. *Gut.* 2000;46:645-50.

[20] Satoh K, Kaneko K, Hirota M, Masamune A, Satoh A, Shimosegawa T. Expression of survivin is correlated with cancer cell apoptosis and is involved in the development of human pancreatic duct cell tumors. *Cancer.* 2001;92:271-8.

[21] Sarela AI, Verbeke CS, Ramsdale J, Davies CL, Markham AF, Guillou PJ. Expression of survivin, a novel inhibitor of apoptosis and cell cycle regulatory protein, in pancreatic adenocarcinoma. *Br J Cancer.* 2002;86:886-892.

[22] Tanaka K, Iwamoto S, Gon G, Nohara T, Iwamoto M, Tanigawa N. Expression of *survivin* and its relationship to loss of apoptosis in breast carcinomas. *Clin Cancer Res* 2000;6:127-34.

[23] Ikeguchi M, Ueta T, Yamane Y, Hirooka Y, Kaibara N. Inducible nitric oxide synthase and survivin messenger RNA expression in hepatocellular carcinoma. *Clin Cancer Res.* 2002;8:3131-6.

[24] Adida C, Berrebi D, Peuchmaur M, Reyes-Mugica M, Altieri DC. Anti-apoptosis gene, survivin, and prognosis of neuroblastoma. *Lancet.* 1998;351:882-883.

[25] Adida C, Haioun C, Gaulard P, Lepage E, Morel P, Briere J, Dombret H, Reyes F, Diebold J, Gisselbrecht C, Salles G, Altieri DC, Molina TJ. Prognostic significance of survivin expression in diffuse large B-cell lymphomas. *Blood.* 2000;96:1921-5.

[26] Kappler M, Kotzsch M, Bartel F, Fussel S, Lautenschlager C, Schmidt U, Wurl P, Bache M, Schmidt H, Taubert H, Meye A. Elevated expression level of survivin protein in soft-tissue sarcomas is a strong independent predictor of survival. *Clin Cancer Res.* 2003;9:1098-104.

[27] Cohen C, Lohmann CM, Cotsonis G, Lawson D, Santoianni R. Survivin expression in ovarian carcinoma: correlation with apoptotic markers and prognosis. *Mod Pathol.* 2003;16:574-83.

[28] Rohayem J, Diestelkoetter P, Weigle B, Oehmichen A, Schmitz M, Mehlhorn J, Conrad K, Rieber EP. Antibody response to the tumor-associated inhibitor of apoptosis protein survivin in cancer patients. *Cancer Res.* 2000;60:1815-7.

[29] Koziol JA, Zhang JY, Casiano CA, Peng XX, Shi FD, Feng AC, Chan EK, Tan EM. Recursive partitioning as an approach to selection of immune markers for tumor diagnosis. *Clin Cancer Res.* 2003;9:5120-6.

[30] Swana HS, Grossmann D, Anthony JN, Weiss RM, Altieri DC. Tumor content of the antiapoptosis molecule survivin and recurrence of bladder cancer. *N Eng J Med* 1999;341:452-3.

[31] Nakanishi K, Tominaga S, Hiroi S, Kawai T, Aida S, Kasamatsu H, Aurues T, Hayashi T, Ikeda T. Expression of survivin does not predict survival in patients with transitional cell carcinoma of the upper urinary tract. *Virchows Arch.* 2002;441:559-63.

[32] Lehner R, Lucia MS, Jarboe EA, Orlicky D, Shroyer AL, McGregor JA, Shroyer KR. Immunohistochemical localization of the IAP protein survivin in bladder mucosa and transitional cell carcinoma. *Appl Immunohistochem Mol Morphol.* 2002;10:134-8.

[33] Gazzaniga P, Gradilone A, Giuliani L, Gandini O, Silvestri I, Nofroni I, Saccani G, Frati L, Agliano AM. Expression and prognostic significance of LIVIN, SURVIVIN and other apoptosis-related genes in the progression of superficial bladder cancer. *Ann Oncol.* 2003;14:85-90.

[34] Smith SD, Wheeler MA, Plescia J, Colberg JW, Weiss RM, Altieri DC. Urine detection of survivin and diagnosis of bladder cancer. *JAMA* 2001;285:324-8.

[35] Hausladen DA, Wheeler MA, Altieri DC, Colberg JW, Weiss RM. Effect of intravesical treatment of transitional cell carcinoma with bacillus Calmette-Guerin and mitomycin C on urinary survivin levels and outcome. *J Urol.* 2003;170:230-4.

[36] Schultz IJ, Kiemeney LA, Witjes JA, Schalken JA, Willems JL, Swinkels DW, de Kok JB. Survivin mRNA expression is elevated in malignant urothelial cell carcinomas and predicts time to recurrence. *Anticancer Res.* 2003;23:3327-31.

[37] Sharp JD, Hausladen DA, Maher MG, Wheeler MA, Altieri DC, Weiss RM. Bladder cancer detection with urinary survivin, an inhibitor of apoptosis. *Front Biosci.* 2002;7:e36-41.

[38] Altieri DC, Marchisio PC, Marchisio C. Survivin apoptosis: an interloper between cell death and cell proliferation in cancer. *Lab Invest.* 1999;79:1327-33.

[39] Reed JC. The survivin saga goes on in vivo. *J Clin Invest.* 2001;108:965-9.

[40] Yamamoto T, Tanigawa N. The role of survivin as a new target of diagnosis and treatment in human cancer. *Med Electron Microsc.* 2001;34:207-12.

[41] Chiou SK, Jones MK, Tarnawski AS. Survivin - an anti-apoptosis protein: its biological roles and implications for cancer and beyond. *Med Sci Monit.* 2003;9:PI25-9.

[42] Ambrosini G, Adida C, Sirugo G, Altieri DC. Induction of apoptosis and inhibition of cell proliferation by survivin gene targeting. *J Biol Chem.* 1998;273:11177-82.

[43] Li F, Altieri DC. The cancer antiapoptosis mouse survivin gene: characterization of locus and transcriptional requirements of basal and cell cycle-dependent expression. *Cancer Res.* 1999;59:3143-51.

[44] Li F, Altieri DC. Transcriptional analysis of human survivin gene expression. *Biochem J.* 1999;344 Pt 2:305-11.

[45] Khochbin S, Lawrence JJ. An antisense RNA involved in p53 mRNA maturation in murine erythroleukemia cells induced to differentiate. *EMBO J.* 1989;8:4107-14.

[46] Vanhee-Brossollet C, Thoreau H, Serpente N, D'Auriol L, Levy JP, Vaquero C. A natural antisense RNA derived from the HIV-1 env gene encodes a protein which is recognized by circulating antibodies of HIV+ individuals. *Virology.* 1995;206:196-202.

[47] Uren AG, Beilharz T, O'Connell MJ, Bugg SJ, van Driel R, Vaux DL, Lithgow T. Role for yeast inhibitor of apoptosis (IAP)-like proteins in cell division. *Proc Natl Acad Sci U S A.* 1999;96:10170-5.

[48] Li F, Ambrosini G, Chu EY, Plescia J, Tognin S, Marchisio PC, Altieri DC. Control of apoptosis and mitotic spindle checkpoint by survivin. *Nature.* 1998;396(6711):580-4.

[49] O'Connor DS, Grossman D, Plescia J, Li F, Zhang H, Villa A, Tognin S, Marchisio PC, Altieri DC. Regulation of apoptosis at cell division by p34cdc2 phosphorylation of survivin. *Proc Natl Acad Sci U S A.* 2000;97:13103-7.

[50] Sun C, Cai M, Gunasekera AH, Meadows RP, Wang H, Chen J, Zhang H, Wu W, Xu N, Ng SC, Fesik SW. NMR structure and mutagenesis of the inhibitor-of-apoptosis protein XIAP. *Nature.* 1999;401(6755):818-22.

[51] Deveraux QL, Takahashi R, Salvesen GS, Reed JC. X-linked IAP is a direct inhibitor of cell-death proteases. *Nature (Lond)* 1997;388:300-4.

[52] Marusawa H, Matsuzawa S, Welsh K, Zou H, Armstrong R, Tamm I, Reed JC. HBXIP functions as a cofactor of survivin in apoptosis suppression. *EMBO J.* 2003;22:2729-40.

[53] Du C, Fang M, Li Y, Li L, Wang X. Smac, a mitochondrial protein that promotes cytochrome c-dependent caspase activation by eliminating IAP inhibition. *Cell.* 2000;102:33-42.

[54] Verhagen AM, Ekert PG, Pakusch M, Silke J, Connolly LM, Reid GE, Moritz RL, Simpson RJ, Vaux DL. Identification of DIABLO, a mammalian protein that promotes apoptosis by binding to and antagonizing IAP proteins. *Cell.* 2000;102:43-53.

[55] Agarwal ML, Taylor WR, Chernov MV, Chernova OB, Stark GR. The p53 network. *J Biol Chem.* 1998;273:1-4.

[56] Liebermann DA, Hoffman B, Steinman RA. Molecular controls of growth arrest and apoptosis: p53-dependent and independent pathways. *Oncogene.* 1995;11:199-210.

[57] Tsujimoto Y, Cossman J, Jaffe E, Croce CM. Involvement of the bcl-2 gene in human follicular lymphoma. *Science.* 1985;228(4706):1440-3.

[58] Skoufias DA, Mollinari C, Lacroix FB, Margolis RL. Human survivin is a kinetochore-associated passenger protein. *J Cell Biol.* 2000;151:1575-82.

[59] Uren AG, Wong L, Pakusch M, Fowler KJ, Burrows FJ, Vaux DL, Choo KH. Survivin and the inner centromere protein INCENP show similar cell-cycle localization and gene knockout phenotype. *Curr Biol.* 2000;10:1319-28.

[60] Ka H, Hunt JS. Temporal and spatial patterns of expression of inhibitors of apoptosis in human placentas. *Am J Pathol.* 2003;163:413-22.

[61] Gianani R, Jarboe E, Orlicky D, Frost M, Bobak J, Lehner R, Shroyer KR. Expression of survivin in normal, hyperplastic, and neoplastic colonic mucosa. *Hum Pathol.* 2001;32:119-25.

[62] Konno R, Yamakawa H, Utsunomiya H, Ito K, Sato S, Yajima A. Expression of survivin and Bcl-2 in the normal human endometrium. *Mol Hum Repro* 2000;6:529-34.

[63] Chiodino C, Cesinaro AM, Ottani D, Fantini F, Giannetti A, Trentini GP, Pincelli C. Communication: expression of the novel inhibitor of apoptosis survivin in normal and neoplastic skin. *J Invest Dermatol* 1999;113:415-8.

[64] Pezzella F, Turley H, Kuzu I, Tungekar MF, Dunnill MS, Pierce CB, Harris A, Gatter KC, Mason DY. bcl-2 protein in non-small-cell lung carcinoma. *N Engl J Med.* 1993;329:690-4.

[65] Bhargava V, Kell DL, van de Rijn M, Warnke RA. Bcl-2 immunoreactivity in breast carcinoma correlates with hormone receptor positivity. *Am J Pathol.* 1994;145:535-40.

[66] Fontanim G, Vignati S, Bigini D, Mussi A, Lucchi M, Angeletti CA, Basolo F, Bevilacqua G. Bcl-2 protein: a prognostic factor inversely correlated to p53 in non-small-cell lung cancer. *Br J Cancer* 1995;71:1003-7.

[67] Lu QL, Abel P, Foster CS, Lalani FN. bcl-2: role in epithelial differentiation and oncogenesis. *Hum Pathol* 1996;27:102-10.

[68] Lauwers GY, Scott GV, Karpeh MS. Immunohistochemical evaluation of bcl-2 protein expression in gastric adenocarcinomas. *Cancer.* 1995;75:2209-13.

[69] Ginsberg D, Mechta F, Yaniv M, Oren M. Wild-type p53 can down-modulate the activity of various promoters. *Proc Natl Acad Sci USA* 1991;88:9979-83.

INDEX

A

B

C

D

E

F

G

H

I

J

K

L

M

N

O

P

S

T

U

V

W

X

Y